TOXICOLOGY OF THE EYE, EAR, AND OTHER SPECIAL SENSES
Target Organ Toxicology Series

Target Organ Toxicology Series

Editor-in-Chief: Robert L. Dixon
U.S. EPA, Office of Health Effects, Washington, D.C.

Target Organ Toxicology Series

Toxicology of the Eye, Ear, and Other Special Senses

Editor

A. Wallace Hayes, Ph.D.

Corporate Toxicologist
R. J. Reynolds Industries, Inc.
Winston-Salem, North Carolina

Raven Press ■ New York

Raven Press, 1140 Avenue of the Americas, New York, New York 10036

Made in the United States of America

Library of Congress Cataloging in Publication Data
Main entry under title:

Toxicology of the eye, ear, and other special senses.

(Target organ toxicology series)
Includes bibliographies and index.
1. Eye—Diseases and defects.   2. Ear—Diseases.
3. Sense-organs—Diseases.   4. Toxicology.   I. Hayes, A.
Wallace (Andrew Wallace), 1939-   .   II. Series.
RE48.T69   1985   617'.51   82-42624
ISBN 0-89004-840-1

Preface

Sight is man's richest sense, his link to the world and the wealth of imagery. Vision begins with light, the abundant rain of the sun's energy falling through space to touch and warm the earth. Light projects value, tone, and shadow into nature. The eye, keen to this kaleidoscopic effect, then relates what it senses to the brain, perception's ultimate seat. Hearing is no less a sense, and for that matter, the same can be said of the other special senses. Each waking second the eyes, the ears, and the other sense organs send billions of pieces of fresh information to the brain. These fragments of information converge in the mind as images of stunning subtlety. Man sees in such detail because in the eye, the diverse physical world comes closest to touching the rare perceptive power of the mind. The eye, the ear, and the other special sense organs are all extensions of the brain. The wonder of these senses is often taken for granted, often abused, and generally neglected in the field of toxicology.

Injury to the organs of special sense by chemicals has been recognized in the workplace, but a toxicologic discipline dealing with such injury has only recently developed. Toxicity to these organs may be manifested as immediate failure or as a more insidious alteration of function that may not become manifested for many years. In either case, the result may be catastrophic, as normal function is essential to quality of life.

These senses comprise a complex and highly dynamic series of organs whose normal function is essential for maintenance of the quality of life that most humans are accustomed to. Unfortunately, real or potential risks to these systems are difficult to assess because of the complexity inherent in them. Some of the problems in assessment are associated with the wide variations in function that can occur and still lie within the classification of normal. Others are associated with the plasticity of the systems as they interconnect to the nervous system, and still others with our incomplete understanding of precisely what is being measured by certain tests. Clearly, no single test or approach will suffice to examine the functional capacity of these organs.

This volume deals, therefore, with an interdisciplinary approach to the toxicology of the eye, ear, and other special senses. The normal morphology, physiology, and biochemistry of these organs are discussed to lay the groundwork for the more applied aspects. The focus then is on animal test procedures for the assessment of toxic effects. Conceptual and methodologic problems are discussed in an effort to show both their usefulness and their limitations.

The volume brings together information previously available only from scattered sources. Although it is written primarily for toxicologists who have a need to enlarge their knowledge in an area often overlooked in routine testing—the toxicology of the eye, ear, and other special senses—scientists and graduate students in related disciplines should find this a valuable textbook of information that will also be useful for their general comprehension of the problems associated with these particular toxic responses.

A. Wallace Hayes

Contents

Structure and Function

Eye

Ear

Contributors

Joseph C. Arezzo
Albert Einstein College of Medicine
1300 Morris Park Avenue
Bronx, New York 10461

Vernon A. Benignus
Environmental Protection Agency
Medical Research Building C-224H
University of North Carolina
Chapel Hill, North Carolina 27514

Patricia M. Blough
Department of Psychology
Brown University
Providence, Rhode Island 02912

Patrick A. Cabe
Route 3, Box 163 A
Apex, North Carolina 27502

Ping-Kwong Chan
Toxicology Department
Rohm & Haas
Springhouse, Pennsylvania 19477

Chia-Shong Chen
Department of Psychology
Monash University
Clayton, Victoria, Australia

Bruce P. Halpern
Uris Hall
Cornell University
Ithaca, New York 14853

A. Wallace Hayes
Bowman Gray Technical Center
R. J. Reynolds Industries
Winston-Salem, North Carolina 27102

Ralph Heywood
Huntington Research Centres
Huntington, Cambridgeshire
PE18 6ES England

Richard M. Hoar
Department of Toxicology and Pathology
Hoffman-La Roche, Inc.
Nutley, New Jersey 07110

Michael R. Isley
Department of Psychology
University of North Carolina
Chapel Hill, North Carolina 27514

Merle Lawrence
Kresge Hearing Research Institute
1301 East Ann Street
Ann Arbor, Michigan 48109

Connie S. McCaa
Division of Ophthalmology
University of Mississippi
School of Medicine
Jackson, Mississippi 39211

John H. Mills
Department of Otolaryngology
Medical University of South Carolina
1 Ashley Avenue
Charleston, South Carolina 29425

Aage R. Møller
Department of Neurological Surgery
University of Pittsburgh School of
* Medicine*
Pittsburgh, Pennsylvania 15213

Daniel W. Nebert
Developmental Pharmacology Branch
National Institute of Child Health &
* Human Development*
National Institutes of Health
Bethesda, Maryland 20205

ix

James D. Prah
U.S. Environmental Protection Agency
Research Triangle Park, North Carolina
   27711

Diane C. Rogers
Department of Psychology
University of North Carolina
Chapel Hill, North Carolina 27514

James C. Saunders
Department of Othorhinolaryngology and
   Human Communication
University of Pennsylvania
Philadelphia, Pennsylvania 19104

Herbert H. Schaumburg
Albert Einstein College of Medicine
1300 Morris Park Avenue
Bronx, New York 10461

Hitoshi Shichi
Institute of Biological Sciences
Oakland University
Rochester, Michigan 48063

Paul G. Shinkman
Department of Psychology
University of North Carolina
121 Davie Hall
Chapel Hill, North Carolina 27514

Peter S. Spencer
Albert Einstein College of Medicine
1300 Morris Park Avenue
Bronx, New York 10461

William G. Thomas
Hearing and Speech Center
N. C. Memorial Hospital
Chapel Hill, North Carolina 27514

John S. Young
Johns Hopkins
615 North Wolfe Street
Baltimore, Maryland 21205

Toxicology of the Eye, Ear, and Other Special Senses, edited by A. W. Hayes. Raven Press, New York © 1985.

Anatomy, Physiology, and Toxicology of the Eye

Connie S. McCaa

Division of Ophthalmology, University of Mississippi School of Medicine, Jackson, Mississippi 39211

The eyes are at risk of environmental injury by direct exposure to airborne pollutants, by splash injury from chemicals, and by exposure via the circulatory system to numerous drugs and blood-borne toxins. In addition, drugs or toxins can destroy vision by damaging the visual nervous system. This chapter describes the anatomy and physiology of the eye and visual nervous system and includes a discussion of some of the more common toxins affecting vision in man.

ANATOMY OF THE EYEBALL

The eye consists of a retinal-lined fibrovascular sphere that contains the aqueous humor, the lens, and the vitreous body, as illustrated in Fig. 1.

The *retina* is the essential component of the eye and serves the primary purpose of photoreception. All other structures of the eye are subsidiary and act to focus images on the retina, to regulate the amount of light entering the eye, or to provide nutrition, protection, or motion. The retina may be considered as an outlying island of the central nervous system, to which it is connected by a tract of nerve fibers, the *optic nerve.*

The retina is within two coats of tissue that contribute protection and nourishment. On the outside of the sphere the *fibrous tunic*, corresponding to the dura mater, serves as a protective envelope. The posterior part of the fibrous tunic, the *sclera*, is white and opaque. The anterior portion, the *cornea*, is clear and transparent.

Immediately internal to the sclera lies the *uvea*, a vascular tunic analogous to the pia-arachnoid of the central nervous system. Primarily, the uvea provides nutrients to the eye. The posterior portion of the uvea is the *choroid*, a tissue composed almost entirely of blood vessels. A second portion of the uvea, the *ciliary body*, lies just anterior to the choroid and posterior to the corneoscleral margin and provides nutrients by forming intraocular fluid, the *aqueous humor*. In addition, the ciliary body contains muscles that provide a supporting and focusing mechanism for the lens. The most anterior portion of the uveal tract, the *iris*, is

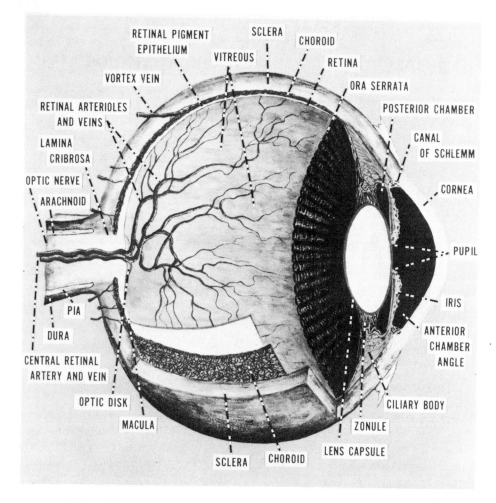

FIG. 1.   Internal structure of the human eye. Illustration by Keith Everett, M.D.

deflected into the interior of the eye. The iris acts as a diaphragm with a central rounded opening, the *pupil*, which dilates to allow more light to the retina in dim lighting and constricts in bright lighting. The iris also has some degree of nutritive function, since it acts to help regulate the fluid flow in the eye.

The *lens*, the focusing mechanism of the eye, is located immediately behind the iris and is supported from the ciliary body by a suspensory ligament, the *zonule*. The space between the iris and the lens is called the *posterior chamber*. The *anterior chamber* consists of the space between the iris and the cornea. Behind the lens is the *vitreous*, a gel-like, transparent body that occupies the space between the lens and the retina.

THE CORNEA

The cornea, the window of the eye, is unique because of its transparency. Corneal transparency is dependent on a special arrangement of cells and collagenous fibrils in acid mucopolysaccharide environment, an absence of blood vessels, and deturgescence (the state of relative dehydration of corneal tissue). Any toxin interfering with any one of these factors may result in corneal opacification.

Structure of the Cornea

As illustrated in Fig. 2, the cornea is composed of five distinct layers: (a) epithelium, (b) Bowman's membrane, (c) stroma, (d) Descemet's membrane, and (e) endothelium. In addition, a tear film always covers the cornea of a healthy eye.

The Tear Film

The tear film is made up of three layers. The portion immediately next to the epithelium is rich in glycoprotein produced by the goblet cells of the conjunctival epithelium; a middle watery layer is secreted by the lacrimal glands; an outside oily layer is produced by the meibomian glands and the glands of Moll and Zeis

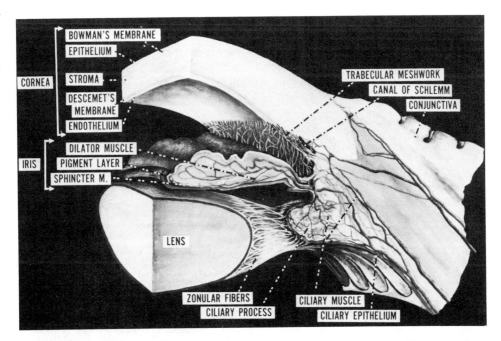

FIG. 2. Structure of the anterior compartment of the human eye. Illustration by Keith Everett, M.D.

of the lid. The tear film is essential for maintenance of the proper optical qualities of the cornea and its deficiency may result in corneal damage.

Corneal Epithelium

The corneal epithelium consists of five or six layers of cells that rest on a basement membrane. It is replaced by growth from its basal cells with perhaps greater rapidity than any other stratified epithelium (29).

Bowman's Membrane

Bowman's membrane is not a true basement membrane but is a clear acellular layer that is a modified portion of the superficial stroma. It is a homogeneous layer without cells and has no capacity to regenerate if injured.

Corneal Stroma

The stroma makes up approximately 90% of the thickness of the cornea. It consists of alternating lamellae of collagenous tissue parallel to the surface of the cornea. The corneal cells, or keratocytes, are relatively few and lie within the collagen lamellae (29).

Descemet's Membrane

Descemet's membrane is a strong, homogeneous, true basement membrane. It is produced by the endothelial cells and can be regenerated if injured. Descemet's membrane is elastic and is more resistant than the remainder of the cornea to trauma and disease.

Corneal Endothelium

The corneal endothelium consists of a single layer of flattened cuboidal cells. The endothelium does not regenerate and is essential for maintaining dehydration of corneal tissue. Therefore, chemical or physical damage to the endothelium of the cornea is far more serious than damage to the epithelium. Destruction of the endothelial cells may cause marked swelling of the cornea and result in loss of its transparency.

Permeability of the Cornea to Drugs or Toxins

The penetration of drugs through the cornea is by differential solubility. The epithelium and endothelium will allow the passage of fat-soluble substances and the stroma will allow the passage of water-soluble substances. All drugs that readily enter into the eye after topical application have the ability to exist in equilibrium in solution as ionized and nonionized forms. In the nonionized form they traverse the endothelium and epithelium and in the ionized form penetrate the stroma (13).

Toxic Agents Affecting the Cornea

Caustic Agents

Accidental splashing of substances into the eyes is the most common cause of toxic eye injuries. Alkalis and acids may result in rapid, deep, penetrating damage to cornea and deeper eye structures. The injuries produced by alkalis and acids are principally a result of extreme change of the pH within the tissue, an almost immediate action that can be treated only by rapid emergency action. There may be rapid dissolution of epithelium and clouding of corneal stroma from alkalis or coagulation of epithelium by acids, but many changes appear later, including edema, further opacification, and vascularization, and degeneration of the cornea. Alkali injury notoriously results in late changes, with extreme corneal injury and opacification.

Recent reports provide evidence that ocular alkali burns result in a decrease in aqueous humor ascorbate concentrations. The corneal ulceration with alkali burns may be based on ascorbate deficiency, which results in the failure of fibroblasts to produce sufficient collagen repair. Animal studies have shown that reversal of ascorbate deficiency by immediate treatment with parenteral or topical ascorbate significantly decreases the incidence of subsequent corneal ulceration and perforation (26), and a randomized clinical trial of ascorbic acid in the treatment of human alkali-burned eyes is now underway.

Organic Solvents

Organic solvents, especially those which are good fat solvents, may cause loss of some or all of the corneal epithelium. Yet even if all the epithelium is lost from the cornea as a result of organic solvents, it generally regenerates in a few days without residual permanent damage (11).

Gases, Vapors, and Dusts

A great many gases, vapors, and dusts induce stinging sensations in the eyes and stimulate tearing. Some of these may cause permanent corneal damage. For example, scarring and distortion of the cornea have disabled workmen many years after chronic industrial exposure to the dusts or vapors resulting from the manufacture of hydroquinone, a chemical used in photographic film development (11).

Deposits in the Cornea

Some drugs, such as chloroquine, hydroxychloroquine, chlorpromazine, and indomethacin, produce deposits in the corneal epithelium. These deposits generally appear as fine granules scattered throughout the epithelium. Usually the deposits do not interfere with vision, but they may defract light and produce an appearance of halos around light. These deposits are generally reversible when the drugs are discontinued.

THE SCLERA

The sclera is hydrated and has large collagen fibrils arranged haphazardly; therefore, it is opaque and white rather than clear. The sclera has three layers: (a) the episclera, the outer layer; (b) the sclera; and (c) the melanocytic layer, the inner lamina fusca. The episclera, a highly vascular connective tissue, attaches Tenon's capsule to the sclera. The sclera is approximately 1 mm thick posteriorly and gradually thins to about 0.3 mm just posterior to the insertions of the recti muscles. Therefore, these sites posterior to the insertion of the muscles are the areas of the eye that are most liable to rupture with trauma to the globe.

THE RETINA

The sensory retina covers the inner portion of the posterior two-thirds of the wall of the globe. It is a thin structure that in the living state is transparent and purplish-red in color due to the visual purple of the rods. The retina is a multilayered sheet of neural tissue closely applied to a single layer of pigmented epithelial cells. The sensory retina is attached only at two regions; the anterior extremity is firmly bound to the pigment epithelium at its dentate termination, the ora serrata. Posteriorly, the optic nerve fixes the retina to the wall of the globe. The potential space between the sensory retina and the retinal pigment epithelium may fill with fluid and result in retinal detachment. The fluid usually comes from the vitreous and enters the subretinal space through a tear or hole in the retina (rhegmatogenous or tear-induced retinal detachment). Less commonly, fluid may leak from blood vessels and cause an exudative retinal detachment.

The retina is 0.1 mm thick at the ora serrata and 0.23 mm thick at the posterior pole. It is thinnest at the fovea centralis, the center of the macula. The fovea may suffer irreparable damage in a brief period of separation from its only blood supply, the underlying choriocapillaris, during retinal detachment.

Composition of the Sensory Retina

The sensory retina is composed of highly organized tissue consisting of nine histologic layers resting on pigment epithelium. From the outside of the eye the layers are in the following order: the layer of rods and cones, the external limiting membrane, the outer nuclear layer, the outer plexiform layer, the inner nuclear layer, the inner plexiform layer, the ganglion cell layer, the nerve fiber layer, and the internal limiting membrane.

The Retinal Pigment Epithelium

The pigment epithelium consists of a single layer of cells that is firmly attached to the basal lamina of the choroid and loosely attached to the rods and cones. Microvilli form the apical parts of the cells and project among the rods and cones. The pigment granules consist of melanoprotein and lipofuscin.

The functions of the pigment epithelium are not completely understood. It produces pigment that acts to absorb light. Also, it has phagocytic functions and provides mechanical support to the processes of the photoreceptors.

Photoreceptor Cells of the Retina

The rods and cones, the light-receptive elements of the retina, transform physical energy into nerve impulses. Transformation of light energy depends on alteration of visual pigments contained in the rods or cones.

Rhodopsin, a derivative of vitamin A, is the visual pigment of the rods. Rhodopsin is composed of retinal (vitamin A aldehyde) bound to a large protein, opsin. The retinal is identical in rods and cones but the protein moiety differs. Light isomerizes the retinal from the 11-*cis* to an all-*trans* shape, releasing the retinal from the opsin. The chemical sequence following the isomerization of retinal produces a transient excitation of the receptor that is propagated along its axon. The bipolar cell transmits this information to the inner plexiform layer where it is modified through connections between amacrine, bipolar, and ganglion cells. The ganglion cells pass this analyzed information to the brain (23).

Toxins Affecting the Retina

Chloroquine and Hydroxychloroquine

Chloroquine and hydroxychloroquine are 4-aminoquinoline drugs used as antimalarial agents and in the treatment of certain chronic inflammatory disorders such as systemic lupus erythematosus and rheumatoid arthritis.

Chloroquines are deposited in richly cellular organs such as kidney, lung, liver, and spleen bound to nucleoproteins and nucleic acids. In addition, they are bound by melanin-containing tissues of the eye: the iris, choroid, and pigment epithelium of the retina.

Clinical Features

In the early stages of chloroquine retinopathy clinical symptoms may be absent. Later stages may result in decreased visual activity, sensitivity to light, night blindness, and light flashes. Pericentral or paracentral scotomas may be detected by Amsler grid exam or visual field testing. Abnormal color vision, mildly decreased dark adaptation, depressed electrooculogram (EOG), and a reduced b-wave on the electroretinogram (ERG) are noted in retinal function studies (5).

Disturbance of the macula is almost always present in chloroquine retinopathy. Initially it may present as edema followed by development of pigmentary changes. The latter may vary from an extremely subtle abnormality to one having a "bull's-eye" appearance to complete loss of macular pigment (8,15,25).

Chloroquine-induced retinal damage primarily occurs at the level of the pigment epithelium and rods and cones. There is loss of the rods and cones with migration of pigment from the adjacent epithelium into the inner retinal layer. Electron microscopic examination has shown additional abnormalities of the ganglion cells consisting of membranous cytoplasmic bodies and clusters of curvilinear tubules (28).

Treatment

Chloroquine retinopathy is not reversible, even after the drug is discontinued, because chloroquine is stored in the tissues. Therefore, the best treatment for chloroquine retinopathy appears to be prevention.

There is a definite relationship between retinopathy and daily total doses. The dosage concentration of chloroquine should be kept to less than 250 mg/day, the hydroxychloroquine concentration to less than 200 to 400 mg/day, and the duration of treatment to less than 1 year. Most cases of chloroquine retinopathy occur at a dosage concentration of 500 mg/day or more. A total dosage of 100 g can be retinopathic. The risk, however, significantly increases as the total dose becomes greater than 300 g (24).

The visual prognosis is guarded when a retinopathy secondary to chloroquine develops. In a significant number of cases there is a progressive loss of visual acuity that can continue for several years following the discontinuation of chloroquine (19). All patients on chloroquine should receive periodic ophthalmologic examinations.

Thioridazine

Thioridazine is one of the most commonly used phenothiazines in the treatment of serious psychiatric illness. Although all phenothiazine derivatives can cause corneal epithelial pigmented deposits and anterior subcapsular epithelial lens deposits, only the piperidines are prone to cause retinotoxic effects. There is a 75% incidence of retinopathy with thioridazine at a daily dosage concentration of 1,200 to 2,100 mg/day (12). A pigmentary mottling of the macula and posterior pole can be observed associated with decreased visual acuity and pericentral and central scotomas (4). Improvement in visual acuity usually occurs after the drug is stopped.

Quinine

Quinine may cause ocular damage when taken in large doses. In the past it was used as an antimalarial agent and more recently has been used as an abortifacient. Retinal vasodilatation develops first and is followed by marked constriction of the retinal arterioles. Retinal edema involving the macula is occasionally seen and the disc is usually pale. In the later stages diffuse pigmentary changes can occur.

A controversy persists regarding the primary site of damage of quinine. Francois et al. (9) concluded that the earliest lesion must be in the ganglion cells or the optic nerve, with later changes occurring at the retinal arterial level.

There is a tendency for visual recovery in most cases but in severe toxicity optic atrophy results.

Quinine retinopathy can be produced if the individual takes quinine hydrochloride in a dosage between 2.5 and 4 g (5).

AQUEOUS HUMOR

Aqueous humor, contained in the anterior compartment of the eye, is produced by the ciliary body and drained through outflow channels into the extraocular venous system. The aqueous circulation is a vital element in the maintenance of normal intraocular pressure (IOP) and in the supply of nutrients to avascular transparent ocular media, i.e., the lens and the cornea. Circulatory disturbance of the aqueous humor leads to abnormal elevation of the IOP, a condition known as glaucoma that can ultimately lead to blindness.

Aqueous Humor Formation

The formation of aqueous humor is dependent on the interaction of complex mechanisms within the ciliary body, such as blood flow, transcapillary exchange, and transport processes in the ciliary epithelium. Maintenance of the IOP is controlled by a delicate equilibration of aqueous humor formation and outflow; aqueous formation and ocular blood flow are in turn influenced by the IOP (22).

Formation of Aqueous by the Ciliary Epithelium

The ciliary epithelium is composed of two layers, the outer pigmented and the inner nonpigmented epithelium. ATPase is responsible for sodium transport to the posterior chamber and for aqueous formation; it is found predominantly in the nonpigmented epithelium (7).

Chemical analysis of the aqueous humor indicates that this fluid is not a simple dialysate or ultrafiltrate of the blood plasma (17). Continuous aqueous production by the ciliary processes requires an active mechanism demanding metabolic energy. Aqueous humor formation is therefore thought to be due to a secretory mechanism in the ciliary epithelium together with ultrafiltration from the capillaries in the ciliary processes. The secretory mechanism involves active transport of electrolytes, coupled fluid transport, and carbonic anhydrase action.

Aqueous Humor Circulation and Drainage

The anterior ocular compartment containing aqueous humor consists of two chambers of unequal volume, the anterior and posterior chambers (Fig. 2). Communication between the anterior and posterior chambers occurs through the pupil. The aqueous humor is secreted by the ciliary processes into the posterior chamber from which it flows into the anterior chamber. It is drained from the anterior chamber into the extraocular venous systems through porous tissue in the iridocorneal angle and Schlemm's canal (in humans and other primates) or venous plexus (in lower mammals). This drainage system is called the conventional drainage route. In humans and other primates, some aqueous leaves the eye by bulk flow via the ciliary body, suprachoroid, and sclera to the episcleral space; this route is called the uveoscleral drainage route or unconventional route.

Effect of Corticosteroids on Intraocular Pressure

Topical application of corticosteroids to normal human eyes occasionally results in IOP elevation accompanied by an increase in the outflow resistance (1). After discontinuation of steroids, the IOP usually returns to normal levels but may remain irreversibly elevated. The hypertensive IOP response to steroids appears to be genetically determined (2).

THE LENS

The lens is a biconvex, transparent, and avascular structure. It is suspended behind the iris by the zonule of Zinn, a suspensory ligament that connects it with the ciliary body. The lens capsule is a semipermeable membrane that will admit water and electrolytes. A subcapsular epithelium is present anteriorly. Subepithelial lamellar fibers are continuously produced throughout life. The nucleus and cortex of the lens are made up of long concentric lamellae, each of which contains a flattened nucleus in the peripheral portion of the lens near the equator.

Function of the Lens

The lens acts to focus light rays on the retina. To focus light from a near object the ciliary muscle contracts, pulling the choroid forward and releasing the tension on the zonules. The elastic lens capsule then molds the pliable lens into a more spherical shape with greater refractive power. This process is known as accommodation. With age, the lens becomes harder and the ability to accommodate for near objects is decreased.

Composition of the Lens

The lens consists of about 65% water and 35% protein (the highest protein content of any tissue of the body). Potassium is more concentrated in the lens than in most body tissues and ascorbic acid and glutathione are both present in the lens. It contains no nerve fibers or blood vessels; therefore, its nutrition is derived from the surrounding fluids. Mechanical injury to the lens or damage from altered nutrient concentration in the aqueous may result in cataract formation.

Cataract

A cataract is a lens opacity. Senile cataract is the most common type and is usually bilateral. Traumatic cataract, congenital cataract, and cataracts secondary to diabetes mellitus, galactosemia, other systemic diseases, and toxins are less common.

Cataract Formation

Cataractous lenses exhibit protein alteration, lens edema, vacuole formation, necrosis, and disruption of the lens fibers. Cataract formation is characterized by a reduction in oxygen uptake and an initial increase in water content followed by dehydration. Sodium and calcium content is increased while potassium, ascorbic acid, protein, and glutathione content is decreased.

Sugar Cataracts

Examples of sugar-type cataracts are those produced by galactose, xylose, and glucose. Galactose and xylose administered in large amounts to animals and blood glucose in excess, as in severe diabetes with persistent severe hyperglycemia, can produce cataract.

Sugars in high concentration in the aqueous humor readily enter the lens and are converted to sugar alcohols by aldose reductase (galactose to dulcitol or galactitol, glucose to sorbitol, and xylose to xylitol). The sugar alcohols accumulate in the lens and have an osmotic effect, causing water to enter the lens and causing lens cells and fibers to swell and become disrupted. These changes lead to formation of cataract (6).

Corticosteroid Cataracts

Posterior subcapsular cataracts have been produced by a variety of glucocorticoids used medically for long periods either systemically or applied to the surface of the eye. The toxicologic mechanism of cataract induction by the corticosteroids has not been defined.

Toxic Cataracts

Many cases of toxic cataract appeared in the 1930s as a result of ingestion of dinitrophenol, a drug taken to suppress appetite. Triparanol (MER/29) was also found to cause cataract. Echothiophate iodide, a strong miotic used in the treatment of glaucoma, has also been reported to cause cataract.

THE VITREOUS

Anatomy of Vitreous

The vitreous is a clear, avascular, gel-like body that comprises two-thirds of the volume and weight of the eye. It fills the space bounded by the lens, retina, and optic disc. Its gelatinous form and consistency are due to a loose syncytium of long-chain collagen molecules capable of binding large quantities of water. The vitreous is about 99% water; collagen and hyaluronic acid make up the remaining 1%.

THE VISUAL PATHWAY

The visual pathway from the retina may be divided into six levels: the optic nerve, the optic chiasm, the optic tract, the lateral geniculate nucleus, the optic radiation, and the visual cortex.

Anatomy of the Optic Nerve

The optic nerve consists of about 1 million axons arising from the ganglion cells of the retina. The nerve fiber layer of the retina is composed of these axons and they converge to form the optic nerve. The orbital portion of the nerve travels within the muscle cone to enter the bony optic foramen to gain access to the cranial cavity. The optic nerve is made up of visual fibers (80%) and afferent pupillary fibers (20%).

The Optic Chiasm

After a 10-mm intracranial course, the optic nerves from each eye join to form the optic chiasm. At the optic chiasm the nasal fibers, constituting about three-fourths of all the fibers, cross over to run in the optic tract of the opposite side.

The Optic Tract

In the optic tract crossed nasal fibers and uncrossed temporal fibers from the chiasm are rearranged to correspond with their position in the lateral geniculate body. All of the fibers receiving impulses from the right visual field are projected to the left cerebral hemisphere, and those from the left field are projected to the right cerebral hemisphere. Each optic tract sweeps around the hypothalamus and cerebral peduncle to end in the lateral geniculate body, with a smaller portion carrying pupillary impulses continuing to the pretectal area and superior colliculi.

The Lateral Geniculate Nucleus

The visual fibers synapse in the lateral geniculate body. The cell bodies of this structure give rise to the geniculocalcarine tract, the final neurons of the visual pathway.

The Optic Radiation

The geniculocalcarine tract passes through the posterior limb of the internal capsule and then fans into the optic radiation, which traverses parts of the temporal and parietal lobes en route to the occipital cortex.

The Visual Cortex

Optic radiation fibers representing superior retinal quadrants terminate on the superior lip of the calcarine fissure, and those representing inferior retinal quadrants end in the inferior lip. The macula is represented in a large region posteriorly, and retinal areas close to the macula are represented more anteriorly.

Toxins Affecting the Visual Nervous System

Methanol

Methyl alcohol (wood alcohol) has long been used as an intoxicating drink either accidentally or as an adulterant of ethyl alcohol. Benton and Calhoun examined 320 cases of methanol toxicity after a mass poisoning with contaminated moonshine whiskey in Atlanta (3). Symptoms appeared within 18 to 48 hr and consisted of decreased visual acuity, papilledema, and scotomas. Optic atrophy was visible in 30 to 60 days.

Histopathologic studies show that myelin is mainly affected, with preservation of axons and retinal ganglion cells (14).

Methyl alcohol is metabolized to formaldehyde and formic acid, which are the toxic agents. Since the same pathways are used for the metabolism of methyl alcohol and ethyl alcohol, the treatment for acute methyl alcohol poisoning includes oral administration of ethyl alcohol 100 proof (50%) as well as alkalinization of the plasma with intravenously administered sodium bicarbonate solution. Most patients show improvement in visual acuity in 4 to 6 days; those who have not improved by that time have a poor visual prognosis.

Nutritional Amblyopia (Tobacco-Alcohol Amblyopia)

Nutritional amblyopia is the preferred term for the entity sometimes referred to as tobacco-alcohol amblyopia. Clinical evidence overwhelmingly favors a dietary deficiency of B-complex vitamins, especially thiamine, rather than the direct toxic effects of tobacco or chronic alcoholism.

Persons with poor dietary habits may develop centrocecal scotomas. Bilateral loss of central vision is present in over 50% of the patients affected, with a resulting visual acuity of 20/200 or less.

Prognosis for recovery is excellent for all but the most chronic cases. Reduction in alcohol and tobacco usage plus adequate diet and B-complex vitamin supplementation is effective in curing the disease.

Drugs or Toxins Causing Papilledema

Papilledema as a toxic manifestation of drugs or chemicals can occur as an accompaniment of optic neuritis or as a manifestation of elevation of intracranial pressure. The substances that have most clearly produced papilledema are the corticosteroids, ethylene glycol, nalidixic acid, tetracycline, and vitamin A.

Drugs or Toxins Associated with Optic Neuropathies

More than 40 substances have been reported to result in optic nerve damage with resulting visual loss, impairment of color vision, and central or centrocecal scotomas. Some of the agents that have been more frequently reported as causing optic neuropathies are the following:

Chloramphenicol

Optic neuropathy associated with ingestion of chloramphenicol is well documented (10). Most of the patients had received prolonged courses of treatment for chronic infections. Histologic examination has shown loss of ganglion cells with demyelination of the corresponding portions of the optic nerve.

Ethambutol

The relationship of this drug to optic nerve disease is established (20). It is thought that optic neuropathy does not occur, or occurs infrequently, with a dosage below 15 mg/kg/day. However, in cases of renal damage with impaired excretion of the drug, optic neuropathy may occur at a lower dose. Quere et al. (27) have suggested the use of dibencoside (coenzyme B), a chelating agent, in treating toxic optic neuropathy from ethambutol.

Isoniazid

Optic neuropathy resulting in optic atrophy has been reported in patients taking isoniazid for pulmonary tuberculosis (16). Kiyosawa and Ishikawa reported resolution of isoniazid-induced optic neuropathy after withdrawal of the drug and initiation of pyridoxine (18).

Lead

Ingestion of lead may cause encephalopathy, papilledema, optic neuropathy, and optic atrophy. Loewe in 1906 reviewed the literature and cited over 60 cases of optic neuropathy resulting from lead intoxication (21). However, this condition is now rare.

ACKNOWLEDGMENTS

Acknowledgment is given to Beth Shannon and Kim Culpepper for assisting in preparing the manuscript. This study was supported in part by NIHR grant G 008103981.

REFERENCES

1. Armaly, M. (1963): Effect of corticosteroids on intraocular pressure and fluid dynamics, I and II. *Arch. Ophthalmol.*, 70:482–491.
2. Becker, B., and Hahn, K. (1964): Topical corticosteroids and heredity in primary open-angle glaucoma. *Am. J. Ophthalmol.*, 57:543–556.
3. Benton, C. D., and Calhoun, F. P., Jr. (1953): The ocular effects of methyl alcohol poisoning: Report of a catastrophe involving 320 persons. *Am. J. Ophthalmol.*, 36:1677–1685.
4. Bernstein, H. N. (1977): Ocular side-effects of drugs. In: *Drugs and Ocular Tissues*, edited by S. Dikstein. S. Karger, Basel.

5. Chen, C. J. (1979): Toxic effects on the retina. In: *Vitreoretinal Disease: A Manual for Diagnosis and Treatment*, edited by P. H. Morse, pp. 591–606. Year Book Medical Publishers, Inc., Chicago.
6. Chylack, L. T., and Kinoshita, J. H. (1969): Biochemical evaluation of a cataract induced in high glucose medium. *Invest. Ophthalmol.*, 8:401–412.
7. Cole, D. F. (1964): Localization of ouabain-sensitive adenosine triphosphatase in ciliary epithelium. *Exp. Eye Res.*, 3:72–75.
8. Crews, S. (1964): Chloroquine retinopathy with recovery in early stages. *Lancet*, 2:436–438.
9. Francois, J., De Rouck, A., and Cambie, E. (1972): Retinal and optic evaluation in quinine poisoning. *Ann. Ophthalmol.*, 4:177–185.
10. Godel, V., Nemet, P., and Lazar, M. (1980): Chloramphenicol optic neuropathy. *Arch. Ophthalmol.*, 98:1417–1421.
11. Grant, W. Morton (1974): *Toxicology of the Eye*. Charles C. Thomas, Springfield, IL.
12. Hagopian, V., Stratton, D., and Busiek, R. (1966): Five cases of pigmentary retinopathy associated with thioridazine administration. *Am. J. Psychiatry*, 123:97–100.
13. Havener, W. H. (1978): *Ocular Pharmacology*. The C. V. Mosby Co., St. Louis.
14. Hayreh, M. S., Hayreh, S. S., Baumbach, G. L., Cancilla, P., and Martin-Amat, G. (1977): Methyl alcohol poisoning. III. Ocular toxicity. *Arch. Ophthalmol.*, 95:1851–1858.
15. Hobbs, H., and Calnan, C. (1958): The ocular complications of chloroquine therapy. *Lancet*, 1:1207–1209.
16. Kass, K., Mandel, W., Cohen, H., and Dressler, S. H. (1957): Isoniazid as a cause of optic neuritis and atrophy. *JAMA*, 164:1740–1743.
17. Kinsey, V. E. (1951): The chemical composition and the osmotic pressure of the aqueous humor and plasma of the rabbit. *J. Gen. Physiol.*, 34:389–401.
18. Kiyosawa, M., and Ishikawa, S. (1981): A case of isoniazid-induced optic neuropathy. *Neuro-Ophthalmology*, 2:67–70.
19. Krill, A., Potts, A., and Johanson, G. (1971): Chloroquine retinopathy, investigation of discrepancy between dark adaptation and electroretinographic findings in advanced stages. *Am. J. Ophthalmol.*, 71:530–543.
20. Liebold, J. E. (1960): The ocular toxicity of ethambutol and its relationship to dose. *Ann. N.Y. Acad. Sci.*, 135:904–909.
21. Loewe, O. (1906): A case of transient lead amaurosis. *Arch. Ophthalmol.*, 35:164–171.
22. Mishima, S., Masuda, K., and Tamura T. (1977): Drugs influencing aqueous humor formation and drainage. In: *Drugs and Ocular Tissues*, edited by S. Dikstein. S. Karger, Basel.
23. Moses, R. A. (1975): *Adler's Physiology of the Eye*. The C. V. Mosby Co., St. Louis.
24. Nylander, U. (1966): Ocular damage in chloroquine therapy. *Acta Ophthalmol.*, 44:335–348.
25. Percival, S., and Behrman, J. (1969): Ophthalmological safety of chloroquine. *Br. J. Ophthalmol.*, 53:101–109.
26. Pfister, R. R., and Paterson, C. A. (1980): Ascorbic acid in the treatment of alkali burns of the eye. *Ophthalmology*, 87:1050–1057.
27. Quere, M. A., Ballereau, L., and Baikoff, G. (1976): Le traitement des nevrites optiques graves a l'ethambutol. *Bull. Soc. Ophtalmol. Fr.*, 76:935–938.
28. Ramsey, M., and Fine, B. (1972): Chloroquine toxicity in the human eye. *Am. J. Ophthalmol.*, 72:229–235.
29. Warwick, R. (1976): *Eugene Wolfe's Anatomy of the Eye and Orbit*. W. B. Saunders Co., Philadelphia and Toronto.

Toxicology of the Eye, Ear, and Other Special Senses, edited by A. W. Hayes. Raven Press, New York © 1985.

Structure and Function of the Ear and Auditory Nervous System

Merle Lawrence

Kresge Hearing Research Institute, University of Michigan Medical School, Ann Arbor, Michigan 48109

Sound conduction and sound conversion to a coded nerve impulse are the two basic peripheral processes of hearing, the latter being the more complicated and mysterious. It is during sound conversion that an extremely minute molecular disturbance is analyzed and a stimulus to a diverse network of fine unmyelinated nerve fibers is produced. A most delicate balance of the chemical environment is required to maintain a living organ in a condition that will achieve this process. The environment for this chemical balance is structured as a fluid system within a fluid system (Fig. 1); the mechanisms of chemical exchange between these two are still far from understood.

THE LABYRINTHS

The bony labyrinth within the petrous portion of the temporal bone is filled with perilymph that is connected with the cerebral spinal fluid (CSF) by the cochlear aqueduct. The patency of this duct varies among species and even during different stages of human life. For example, during fetal life and in neonates this aqueduct remains wide open, whereas in the adult it becomes quite narrow, having passed through a long bony channel.

At the labyrinthine end, the cochlear aqueduct opens into the scala tympani of the inner ear in the region of the round window beneath the basilar membrane. The scala tympani comprises the space between the basilar membrane and the bony wall of the otic capsule. While twisting with the spirals of the cochlea, the scala tympani joins the scala vestibuli at the apex through the helicotrema opening. The perilymph continues to fill these scalae as it winds back down the turns of the cochlea between the bony separation and Reissner's membrane. The bony labyrinth of the scala vestibuli widens at the base to surround the membranous utricle and saccule and then continues around the semicircular canals. The footplate of the stapes borders this enlarged vestibule of perilymph and conveys its minute motion to the endolymph through the perilymph and Reissner's membrane.

Because the cochlear aqueduct enters the perilymphatic channels at one end of the bony labyrinth, it seems unlikely that CSF will flow into the inner ear. Instead,

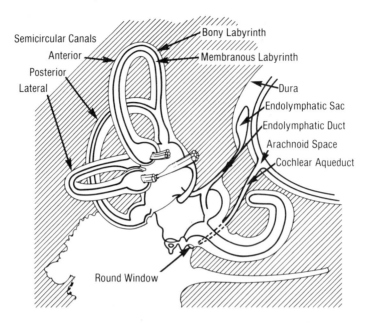

FIG. 1. Labyrinths of inner ear, creating the two fluid systems. The membranous labyrinth, which houses the endolymphatic duct, utricle, saccule, and semicircular ducts, is lodged within the bony labyrinth and contains endolymph. Perilymph fills the space separating the membranous from the bony labyrinth.

it is more likely that the perilymph produced within the inner ear is slowly absorbed into the CSF system.

More sodium and protein are added to perilymph somewhere within the perilymphatic system. In the region of the spiral ligament above Reissner's membrane (Fig. 2), there is a capillary network that may well be responsible for providing perilymph with those chemical characteristics that make it different from CSF. The capillaries are close to the surface and are arranged in a way to suggest the formation of a plasma filtrate.

The endolymphatic fluid is a closed system separated from perilymph by Reissner's membrane, the basilar membrane, and the membranous walls of the utricle, saccule, and semicircular canals. The endolymphatic duct is located midway between the cochlear and vestibular complexes and is continuous with the duct connecting the utricle and saccule. Like the perilymphatic aqueduct, the endolymphatic duct passes through bone and ends in a closed sac within the folds of the dura. Like perilymph, endolymph is not a stagnant pool. The fluid is generated and its ionic contents are controlled within the membranous labyrinth, all the while slowly moving in the direction of the endolymphatic duct to be absorbed in the endolymphatic sac.

The blood supply to the membranous labyrinth is separate from that of the otic capsule. The cochlear artery is a terminal branch of the vertebral-basilar artery complex and enters through the internal auditory meatus. After entering the modiolus the artery coils around the nerve, giving off branching arterioles that supply capillaries to the various parts of the labyrinthine structures.

THE STRIA VASCULARIS

In a spiral groove (Fig. 2) of the otic capsule around the coils of the cochlea is the spiral ligament. This forms one boundary of the triangle-shaped scala media. Along the surface facing the endolymph is the stria vascularis—a specialized structure that provides for the peculiar characteristics of the endolymph.

The stria vascularis is a unique structure with specialized cells. These have been described mostly from guinea pig observations made by both light and electron microscopy. Kimura and Schuknecht (7) describe, in humans, the ultrastructure of the three types of cells making up the stria vascularis: marginal (or dark), intermediate (or light), and basal cells. The cells on the endolymphatic surface are the marginal cells whose nuclei are close to the surface. On the opposite surface of these cells, the membrane is deeply corrugated, interlocking with the cells of the intermediate and basal cells. The intermediate cells are fewer in number than the

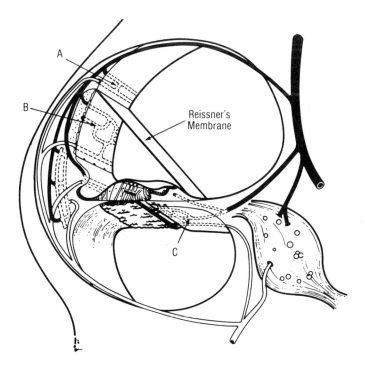

FIG. 2. Cross section of cochlear duct showing the various capillary areas. Regions include (A) the capillaries in the spiral ligament above Reissner's membrane, (B) the stria vascularis, and (C) the spiral capillaries beneath the tunnel of Corti.

marginal cells with which they interlock. Basal cells lie next to the spiral ligament. They are flat and long with cell processes that extend a short distance toward the marginal cells. The luminal surface of the marginal cells shows varying numbers of microvilli and pinocytotic invaginations, whereas the intermediate cells contain a large number of mitochondria. An extensive network of tubules filled with a diffuse substance lies close to the luminal surface, and the marginal cells adjacent to each other are interlocked with numerous infoldings.

Jahnke (6), using freeze-fracture techniques in the guinea pig, adds that the marginal cells appear to provide a barrier between the endolymphatic and the intracellular spaces. However, these spaces are tightly sealed to the spiral ligament so that the spaces appear to make up a compartment.

The capillaries of this area enter through the basal cell layer and pass among the intermediate and marginal cells. Smooth muscle cells and neural elements are absent in these capillaries, whose endothelial cell walls are extremely thin but not fenestrated.

The stria vascularis, whose marginal cells lie between the capillaries and endolymph, is responsible for maintaining the high potassium content of the endolymph. Along with this high potassium, endolymph has a positive electrical charge (approximately $+80$ mV) with respect to perilymph. The source of this potential has been localized to the stria vascularis (15) and is believed to be the result of the combined effect of an electrogenic pump and a potassium diffusion potential (14): the electrogenic component generating $+100$ mV and the potassium diffusion potential accounting for -20 mV. It is further theorized that the pump is located in the membrane of the marginal cells facing the endolymph.

It appears then that the stria vascularis is an organ in its own right. It has a high rate of metabolism and requires oxygen from its own capillaries. The oxygen that can be measured by an electrode in the scala media diffuses out from the stria.

THE SENSORY CELLS

The sensory cells of the organ of Corti are protected from endolymph, and their oxygen and nutrients are provided by the spiral vessels.

The capillaries of the osseous spiral lamina emerge beneath the organ of Corti to form two parallel systems lying beneath the feet of the pillar cells, thus bordering the tunnel. The distance between these capillaries and the hair cells is generally less than 50 μm, while the distance from capillary to tunnel fluid is only a few microns (9). The basilar membrane, the organ of Corti, and these capillaries are so situated that fluid exchange is facilitated. The feet of the inner pillar cells rest on the edge of the spiral lamina between the habenula perforata and the attachment of the basilar membrane. From this attachment to a point beneath the outer pillars there is only a thin fibrous layer separating the fluid spaces of the tunnel and the lamella cells on the scala tympani side.

As described, perilymph fills the scala tympani beneath the basilar membrane and passes easily through the thin area of the basilar membrane, named by Corti as the zona arcuata, between the pillars. This cortilymph (3) within the organ of Corti differs from perilymph by the oxygen and nutrients that diffuse from the spiral capillaries.

Several lines of evidence have indicated the role of the spiral vessels in the maintenance of cortilymph. Vosteen (17) reviewed a number of experiments that indicate the spiral vessels as the main source of oxygen for the sensory cells. In other studies, direct measures of oxygen availability were made simultaneously (11) in the tunnel fluid and endolymph as animals were made anoxic by shutting off their respiratory air. Oxygen concentration in the tunnel changed rapidly with the anoxic condition of the animal, whereas the oxygen concentration of the endolymph responded much more slowly. Apparently the spiral vessels provide oxygen directly to the sensory cells.

Adequate function of these sensory cells, the *sine qua non* of hearing, requires more than a sufficient oxygen supply. Even though the sensory cells are protected from endolymph, the positive endolymphatic potential plays an important role. Thus, the capillary blood supply to both the tunnel of Corti and the stria vascularis plays still a more important role (Fig. 3). However, the oxygen released by the

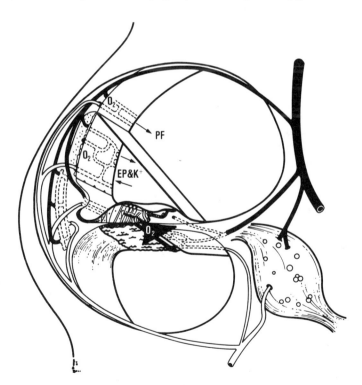

FIG. 3. Capillary areas vulnerable to attack by toxins: PF, plasma filtrate providing perilymph with its chemical constituents; EP and K^+, endolymphatic potential and high potassium controlled by the stria vascularis; O_2, oxygen sources for the areas maintaining microhomeostasis.

stria vascularis capillaries is utilized by the stria vascularis itself (2,16) and is not a supply for the sensory cells.

AREAS OF VULNERABILITY

There are then several capillary areas and transport functions that can be affected by toxic agents. An absence of blood cells has been reported (10) in both the stria vascularis and the spiral vessels following an acoustic overstimulation in the guinea pig. Hawkins (4) has reported that for adequate dosages of both quinine (quinine dihydrochloride) and salicylates (sodium salicylate) there results a partial occlusion of the spiral capillaries by the swollen endothelial cells that block the passage of blood cells.

Pike and Bosher (13) have shown that intravenous furosemide in guinea pigs produces ultrastructural abnormalities in the marginal cells of the stria vascularis with shrinkage of intermediate cells and enlargement of the intercellular spaces. These changes are correlated with changes in the ion-transporting mechanism of the stria (1).

Ototoxic drugs may also affect the capillaries above Reissner's membrane (5), and changes in the ionic content of the endolymph may affect the tectorial membrane, thus changing the adequate performance of the organ of Corti itself (8).

It is apparent, then, that both the morphology and function of the ear and its physiologic processes are subject to changes resulting in alterations of the micro-homeostatic conditions of the organ of Corti. Some drugs, such as the salicylates, will produce a partial hearing loss that may exist as long as the drug is taken, but when the drug is stopped, hearing returns to normal. Of the physiologic processes just described one might ask which ones are able to function at "half normal." Perhaps all of them, but most ototoxic effects from the antibiotics and diuretics seem to be permanent. However, the endolymphatic potential on which adequate function of the organ of Corti seems to depend can be reduced and maintained at lowered levels by reduction in blood oxygen.

Experiments (12) have shown that the reduced endocochlear potential from partial anoxia can be maintained over relatively long periods of time. Perhaps such an effect can account for the reversible hearing loss seen in some deafnesses resulting from toxins.

This brief outline of the morphology and possible physiologic functions of capillary areas and cell groups covers only in a very sketchy way the processes that are currently known. The reason why certain toxins have an affinity for the ear may be related to the lack of replaceable cell groups and the poor redundancy of the blood supply.

REFERENCES

1. Bosher, S. K. (1980): The nature of the ototoxic action of ethacrynic acid upon the mammalian endolymph system. II. Structural-functional correlates in the stria vascularis. *Acta Otolaryngol.*, 90:40–54.

2. Chou, J. T. Y., and Rodgers, Y. (1962): Respiration of tissues lining the mammalian membranous labyrinth. *J. Laryngol. Otol.*, 76:341–351.
3. Engstrom, H., and Wersall, J. (1953): Is there a special nutritive cellular system around the hair cells of the organ of Corti? *Ann. Otol.*, 62:507–512.
4. Hawkins, J. E., Jr. (1967): Iatrogenic toxic deafness in children. In: *Deafness in Children*, edited by F. McConnell and P. H. Ward. Vanderbilt University Press, Nashville, Tn.
5. Hawkins, J. E., Jr. (1973): Comparative otopathology: Aging, noise, and ototoxic drugs. *Adv. Otorhinolaryngol.*, 20:125–141.
6. Jahnke, K. (1975): The fine structure of freeze-fractured intercellular junctions in the guinea pig inner ear. *Acta Otolaryngol. (Suppl.)*, 336.
7. Kimura, R. S., and Scuknecht, H. F. (1970): The ultrastructure of the human stria vascularis. Part I. *Acta Otolaryngol.*, 69:415–427.
8. Kronester-Frei, A. (1979): The effect of changes in endolymphatic ion concentration on the tectorial membrane. *Hearing Res.*, 1:81–94.
9. Lawrence, M., and Clapper, M. P. (1972): Analysis of flow pattern in vas spirale. *Acta Otolaryngol.*, 73:94–103.
10. Lawrence, M., Gonzalez, G., and Hawkins, J. E., Jr. (1967): Some physiological factors in noise-induced hearing loss. *Am. Ind. Hyg. Assoc. J.*, 28:425–430.
11. Lawrence, M., and Nuttall, A. L. (1972): Oxygen availability in tunnel of Corti measured by microelectrode. *J. Acoust. Soc. Amer.*, 52:566–573.
12. Nuttall, A. L., and Lawrence, M. (1980): Endocochlear potential and scala media oxygen tension during partial anoxia. *Am. J. Otolaryngol.*, 1:147–153.
13. Pike, D. A., and Bosher, S. K. (1980): The time course of the strial changes produced by intravenous furosemide. *Hearing Res.*, 3:79–89.
14. Sellick, P. M., and Johnstone, B. M. (1975): Production and role of inner ear fluid. *Progr. Neurobiol.*, 5:337–362.
15. Tasaki, I., and Spyropoulus, C. (1959): Stria vascularis as source of endocochlear potential. *J. Neurophysiol.*, 22:149–155.
16. Thalmann, I., Matschinsky, F. M., and Thalmann, R. (1970): Quantitative study of selected enzymes involved in energy metabolism of cochlear duct. *Ann. Otol. Rhinol. Laryngol.*, 79:12–29.
17. Vosteen, K.-H. (1970): Passive and active transport in the inner ear. *Arch. Klin. Exp. Ohr. Nas. Kehlk. Heilk.*, 195:226–245.

Toxicology of the Eye, Ear, and Other Special Senses, edited by A. W. Hayes. Raven Press, New York © 1985.

Olfaction: Anatomy, Physiology, and Behavior[1]

James D. Prah and Vernon A. Benignus

United States Environmental Protection Agency, Neurotoxicology Division, Neurophysiology Branch; and University of North Carolina, Psychology Department, Chapel Hill, North Carolina 27514

> It is true the sense of smell is of all the least necessary, and still it is a tyrant like the others, and plays its part as such openly or behind the scene. It, too, moulds our disposition, awakens desires—most material desires, too—and these are followed by actions which, when speaking of man, we boldly designate as entirely voluntary (because they can be prevented by our will), and when of animals, we put to the account of that universal wizard called instinct. (1)
>
> ANONYMOUS

The sense of smell has been neglected in comparison to other senses. Among the reasons for this are (a) inaccessibility of anatomic structures, (b) poor theoretical knowledge about the nature of the physical stimulus, (c) difficulty with generating and presenting stimuli, and (d) the belief that the olfactory sense is not important to humans. Some of these (a, b, and c) remain problems, but techniques for dealing with them are being devised (2–4). No recent major advance in olfactory stimulus theory has occurred. The belief that olfaction has little significance for humans has been questioned recently and will be discussed in this paper.

The major reason for reviewing olfaction in a toxicologic/environmental context is that this neural tissue is directly exposed to air pollutants. Since these olfactory receptors appear to function by retaining molecules on their surface, airborne pollutants and toxic substances have a high potential for producing olfactory damage. The olfactory system is perhaps the most vulnerable neural tissue in terms of airborne pollutants, since the receptors are (a) directly exposed and (b) exposed via the circulatory system to blood-borne toxicants.

This review will describe the anatomy and physiology of the olfactory system and will also discuss the behavioral implications of this sense. In the limited space

---

[1]This chapter has been reviewed by the Health Effects Research Laboratory and has been approved for publication. Mention of trade names or commercial products does not constitute endorsement or recommendation for use.

available only overall conclusions can be given. Key references will be cited for further study.

OLFACTORY ANATOMY

Peripheral Anatomy and Physiology

Nasal Passages

Peripheral features of the olfactory system are illustrated in Figs. 1 and 2. Because of the shape of the three to four turbinates, only about 2% of inspired air reaches the olfactory epithelium during normal respiration (5). During passage over the nasal epithelium, temperature and humidity of inspired air are altered to body temperature and nearly aqueous saturation (6). Particulate matter in inspired air is deposited on nasal mucosa and swept toward the pharynx by the respiratory cilia (7). Mucus is supplied to the nasal epithelium by glands and goblet cells within the mucosa (8).

There is a daily cyclic variation in the flow resistance of each nasal passage (9,10) that is caused by the regular constriction and dilation of the mucosal venous cavernous tissue (11) and is thought to be hypothalamically regulated (12) via the vidian nerve (13). At the peak of the cycle one nasal cavity has low flow resistance and the mucosa is moist, while the other has high flow resistance and dry nasal mucosa (14).

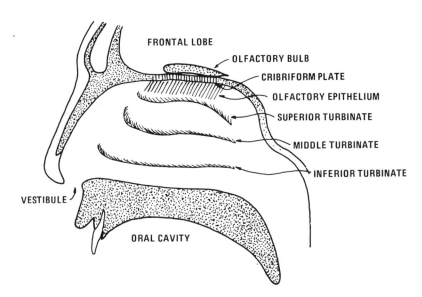

FIG. 1.   Midsagittal view of nasal cavity, showing location of olfactory structures and turbinates. (Adapted from Proetz, ref. 109.)

FRONTAL LOBES

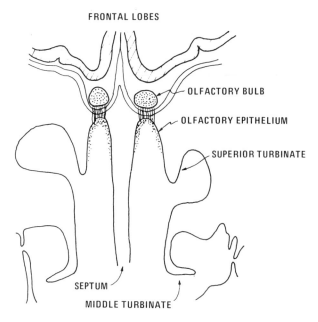

OLFACTORY BULB

OLFACTORY EPITHELIUM

SUPERIOR TURBINATE

SEPTUM

MIDDLE TURBINATE

FIG. 2. Coronal section through nasal cavity showing the location of olfactory structures with respect to the brain. The convoluted shape of the turbinates is also shown. (Adapted from Schneider, ref. 110.)

Olfactory Epithelium

The human olfactory epithelia, located at the apex of the nasal cavities (Figs. 1 and 2), encompass about 2 cm² and contain approximately 6×10^6 receptor cells (15). In contrast, the rabbit olfactory epithelia cover about 9 cm² and contain about 100×10^6 cells (16). The olfactory epithelium is covered by a mucous layer secreted by Bowman's glands. This sensory epithelium is about 70 μm thick, in contrast to the 45-μm thickness of the surrounding respiratory epithelium (15).

The olfactory epithelium (Fig. 3) is composed of receptor, basal, and sustentacular cells. The receptors are bipolar sensory cells and are often compared morphologically and functionally to the bipolar retinal cells. They are capped by 10 to 30 immotile cilia (17), in the typical 9 + 2 microtubule configuration (18), which extend about 160 μm into the mucus. It is presumed that the receptor sites are located on the cilia (19). The small axons, about 0.2 μm in diameter, are grouped in fascicles of 10 to 100 and enwrapped by Schwann cells (19) before penetrating the cribriform plate. These axons synapse in the olfactory bulb (OB) in a loose topographic mapping from the olfactory epithelium to the OB.

The sustentacular cells, as the name implies, support the receptor cells, provide a secretion with an unknown role and composition, and insulate the receptor cells from each other (20–22). They are capped with microvilli.

The basal cells, located at the base of the epithelium, are apparently the source for replacement receptor cells (23). The olfactory sensory neurons are unique in

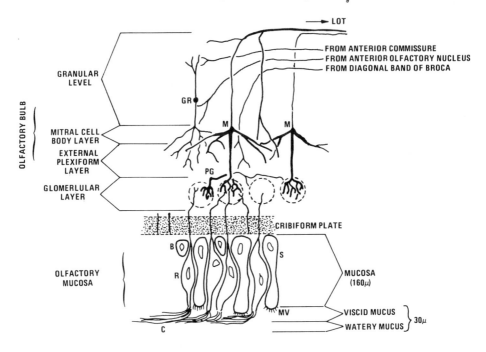

FIG. 3. Cells and connections of the olfactory epithelium and olfactory bulb. B, Basal cell; C, olfactory cilia; GR, granular cell; LOT, lateral olfactory tract; M, mitral cell; MV, microvilli; PG, periglomerular cell; R, receptor cell; S, sustentacular cell.

their ability to regenerate and reestablish functional synapses with the OB after destruction. Regeneration has been demonstrated in frogs, pigeons, mice, rabbits, rhesus monkey, squirrel monkey, and catfish (23–28). Regeneration of the olfactory receptors has not been demonstrated in humans. There is some evidence in humans that after 2 years of age the olfactory epithelium begins to atrophy (29–31). This progressive deterioration was not found in all specimens and was highly variable; nonetheless it may be the origin of the loss of olfactory sensitivity in the elderly (32–34). Interestingly, in geriatric rats the same developmental phenomenon is noted (35,36) after about 27 months of age.

Trigeminal Innervation

The nonolfactory nasal cavity is innervated by the free nerve endings of the ophthalmic and maxillary branches of the trigeminal nerve (37). It mediates what has been referred to as the common chemical sense and responds to chemical stimulation as irritation or pain (38). These endings are found in the epithelium of the pharynx as well. The sensory nuclei of the trigeminal nerve extend from the spinal cord to the mesencephalon.

Central Olfactory Structures

The connection and ultrastructure of the central aspects of the olfactory system have been reviewed by Shepherd (39,40). Other reviews (41–43) provide complementary information.

Olfactory Bulb

The major intrinsic connections of the OB are illustrated in Fig. 3. In the rabbit the receptor cell axons are unbranched until they ramify within the OB glomeruli (spherical areas of dense neuropil) and synapse with the mitral, periglomerular, and tufted cells. According to Allison and Warwick (16) about 25×10^3 receptor axons synpase with each of the 1,900 glomeruli. About 25 mitral cells contribute to each glomerulus, resulting in a convergence ratio of 1,000 receptors to 1 mitral cell. In humans, with about 3×10^6 receptors per olfactory epithelium and about 1×10^4 glomeruli per OB (44), there are about 300 receptors per glomerulus. The dimensions of the OB in man are about $11 \times 5 \times 2$ mm (44). Myelinated axons of the mitral and tufted cells form the lateral olfactory tract (LOT), which transmits sensory information to the central nervous system. The mitral cells also make secondary dendrodendritic connections with the granule cells. Connections made at this level include other intrinsic and extrinsic synapses. Periglomerular cells, which outnumber the mitral cells by about 20:1, make horizontal connections between glomeruli.

Granule cells in the external plexiform layer of the OB make dendrodendritic synapses with mitral cells and with each other as well as axodendritic connections with centrifugal neurons. Centrifugal neurons synapsing mainly with granule cells originate in the contralateral OB, via the anterior limb of the anterior commissure, in the ipsilateral anterior olfactory nucleus, and in the ipsilateral diagonal band of Broca. The latter fibers extend to synapse with the periglomerular cells.

Neurotransmitters

The neurotransmitters of the olfactory bulb are not well established. Table 1 lists the putative intrinsic neurotransmitters. More than one transmitter for a given cell

TABLE 1. *Cell types and their putative neurotransmitters*

Cell type	Putative transmitter
Receptor	Carnosine, GABA[a]
Granule	GABA, glutamate
Periglomerular	Dopamine, Glutamate, GABA
Mitral	Aspartate
Tufted	Dopamine

[a]GABA = γ-Aminobutyric acid.

type may be listed, reflecting, perhaps, different populations of that cell type. In addition, there are serotonergic innervation to the glomerular region from the brainstem raphe and noradrenergic innervation from the locus coeruleus to the internal granule layer. Further information may be found in Margolis (45), Fallon and Moore (46), Jaffe and Cuello (47), and Halasz, Ljungdahl, and Hokfelt (48).

Olfactory Cortex

A simplified ventral view of the human brain is shown in Fig. 4, showing the approximate area of LOT termination. The principal centripetal cortical connections are shown schematically in Fig. 5. The LOT courses ventrally over the prepiriform cortex toward the amygdaloid body. Along its course fibers branch from it and spread across the ventral cortical surface to synapse in the anterior olfactory nucleus, the piriform lobe (consisting of the prepiriform, piriform, and entorhinal cortices), the nucleus of the LOT, the cortical and medial amygdaloid nuclei, and the hypothalamus. Mitral and tufted cell axons from the LOT form axodendritic synpases with pyramidal cells in the outer molecular layer of the paleocortex, but not the deeper layers.

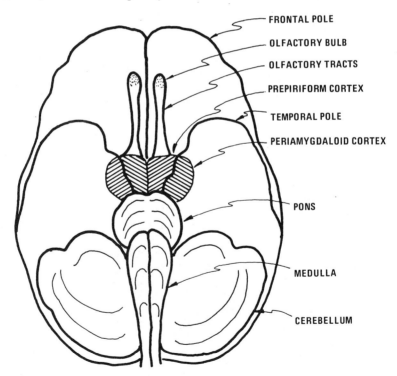

FRONTAL POLE

OLFACTORY BULB

OLFACTORY TRACTS

PREPIRIFORM CORTEX

TEMPORAL POLE

PERIAMYGDALOID CORTEX

PONS

MEDULLA

CEREBELLUM

FIG. 4. Ventral view of the human brain. Crosshatched areas show approximate area of termination of primary olfactory fibers. Structures to which synapses are made underlie these areas.

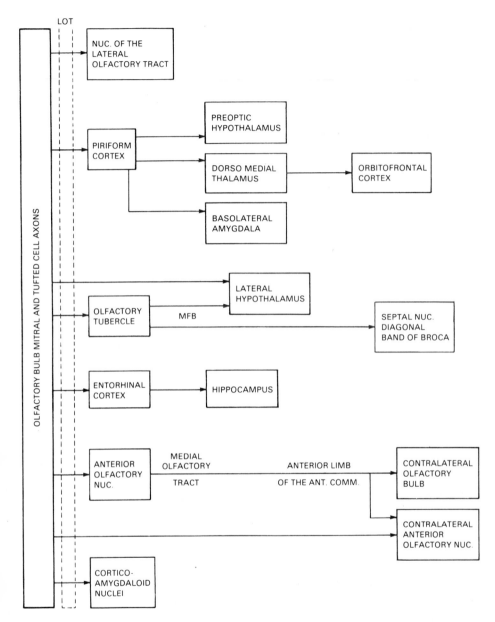

FIG. 5. Schematic of principal centripetal connections of the olfactory bulb. ANT. COMM., Anterior commissure; LOT, lateral olfactory tract; MFB, medial forebrain bundle.

The paleocortical structures send secondary olfactory fibers to other central nervous system sites. The anterior olfactory nucleus contributes fibers to the medial forebrain bundle, which terminates in the hypothalamus, as well as sending centrifugal fibers to the granule cells of the ipsilateral OB. Piriform lobe fibers are traceable to the amygdala, hypothalamus, thalamus, and hippocampus. Amygdaloid cells send axons to the hypothalamus, prepiriform cortex, hippocampus, OB, brainstem, and septum. This is not an exhaustive list of secondary fiber connections; only the major connections are noted.

Other multisynaptic CNS olfactory connections have been recently reported (49–51). These involve pathways originating in the amygdala and prepiriform cortex, which synapse thalamically and then postthalamically in the orbitofrontal cortex. This represents a neocortical projection, as opposed to the allocortical limbic projections.

PHYSIOLOGY AND FUNCTION

Psychophysiology

An olfactory stimulus consists of airborne chemical molecules within the molecular weight range of approximately 15 to 300. The intensity of the stimulus is a function of the number of molecules of odorous substance contacting the olfactory epithelium. The rate of perceived increase in intensity with increased odorant concentration is not constant across different odorants but is a log function of concentration, with the slope being influenced by water solubility of the odorant (52) and chemical functional group (53).

Threshold, usually defined as the stimulus concentration that the subject detects 50% of the time, is somewhat more difficult to study. The problem of adaptation (reduced sensitivity) to the stimulus can occur with multiple presentations of the same stimulus. Cross-adaptation may also occur with successive presentations of different stimuli. Measurement of thresholds presents the additional problems of individual variability and technique (54), of subjects' practice (55), and of instrumentation (56).

The construction of a classification scheme of odor quality has intrigued researchers for centuries (57). Numerous theories have been created to explain olfactory quality (58). Amoore (59) postulated and Beets (60) elaborated upon a stereochemical theory of olfaction based on receptor sites on the cilia. These hypothesized sites had different shapes to receive complementarily shaped primary odor molecules. Their hypothesized primary odors were deduced from organic chemistry and were analogous to primary colors in vision. Unfortunately, evidence for such receptor sites and primary odors is poor, correlations with actual perceived odor qualities are far from perfect, and there are notable exceptions to their rules.

Davies (61) proposed a puncture and penetration theory of olfaction whereby the odorant molecules actually enter the receptor cell and precipitate depolarization. Odor quality was hypothesized to be determined partly by the rate of diffusion through the membrane and the resistance of the individual receptor membranes to puncturing. There is no evidence that odorant molecules actually penetrate a receptor or that they have different diffusion rates.

Wright (62) proposed a molecular vibration theory of odor quality. In this theory the vibrational frequency of molecules in the far-infrared determines the quality while volatility, adsorbability, and water-lipid solubility determine the potency of the odor. This idea has been widely criticized (58,63,64).

A spatiotemporal model of olfaction has been proposed (65). In this analogy to gas chromatography the pattern of spread of odorant molecules across the olfactory epithelium in time determines olfactory quality. There is some solid evidence in support of this new theory. Studies with 2-deoxyglucose (66), transneuronal degeneration (67), mitral cell specificity (68), glomerular specificity (69), and receptor degeneration (70) support the spatial aspect of this theory at the epithelial and bulbar levels. At the level of the piriform cortex the organization of projections is more broadly distributed but statistically discriminable (71). There has been no evidence supporting the temporal aspect.

In sum, while there are many theories about olfaction, most seem to lack hard evidence in their favor. While most involve the structure of the molecule, it is not clear what physicochemical attribute of molecules makes them odoriferous. The unknown nature of the receptor mechanism further complicates the problem.

CNS Olfactory System

Olfactory Bulb

The anatomy of the OB suggests that this structure is more than a simple "telephone repeater" station. At the glomerular level, sensory cells fire into a synaptic neuropil of mitral and periglomerular cell dendrites. Since mitral and tufted cells are the principal neurons in the OB, their apparent function is transmission of sensory data. Even at the glomerular level, however, there is considerable data processing carried on by the network of periglomerular cells. There appears to be odor specificity at the glomerular level (69,72), and as a result of inhibitory synaptic processes there is considerable spatial and temporal sharpening of input data (73,74).

As seen in Fig. 3, connections in the inner three layers of the OB deal with interactions of sensory input data with the output from the CNS. These interactions occur in synapses of mitral and granule cells with axons from centrifugal cells. Granule and periglomerular cells also receive centrifugal influence. It has been demonstrated that the synaptic connections in the inner layers of the OB form recurrent inhibitory loops (75–77) that are responsible for the generation of the oscillatory electroencephalogram (EEG) that can be measured with macroelectrodes in the OB (78). The inner layers of the OB, therefore, seem to integrate sensory stimuli with centrifugal impulses and thus perform higher-level data processing to aid in olfactory perception and control of olfactory-guided behavior.

Odor Code

The question of how odor information is coded and transmitted to the brain is largely unanswered. There are several lines of evidence (see below), but the basic problems with all of them are (a) salient stimulus dimensions are not understood, and (b) perhaps as a consequence of these problems, correlations of electrophysiological responses with stimulus properties are rather low, even though statistically significant.

There is mounting evidence for an odor specificity in the mitral cells of the OB (69,72,79), which might be due to spatially organized projections from the olfactory epithelium (80–82). Some evidence for olfactory coding in OB EEG has also been reported (83). In both the EEG and single unit response data, however, it has been shown that the putative codes also are influenced by habituation and learning (84–87).

Variations in the saliency of odorants to the organism and the effects of arousal states of the organism can easily be confused for odor codes unless these variables are controlled. Similarly, unless intensity of stimulation is controlled for the various odors, a code for intensity might be mistaken for an odor code. Although the cited research provides suggestions for further work, there were many uncontrolled variables in these studies and results contained high residual variance. At this time no really firm groundwork has been laid to aid theorists in untangling pure sensory information from processed and interpreted data. Perhaps the CNS multiplexes these data and generates signals in which interpretational modifiers are appended to sensory data "words."

Brain Olfactory Mechanisms

The structures in the brain that receive olfactory input data are also known to be involved in the regulation of basic behaviors, which are well reviewed by Thompson (88). Laboratory animals will work to receive electrical stimulation to the medial forebrain bundle. The hypothalamus is intimately involved in the regulation of hunger, thirst, sexual activity, sleep, and hormonal control.

Evidence for the possible direct control of the hypothalamus by the olfactory system is found in several studies. Russell, Switz, and Thompson (89) demonstrated the modification of the human menstrual cycle of other women by odor collected from the axillary region of a female donor who had previously demonstrated a "driving" phenomenon on other women's menstrual cycles.

Ovulation was prevented in 87 women by the intranasal administration of luteinizing hormone-releasing factor agonist. Whether this contraceptive effect was olfactorily mediated is unclear (90). Steroids (estradiol, progesterone, or noresthisterose) were shown to arrest spermatogenesis and reduce serum testosterone in rhesus monkeys when given intranasally (91). The levels required were much lower than the levels needed if the steroids were given systemically. Electrical stimulation of the olfactory epithelium was shown to increase the level of plasmatic cortisol in 25 normal humans. This increase was presumably mediated by the hypothalamic neurosecretion of corticotropin-releasing factor and its influence on the pituitary. This effect was not seen in anosmics (92).

Lesions in the amygdala and surrounding structures produced alterations in sexual and social behaviors. All of these areas receive impulses from the OB and, indeed, the electrical activity of these centers is sometimes almost completely dominated by such inputs. It is not clear how much of the information transmitted to these CNS centers is sensory data and how much of it has been processed into signals for action. Whatever the nature of the signals that are sent to the CNS, the signals are sent to widespread and important sites. There are recent data indicating that human amygdala EEG correlates somewhat with odor qualities (93).

Behavior

For neurotoxicologists, the importance of anatomy and physiology rests upon the consequences of disturbances in the CNS on behavior. Behavior is the final common pathway. In nonhuman species it is well known that olfactory stimulation can very strongly influence sexual behavior (94,95) as well as social behaviors between and within species, such as aggression, territorial defense, and identification (96,97). It is usually assumed, however, that olfactory stimuli play only minor roles in influencing the behavior of humans. This assumption is based largely upon introspection about the causes of behavior rather than empirical evidence. In the case where sensory information is distributed to limbic system centers, however, it is questionable whether introspection would yield any information. Such subcortical input might in fact exert so-called "unconscious" influence. If this is the case, odor influences on human behavior could be quite important, especially because of their unobtrusive nature. With the attempts in society to control olfactory environmental pollution, it seems especially important to understand the effects of odors on human behavior.

Evidence is beginning to emerge on the role of the olfactory sense in human behavior. Humans can use odors to identify individuals (98,99), although it is unknown to what extent they normally do so. Humans generate pheromone-like compounds (100,101) and such pheromones affect sexual attractiveness in both males and females (102,103). Other social behaviors in addition to sexual attraction may well be affected by odor cues (104). There are correlations between olfactory acuity in women and menstrual variations (105,106). See Doty (94) for a review of these relationships. There is also evidence that jasmine flowers inhibit lactation in human females (107).

Although the findings regarding olfactory effects on human behavior are only suggestive, it is certainly logical on anatomical and physiological grounds that such effects should exist, since olfactory connections are made to widespread and important CNS sites (108). To assume that the effects are not important might be to overlook a strong and yet unobtrusive effect of the olfactory environment on everyday human behavior. More research on this issue is required.

REFERENCES

1. Anonymous (1866): The sense of smell. *Smithsonian Report.* Government Printing Office, Washington, D.C.
2. Benignus, V. A., and Prah, J. D. (1980): A computer controlled vapor dilution olfactometer. *Behav. Res. Meth. Instrumt.*, 12:535–540.
3. Benignus, V. A., and Prah, J. D. (1980): Flow thresholds of nonodorous air through the human naris as a function of temperature and humidity. *Percept. Psychophys.*, 27:569–573.
4. Prah, J. D., and Benignus, V. A. (1984): Trigeminal sensitivity to contact stimulation: A new method and some results. *Percept. Psychophys.*, 35:65–68.
5. DeVries, H., and Stuiver, M. (1961): The absolute sensitivity of the human sense of smell. In: *Sensory Communications*, edited by W. A. Rosenblith. John Wiley, New York.
6. Seeley, L. E. (1940): Study of changes in the temperature and water vapor content of respired air in the nasal cavity. *Heat Pipe Air Cond.*, 12:377–383.
7. Mygind, N., Petersen, M., and Nielsen, M. H. (1982): Morphology of the upper airway epithelium. In: *The Nose*, edited by D. F. Proctor and I. Andersen. Elsevier, New York.
8. Tos, M. (1982): Goblet cells and gland in the nose and paranasal sinuses. In: *The Nose*, edited by D. F. Proctor and I. Andersen. Elsevier, New York.
9. Stoksted, P. (1952): The physiologic cycle of the nose under normal and pathologic conditions. *Acta Otolaryngol.*, 42:175–179.
10. Eccles, R. (1978): The central rhythm of the nasal cycle. *Acta Otolaryngol.*, 86:464–468.
11. Bojsen-Moller, F., and Fahrenkrug, J. (1971): Nasal swelling-bodies and cyclic changes in the air passages of the rat and rabbit nose. *J. Anat.*, 110:25–37.
12. Stoksted, P. (1953): Rhinometric measurements for determination of the nasal cycle. *Acta Otolaryngol. (Suppl.)*, 109:159–175.
13. Malcomson, K. G. (1959): The vasomotor activities of the nasal mucous membrane. *J. Laryngol. Otol.*, 73:73–98.
14. Stoksted, P. (1953): Measurement of resistance in the nose during respiration at rest. *Acta Otolaryngol. (Suppl.)*, 109:143–158.
15. Moran, D. T., Rowley, J. C., Jafek, B. W., and Lovell, M. A. (1982): The fine structure of the olfactory mucosa in man. *J. Neurocytol.*, 11:721–746.
16. Allison, A. C., and Katz, R. T. T. (1949): Quantitative observations on the olfactory system of the rabbit. *Brain*, 72:186–197.
17. Ohno, I., Ohyama, M., Hanamure, Y., and Ogawa, K. (1981): Comparative anatomy of the olfactory epithelium. *Biomed. Res.*, 2:455–458.
18. Kauer, J. S. (1983): Surface morphology of olfactory receptors. *J. Submicrosc. Cytol.*, 15:167–171.
19. Graziadei, P. P. C. (1971): The olfactory mucosa of vertebrates. In: *Handbook of Sensory Physiology, Vol. 4*, edited by L. M. Beidler. Springer-Verlag, New York.
20. Moulton, D. C., and Beidler, L. M. (1967): Structure and function in the peripheral olfactory system. *Physiol. Rev.*, 47:1–52.
21. Douek, E. (1974): *The Sense of Smell and its Abnormalities.* Churchill Livingstone, Edinburgh.
22. Polyzonis, B. M., Katandaris, P. M., Grigis, P. I., and Demetriov, T. (1979): An electron microscopic study of human olfactory mucosa. *J. Anat.*, 128:77–83.
23. Graziadei, P. P. C., DeHan, R. S., and Metcalf, J. F. (1982): Cell dynamics in the olfactory mucosa of vertebrates. Society for Neuroscience, 2d Annual Meeting, Houston, Texas.
24. Wright, J. W., and Harding, J. W. (1982): Recovery of olfactory function after bilateral bulbectomy. *Science*, 216:322–324.
25. Mulvaney, B. D., and Heist, H. E. (1971): Regeneration of rabbit olfactory epithelium. *Am. J. Anat.*, 131:241–252.
26. Schultz, E. W. (1960): Repair of the olfactory mucosa. *Am. J. Pathol.*, 37:1–19.
27. Monti-Graziadei, G. A., Karlan, M. S., Bernstein, J. J., and Graziadei, P. P. C. (1980): Reinnervation of the olfactory bulb after section of the olfactory nerve in monkey *(Saimiri sciureus)*. *Brain Res.*, 189:343–354.
28. Cancalon, P. (1982): Degeneration and regeneration of olfactory cells induced by $ZnSO_4$ and other chemicals. *Tissue Cell*, 14:717–733.
29. Naessen, R. (1970): The identification and topographical localizations of the olfactory epithelium in man and other mammals. *Acta Otolaryngol*, 70:51–57.

30. Naessen, R. (1971): An enquiry on the morphological characteristics and possible changes with age in the olfactory region of man. *Acta Otolaryngol.*, 71:49–62.
31. Smith, C. G. (1962): Age incidence of atrophy of olfactory nerves in man. *J. Comp. Neurol.*, 77:589–595.
32. Murphy, C. (1983): Age-related effects on the threshold, psychophysical function, and pleasantness of menthol. *J. Gerontol.*, 38:217–222.
33. Stevens, J. C., Plantiga, A., and Cain, W. S. (1982): Reduction of odor and nasal pungency associated with aging. *Neurobiol. Aging*, 3:125–132.
34. Schiffman, S. (1979): Changes in taste and smell with age: Psychophysical aspects. In: *Aging, Vol. 10: Sensory Systems and Communication in the Elderly*, edited by J. M. Ordy and K. R. Brizzee. Raven Press, New York.
35. Smith, C. G. (1935): The change in volume of the olfactory and accessory olfactory bulb of the albino rat during postnatal life. *J. Comp. Neurol.*, 61:477–508.
36. Hinds, J. W., and McNelly, N. A. (1981): Aging in the rat olfactory system: Correlation of changes in the olfactory epithelium and olfactory bulb. *J. Comp. Neurol.*, 203:441–453.
37. Ottoson, D., and Shepherd, G. M. (1967): Experiments and concepts in olfactory physiology. In: *Progress in Brain Research, Vol. 23: Sensory Mechanisms*, edited by Y. Zotterman. Elsevier, New York.
38. Parker, G. H. (1912): The relation of smell, taste and the common chemical sense in vertebrates. *J. Acad. Sci., Phila.*, 15:221–234.
39. Shepherd, G. M. (1979): Olfactory bulb. In: *The Synaptic Organization of the Brain*. Oxford University Press, New York.
40. Shepherd, G. M. (1979): Olfactory cortex. In: *The Synaptic Organization of the Brain*. Oxford University Press, New York.
41. Wenzel, B. M., and Sieck, M. H. (1966): Olfaction. *Annu. Rev. Physiol.*, 28:381–434.
42. Lohman, A. H. M., and Lammers, H. J. (1967): On the structure and fiber connections of the olfactory centres in mammals. In: *Progress in Brain Research, Vol. 23: Sensory Mechanisms*, edited by Y. Zotterman. Elsevier, New York.
43. Allison, A. C. (1953): The morphology of the olfactory system in the vertebrates. *Biol. Rev.*, 28:195–244.
44. Smith, C. G. (1941): Incidence of atrophy of the olfactory nerves in man. *Arch. Otolaryngol.*, 34:533–539.
45. Margolis, F. L., Keller, A., and Ferriero, D. (1974): The olfactory pathway as a model cerebral system. In: *Metabolic Compartmentation and Neurotransmission: Relation to Brain Structure and Function*, edited by S. Berl, D. D. Clarke, and D. Schneider. Plenum Press, New York.
46. Fallon, J. H., and Moore, R. Y. (1978): Catecholamine innervation of the basal forebrain. II. Olfactory bulb, anterior olfactory nuclei, olfactory tubercle and piriform cortex. *J. Comp. Neurol.*, 180:533–544.
47. Jaffe, E. H., and Cuello, A. C. (1980): The distribution of catecholamines, glutamate decarboxylase and choline acetyltransferase in layers of the rat olfactory bulb. *Brain Res.*, 186:232–237.
48. Halasz, N., Ljungdahl, A., and Hokfelt, T. (1978): Transmitter histochemistry of the rat olfactory bulb. II. Fluorescence histochemical, autoradiographic and electron microscopic localization of monoamines. *Brain Res.*, 154:253–271.
49. Keverne, E. B. (1978): Olfaction and taste—Dual systems for sensory processing. *Trends Neurosci.*, 1:32–34.
50. Takagi, S. F. (1979): Dual systems for sensory olfactory processing in higher primates. *Trends Neurosci.*, 2:313–316.
51. Yarita, H., Iino, M., Tanabe, T., Kogure, S., and Takagi, S. F. (1980): A transthalamic olfactory pathway to orbitofrontal cortex in the monkey. *J. Neurophysiol.*, 43:69–85.
52. Tucker, D. (1963): Physical variables in the olfactory stimulation process. *J. Gen. Physiol.*, 46:453–489.
53. Klopping, H. (1971): Olfactory theories and the odors of small molecules. *J. Agri. Food Chem.*, 10:999–1004.
54. Cain, W. S. (1969): Odor intensity: Differences in the exponent of the psychophysical function. *Percept. Psychophys.*, 6:349–354.
55. Berglund, B., Berglund, U., Engen, T., and Ekman, G. (1970): Psychophysical functions of twenty-eight odorants. *Report from Psychology Laboratory (University of Stockholm)*, No. 291.

56. Pangborn, R. M., Berg, H. W., Roessler, E. B., and Webb, A. D. (1964): Influence of methodology on olfactory response. *Percept. Mot. Skills*, 18:91–103.
57. Cain, W. S. (1978): History of research on smell. In: *Handbook of Perception, Vol. 4A*, edited by E. C. Carterette and M. P. Friedman. Academic Press, New York.
58. Harper, R., Smith, E. C. B., and Land, D. B. (1968): *Odour Description and Classification.* American Elsevier, New York.
59. Amoore, J. A. (1970): *Molecular Basis of Odor.* Charles C. Thomas, Springfield, IL.
60. Beets, M. G. J. (1971): Olfactory response and molecular structure. In: *Handbook of Sensory Physiology, Vol. 4*, edited by L. M. Beidler. Springer-Verlag, New York.
61. Davies, J. T. (1953): L'Odeur et la morphologie des molecules. *Indust. Parfum.*, 8:74.
62. Wright, R. H. (1957): In: *Molecular Structure and Organoleptic Quality.* S.C.I. Monograph No. 1. Society of Chemical Industry, London.
63. Roderick, W. R. (1966): Current ideas on the chemical basis of olfaction. *J. Chem. Ed.*, 43:515–520.
64. Davies, J. T. (1971): Olfactory theories. In: *Handbook of Sensory Physiology, Vol. 4*, edited by L. M. Beidler. Springer-Verlag, New York.
65. Mozell, M. M. (1970): Evidence for a chromatographic model of olfaction. *J. Gen. Physiol.*, 56:46–63.
66. Lancet, D., Kauer, J. S., Greer, C. A., and Shepherd, G. M. (1981): High resolution 2-deoxyglucose localization in olfactory epithelium. *Chem. Senses*, 6:343–349.
67. Pinching, A. J., and Powell, T. P. S. (1971): Ultrastructural features of transneural cell degeneration in the olfactory system. *J. Cell Sci.*, 8:253–287.
68. Mair, R. G., and Gesteland, R. C. (1982): Response properties of mitral cells in the olfactory bulb of the neonatal rat. *Neuroscience*, 7:3117–3125.
69. Leveteau, J., and MacLeod, P. (1966): Olfactory discrimination in the rabbit olfactory glomerulus. *Science*, 153:175–176.
70. Land, L. J. (1973): Localized projection of olfactory nerves to rabbit olfactory bulb. *Brain Res.*, 63:153–166.
71. Scott, J. W., McBride, R. L., and Schneider, S. D. (1980): The organization of projections from the olfactory cortex in the piriform cortex and olfactory tubercle. *J. Comp. Neurol.*, 194:519–534.
72. Sharp, F. R., Kauer, J. S., and Shepherd, G. M. (1977): Laminar analysis of 2-deoxyglucose uptake in olfactory bulb and olfactory cortex of rabbit and rat. *J. Neurophysiol.*, 40:800–813.
73. Shepherd, G. M. (1971): Physiological evidence for dendrodendritic synaptic interactions in the rabbit's olfactory glomerulus. *Brain Res.*, 32:212–217.
74. Getchell, T. V., and Shepherd, G. M. (1975): Short-axon cells in the olfactory bulb: Dendrodendritic synaptic interactions. *J. Physiol. (Lond.)*, 251:523–548.
75. Nicoll, R. A. (1969): Inhibitory mechanisms in the rabbit olfactory bulb. *Brain Res.*, 14:157–172.
76. Getchell, T. V., and Shepherd, G. M. (1975): Synaptic actions on mitral and tufted cells elicited by olfactory nerve volleys in the rabbit. *J. Physiol. (Lond.)*, 251:497–522.
77. Mori, K., and Takagi, S. F. (1978): Activation and inhibition of olfactory bulb neurones by anterior commissure volleys in the rabbit. *J. Physiol. (Lond.)*, 279:589–604.
78. Bressler, S. L., and Freeman, W. J. (1980): Frequency analysis of olfactory system EEG in cat, rabbit, and rat. *Electroenceph. Clin. Neurophysiol.*, 50:19–24.
79. Kauer, J. S., and Moulton, D. G. (1974): Responses of the olfactory bulb neurones to odour stimulation of small nasal areas in the salamander. *J. Physiol. (Lond.)*, 243:717–737.
80. Pinching, A. J., and Doving, K. B. (1974): Selective degeneration in the rat olfactory bulb following exposure to different odors. *Brain Res.*, 82:195–204.
81. Moulton, D. G. (1976): Spatial patterning of response to odors in the peripheral olfactory system. *Physiol. Rev.*, 56:578–593.
82. Costanzo, R. M., and O'Connell, R. J. (1980): Receptive fields of second-order neurons in the olfactory bulb of the hamster. *J. Gen. Physiol.*, 76:53–68.
83. Hughes, J. R., Hendrix, D., Wetzel, N., and Johnston, J. (1969): Correlations between electrophysiological activity from the human olfactory bulb and the subjective response to odoriferous stimuli. In: *Olfaction and Taste III*, edited by C. Pfaffmann. Pergamon, Oxford.
84. Cattarelli, M., Pager, J., and Chanel, J. (1977): Modulation des réponses du bulbe olfactif et de l'activité respiratoire en la signification des odeurs chez le rat non constraint. *J. Physiol. (Paris)*, 73:963–984.

85. Freeman, W. J. (1979): Nonlinear dynamics of paleocortex manifested in the olfactory electro-encephalogram. *Biol. Cybern.*, 35:21–38.
86. Freeman, W. J. (1979): EEG analysis gives model of neuronal template-matching mechanism for sensory search with olfactory bulb. *Biol. Cybern.*, 35:221–234.
87. Magnavacca, C., and Chanel, J. (1979): Modulation des réponses du bulbe olfactif à l'odeur du mâle. Étude de l'activité multiunitaire chez la ratte au cours du cycle oestral. *J. Physiol. (Paris)*, 75:815–824.
88. Thompson, R. F. (1967): Hypothalamus and limbic system: The neural substrates of emotion and motivation. In: *Foundations of Physiological Psychology*. Harper and Row, New York.
89. Russell, M. J., Switz, G. M., and Thompson, K. (1980): Olfactory influence in the human menstrual cycle. *Pharmacol. Biochem. Behav.*, 13:737–738.
90. Bergquist, C., Nillius, S. J., and Wide, L. (1979): Intranasal gonadotropin-releasing hormone agonist as a contraceptive agent. *Lancet*, 8136:215–216.
91. Kumar, T. C. A., Sehgal, A., David, G. F. X., Bajaj, J. S., and Prasad, M. R. N. (1980): Effects of intranasal administration of hormonal steroids on serum testosterone and spermatogenesis in rhesus monkey *(Macaca mulatta)*. *Biol. Reprod.*, 22:935–940.
92. Orlandi, F., Serra, D., and Sotgiu, G. (1973): Electrical stimulation of the olfactory mucosa: A new test for the study of the hypothalamic functionality. *Horm. Res.*, 4:141–152.
93. Hughes, J. R., and Andy, O. J. (1979): The human amygdala, Part 2; Neurophysiological correlates of olfactory perception before and after amygdalotomy. *Electroenceph. Clin. Neurophysiol.*, 46:444–451.
94. Doty, R. L. (1976): *Mammalian Olfaction, Reproductive Processes, and Behavior*. Academic Press, New York.
95. Aron, C. (1979): Mechanisms of control of the reproductive function by olfactory stimuli in female mammals. *Physiol. Rev.*, 59:229–284.
96. Cheal, M. L., and Sprott, R. L. (1971): Social olfaction: A review of the role of olfaction in a variety of animal behaviors. *Psych. Rep.*, 29:195–243.
97. Thiessen, D. D., and Rice, M. (1976): Mammalian scent gland marking and social behavior. *Psychol. Bull.*, 83:505–539.
98. Russell, M. J. (1976): Human olfactory communication. *Nature*, 260:520–522.
99. Wallace, P. (1977): Individual discrimination of humans by odor. *Physiol. Behav.*, 19:577–579.
100. Comfort, A. (1971): Likelihood of human pheromones. *Nature*, 230:432–433.
101. Brooksband, B. W. L., Brown, R., and Gustafsson, J. A. (1974): The detection of 5-α-androst-16-en-3α-ol in human male axillary sweat. *Experientia*, 30:864–865.
102. Cowley, J. J., Johnson, A. L., and Brookshank, B. W. L. (1977): The effect of two odorous compounds on performance in an assessment of people test. *Psychoneuroendocrinology*, 2:159–172.
103. Kirk-Smith, M., Booth, D. A., Carroll, D., and Davies, P. (1978): Human social attitudes affected by androstenol. *Res. Commun. Psychol. Psychiatry Behav.*, 3:379–384.
104. Wiener, H. (1966): External chemical messengers. *N.Y. State J. Med.*, 66:3153–3170.
105. Schneider, R. A., Costiloe, J. P., Howard, J. P., and Wolf, S. (1958): Olfactory perception thresholds in hypogonadal women: Changes accompanying administration of androgen and estrogen. *J. Clin. Endocrinol. Metab.*, 18:379–390.
106. Marshall, J. R., and Henkin, R. I. (1971): Olfactory acuity, menstrual abnormality and oocyte status. *Ann. Int. Med.*, 75:207–211.
107. Abraham, M., Devi, N. S., and Sheela, R. (1979): Inhibiting effect of jasmine flowers on lactation. *Indian J. Med. Res.*, 69:88–92.
108. Schneider, R. A. (1974): Newer insights into the role and modifications of olfaction in man through clinical studies. *Ann. N.Y. Acad. Sci.*, 237:217–223.
109. Proetz, A. W. (1941): *Essays on the Applied Physiology of the Nose*. Annals Publishing Co., St. Louis.
110. Schneider, R. A. (1967): The sense of smell in man—Its physiologic basis. *N. Engl. J. Med.*, 277:229–303.

Toxicology of the Eye, Ear, and Other Special Senses, edited by A.W. Hayes. Raven Press, New York © 1985.

Structure and Function of the Somatosensory System: A Neurotoxicologic Perspective

Joseph C. Arezzo, Herbert H. Schaumburg, and Peter S. Spencer

Institute of Neurotoxicology, Departments of Neuroscience, Neurology, and Pathology (Neuropathology), Rose F. Kennedy Center, Albert Einstein College of Medicine, Bronx, New York 10461

The somatosensory system is defined as those elements of the peripheral nervous system (PNS) and the central nervous system (CNS) subserving the modalities of touch, vibration, temperature, pain, and kinesthesia. Specific modalities are associated with unique peripheral receptors, peripheral axons of stereotyped diameter, and specific central projection pathways. Several features of the somatosensory system render regions of it vulnerable to a wide variety of toxicants. The present report highlights these features and, furthermore, suggests that analysis of these regions is invaluable in studying the three most common varieties of toxic neuropathy: toxic distal axonopathies, toxic myelinopathy, and toxic sensory neuronopathy.

RECEPTORS

Structure and Function

Since the early nineteenth century various specialized receptors have been associated with the somatosensory system. These receptors, located in skin, hair follicles, joints, and muscles, transduce mechanical or thermal energy. Minimally, a receptor includes a peripheral axon terminal of one primary afferent neuron, whose cell body is sited proximally in the dorsal root ganglion. Receptors often include nonneural elements that incorporate and interact with the axon terminal in initiating generator potentials. Multiple generator potentials may summate to the threshold necessary for triggering a nerve impulse. Three major categories of somatosensory receptors can be identified: mechanoreceptors, thermoreceptors, and nociceptors. These categories are further subdivided on the basis of location and rate of adaptation.

Mechanoreceptors are sensitive to pressure resulting in deformation of the accessory receptor structure. An example of a slowly adapting mechanoreceptor is a Merkel-cell complex consisting of a myelinated axon terminating at the base of a small dome-like elevation in the skin. Displacement of the dome by as little as 5 μm can result in a suprathreshold generator potential within the Merkel cell-axon terminal complex. Rapidly adapting mechanoreceptors are principally sensitive to rapid or sinusoidal transients in pressure and are exemplified by the pacinian corpuscles. The pacinian corpuscle is composed of an outer capsule formed of connective tissue lamellae separated by fluid-filled interlamellar spaces and an inner core of tightly spaced lamellae (Fig. 1). Proximally, the outer core is penetrated by a canal that contains a single myelinated preterminal axon (7–11 μm across), continuous with a long naked axon terminal deep in the center of the corpuscle. The long terminal axon is elliptical in section, is provided with juxtaposed filopod processes, and has a bulbous ultraterminal ending from whose entire surface filopod processes emanate in a hydra-like array. Filopod processes appear to contact the inner core lamellae. This physical relationship may provide the substrate for transmitting fast pressure changes characteristic of these rapidly adapting vibration receptors (11).

Cutaneous thermoreceptors display three consistent properties: (a) static discharge at constant temperature, (b) dynamic response to temperature change, and (c) relative insensitivity to mechanical stimuli. Punctate regions of the skin, approximately 1 mm in diameter, have been consistently identified as sensitive to

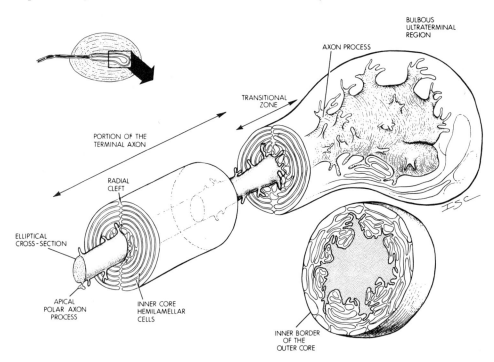

FIG. 1. Three-dimensional diagram of a pacinian corpuscle indicated by the boxed area in the **upper left** diagram, illustrating the distal end of the terminal segment, the transitional zone, and the ultraterminal region. **Lower right**: Cross-sectional view of the ultraterminal chamber. (From Spencer and Schaumburg, ref. 11, reproduced by permission.)

either warm or cold stimuli; however, these modalities have not been reliably associated with specific encapsulated or corpuscular receptors. Temperature sensitivity is conveyed in small-diameter myelinated and unmyelinated fibers. Thermoreceptors most likely are branching matrices of naked axons terminating in the stratum papillare. These terminations contain numerous small vesicles and mitochondria.

Nociceptors, mediating pain, are sensitive to mechanical, thermal, or chemical energy; however, they are selective for stimuli that may cause tissue or neural damage. Morphologically, these receptors also appear to be free nerve endings in the skin and muscle.

Neurotoxicology

Central-peripheral distal axonopathy characterized by degeneration in the distal segments of large-diameter axons is a common morphologic reaction of the nervous system to exogenous toxins (13,14). The neural elements of somatosensory receptors in the hands and feet represent the distal extreme of long afferent fibers, and are particularly vulnerable in these disorders. Selective receptor inactivation is an early change following exposure to certain neurotoxins; e.g., failure of the generator potential followed by loss of the axon filopod processes in pacinian corpuscles are early physiologic and morphologic alterations following acrylamide intoxication (10,12). Toxic sensory neuronopathy, characterized by degeneration of dorsal root ganglion cells, also produces degeneration in sensory axons of peripheral nerve and, presumably, of their axon terminals in receptors (15).

PERIPHERAL NERVE

Structure and Function

Large nerves, such as the tibial, consist of several fascicles containing numerous myelinated and unmyelinated axons (Fig. 2). Each fascicle is enclosed by a perineurial ensheathment, which serves as a diffusion barrier and accounts for much of the tensile strength of the nerve. Distally, the perineurium fuses with the connective tissue of encapsulated sensory receptors but does not cover free nerve endings. Proximally, the perineurium surrounds the dorsal root ganglia, which contains the cell body of the primary afferent fiber and is continuous with the root sheaths. The axon of nerve fibers is ensheathed by a chain of Schwann cells. In myelinated fibers, this ensheathment takes the form of a multilayered membranous structure (myelin), a product of the Schwann cell. Interruptions between each length of myelin sheath, called nodes of Ranvier, occur at regularly spaced intervals along the length of the nerve fiber.

Afferent fibers of the somatosensory system vary in cross-sectional diameter from approximately 0.4 to 20 μm. The rate of impulse conduction varies directly with the diameter of the axon. Heavily myelinated axons are fast conductors while thinly myelinated and unmyelinated axons conduct less rapidly. Subpeaks of the

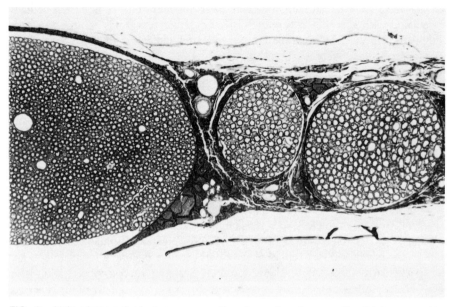

FIG. 2. Light micrograph of a transverse section of a portion of mammalian tibial nerve and its branches, each containing numerous myelinated axons. One-micrometer epoxy section stained with toluidine blue. × 145.

compound action potential can be used to classify axons as to size and conduction velocity. Mechanoreceptors are predominantly subserved by medium- and large-sized myelinated fibers, whereas thermoreceptors and nociceptors rely on relatively small myelinated and unmyelinated fibers. However, there is considerable overlap, and no conduction velocity uniquely specifies a receptor class.

Neurotoxicology

The bipolar dorsal root ganglion cell (DRG) and its long, heavily myelinated axons are exquisitely vulnerable to each of the three common types of neurotoxic injury. Center-peripheral distal axonopathies (e.g., acrylamide, *n*-hexane) are characterized by selective degeneration of long large-diameter axons in both the peripheral and central nervous system. Therefore, bipolar DRG neurons whose peripheral processes extend the length of the sciatic nerve, and whose central processes traverse the length of the spinal cord to the gracile nucleus, are early affected. Toxic myelinopathies (e.g., hexachlorophene, acetyl ethyl tetramethyl tetralin) are associated with bubbling of PNS and CNS myelin sheaths. The long, heavily myelinated axons of the bipolar DRG neuron, extending for great lengths both to CNS and PNS, are consistently involved (9,16). Substances producing neuronopathies (e.g., doxorubicin, pyridoxine) presumably act directly on the soma of neurons (6). Such substances have limited or no access to most nerve cells because the tight junctions of the endothelial cells of nervous system blood vessels (blood-brain and blood-nerve barrier) prevent leakage. The blood vessels of the DRG are fenestrated, permitting such substances to leak out and selectively damage these neurons (toxic sensory neuronopathy). This produces rapid degeneration throughout the length of peripheral sensory axons and dorsal columns. Sensory nerves in upper and lower extremities are equally affected.

SPINAL PATHWAYS

Structure and Function

The spinal cord contains a number of well-defined, modality-specific fiber tracts that ascend from the segmental levels to the brainstem and diencephalon (Fig. 3). The largest of these tracts is the dorsal column system, which forms the dorsal and medial boundaries of the spinal cord. The central projections of dorsal root ganglia course in the medial division of the dorsal root, enter the spinal cord, and divide into a long ascending and a short descending branch (Fig. 4). Fibers from caudal-

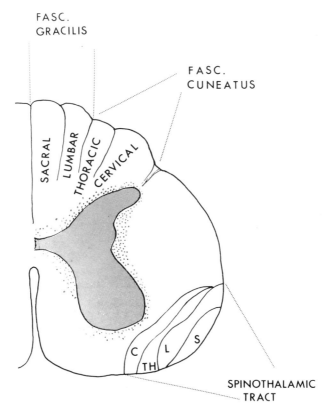

FIG. 3. Schematic diagram of a cervical segment of the human spinal cord outlining the dorsal column and spinothalamic fiber tracts.

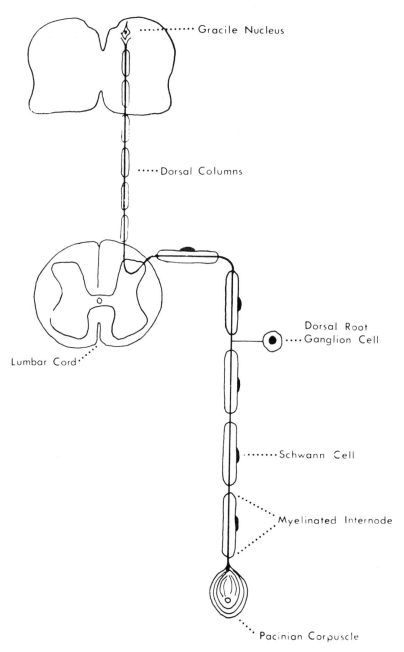

FIG. 4. Diagram of a dorsal root ganglion cell, depicting the ascending (central) branch of the bipolar axon terminating in the gracile nucleus and the descending (peripheral) branch ending in a pacinian corpuscle.

most levels become located medially in the dorsal columns at progressively higher levels, as entering axons are laid down at the lateral margin of the tracts. Thus the medial bundle of fibers (fasciculus gracilis) originates from segments below the midthoracic region, while the lateral portion (fasciculus cuneatus) contains fibers from upper thoracic and cervical segments. In addition to the large-diameter fibers entering directly from DRG neurons (primary afferents), the dorsal columns contain many small-diameter primary afferents (conducting under 25 m/sec). Approximately 10% of the dorsal column fibers originate from cells within the spinal cord (nonprimary afferents). Sensations of touch, vibration, and kinesthesia are conveyed by the dorsal columns. The termination of this system is in the ipsilateral dorsal column nuclei of the medulla oblongata.

The anterior and lateral spinothalamic tracts convey modalities of pain and temperature, as well as touch. Primary afferents of this system course through the lateral division of the dorsal root and enter the spinal gray matter where they contact several interneurons. Axons of the last neuron in the local relay obliquely cross the cord, within one segment of entry, and ascend in the spinothalamic tract. There is both topographic and modality-specific organization within the spino-thalamic tracts. The most lateral fibers represent the caudal segments of the body, and fibers concerned with pain are, in general, anterior to those conveying temperature. The central projections of the spinothalamic tracts are complex and include several thalamic nuclei (ventral posterior lateral, intralaminar, posterior complex) as well as reticular nuclei of the brainstem.

The spinocervical tract, a recently discovered pathway in man, conveys specific cutaneous information and is characterized by the rapid conduction velocity of its axons. This tract arises entirely within the spinal cord from cells in the dorsal horn of the gray matter. Small fibers of the dorsal root enter the cord and synapse on dorsal horn neurons. Axons of these cells ascend as spinocervical tract fibers within the dorsolateral fasciculus on the side of root entry, terminating in the lateral cervical nucleus at the uppermost level of the spinal cord. Axons from cells in the lateral cervical nucleus cross the midline and terminate within the ventral posterior lateral (VPL) nucleus of the thalamus.

Additional ascending somatosensory spinal pathways include the spinoreticular tract, the spinotectal tract, and the spinocerebellar tract.

Neurotoxicology

Many of the dorsal column fibers represent central projections of bipolar DRG cells and, as described in the previous section, are exquisitely vulnerable to the three common forms of neurotoxic injury. Myelinopathic agents may cause bubbling of myelin throughout the length of the dorsal columns. Toxins producing central-peripheral distal axonopathy cause degeneration that is initially confined to the rostral ends of the long fibers ascending the gracile fasciculi and distal regions of peripheral axons. The shorter fibers of the cuneate fasciculi are relatively spared in these disorders (Fig. 5). Toxins producing exclusively central distal axonopathy,

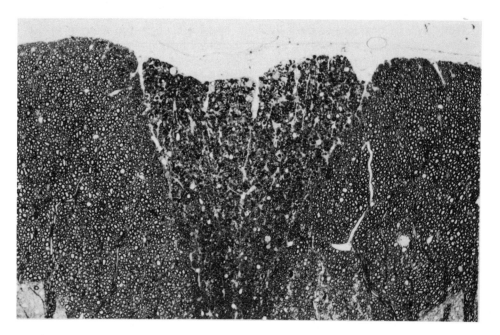

FIG. 5. Medulla oblongata of a rat with hexacarbon distal axonopathy showing selective degeneration of the gracile tracts **(center)**. ×204. (From Spencer and Schaumburg, ref. 13, reproduced by permission.)

e.g., clioquinol, cause degeneration that is also confined to the distal ends of the long fibers ascending in the gracile fasciculi but spares the peripheral nervous system. Neuronopathic agents affect DRG cells at multiple levels resulting in virtually simultaneous axonal degeneration throughout the length of the gracile and cuneate fasciculi.

The remaining ascending spinal somatosensory pathways appear relatively unaffected in neurotoxic conditions.

RELAY NUCLEI

Structure and Function

Neurons in somatosensory relay nuclei (dorsal column, ventral thalamic, lateral cervical) receive projections from ascending spinal tracts, then project to more rostral structures in the neuraxis. Integration of activity and modification of the ascending volley by corticofugal influences occur at these sites. Pre- and postsynaptic feedback inhibition characterizes all levels of the somatosensory system and significantly alters the afferent volley.

The dorsal column nuclei (gracile and cuneate) maintain a remarkable degree of topographic and modality specificity. Axons from cells in these nuclei cross as internal arcuate fibers in the low medulla and ascend in the medial lemniscus to the ventral thalamus. The ventral and posterior tiers of the thalamus are subdivided into a number of nuclear aggregates. The ventral posterior lateral nucleus is the principal somatosensory relay, and it is at this site that somatosensory information conveyed in the anteriolateral and dorsal column-medial lemniscal system converges and is in turn relayed to the cortex.

Neurotoxicology

Changes in the dorsal column and lateral cervical nuclei following various types of neurotoxic injury mirror those of the dorsal columns and spinocervical tracts described in the previous section. There are no reports of neurotoxin-induced degeneration in the human thalamic relay nuclei.

CEREBRAL CORTEX

Structure and Function

The cerebral cortex controls conscious perception of somatosensory events. The previous simple division of the sensorimotor cortex into precentral (motor) and postcentral (sensory) strips has been replaced by a broad-based multiple mapping of the body surface onto the cortex. Serial and parallel processing of somatosensory information occurs at disparate cortical locations and involves extensive interneuron pools, making it difficult to localize the site of action of neurotoxic agents on cortical activity.

The first somatic sensory area (SI) comprises three cytoarchitectonic subfields, Brodmann's areas 3, 1, and 2 (Fig. 6). Area 3 receives a dense projection of large fibers from the ventral tier of the thalamus, whereas areas 1 and 2 receive less

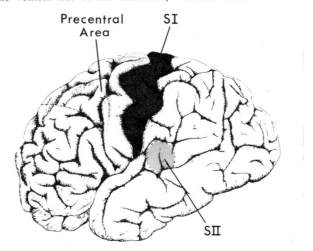

FIG. 6. Lateral view of the human cerebral cortex outlining the location of the SI, SII, and pre-central somatosensory regions. Additional somatosensory areas can be found on the medial surface and within the banks of the central and sylvian tissues.

dense input of fine fibers from this region. Area 3 and the anterior portion of area 1 principally process short-latency cutaneous and muscle-spindle afferents, whereas the posterior portion of area 1 and all of area 2 receive inputs from deep-lying receptors. There are at least two independent mirror-image representations of body surface within SI. For each body representation the caudal dermatomes are represented medially; progressively rostral regions project to more lateral cortical areas. The extent of cortical representation of a body region is proportional to the use of that region and not to its size. Thus, in the sensory homunculus the thumb area exceeds that of the remainder of the arm.

Electrophysiological studies have documented short-latency somatosensory activity within the cortex forming the precentral gyrus (1,8). Independent direct projections from the ventral thalamus can be traced to this region, terminating within the anterior bank of the central sulcus (area 4). Additional cortical somatosensory regions include the superior and inferior parietal lobule, the SII region within the sylvian fissure, the retroinsular field, and polysensory frontal cortex.

Neurotoxicology

It is clear that many neurotoxicants diffusely affect the cerebral cortex by provoking a variety of morphologic, pharmacologic, and physiologic reactions. The reactions are especially common following acute exposure to these agents; however, they do not appear to selectively involve the somatosensory cortex. Similarly, among substances that produce CNS degeneration only after prolonged or subacute exposure, few predominantly affect the somatosensory cortex. However, methylmercury frequently produces widespread selective degeneration of small neurons in the pre- and postcentral gyrus, with only minor involvement of the regions of the frontal and parietal lobe. Mercury also affects small neurons of the calcarine cortex granule cell layer of the cerebellum and dorsal root ganglion cells.

MONITORING OF THE SOMATOSENSORY SYSTEM: ITS RELEVANCE FOR NEUROTOXICOLOGY

A salient feature of the somatosensory system is the remarkable length and heavy myelination of its lower conduction pathways. The length of these fibers allows noninvasive physiological monitoring at several points. For example, human sensory nerve and spinal cord conduction velocity measurements are routine clinical procedures. Unfortunately, axonal neuropathies, in their early stages, generally produce only slight slowing of motor and sensory conduction that may be limited to a specific subset of axons (e.g., large-diameter myelinated fibers). In addition, many common neurotoxic substances initially produce distal axonal degeneration, so that nerve conduction studies at proximal sites are of limited value for the early detection of these disorders.

FIG. 7. Averaged somatosensory evoked potentials recorded overlying sural nerve, cauda equina, spinal cord, and brainstem. Activity was elicited by a suprathreshold electric shock delivered to the sural nerve.

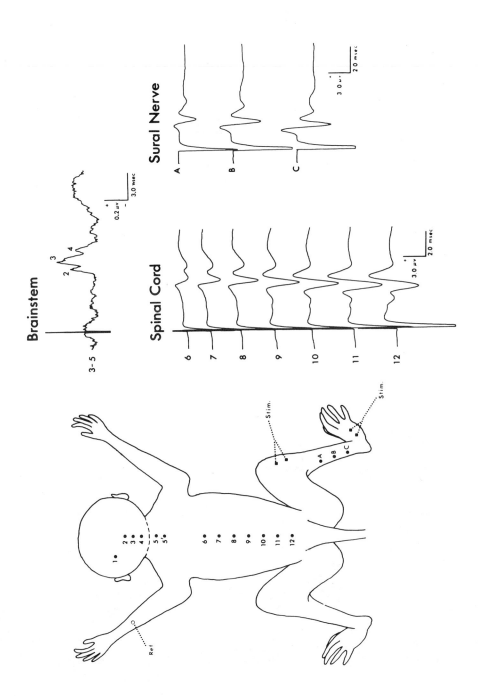

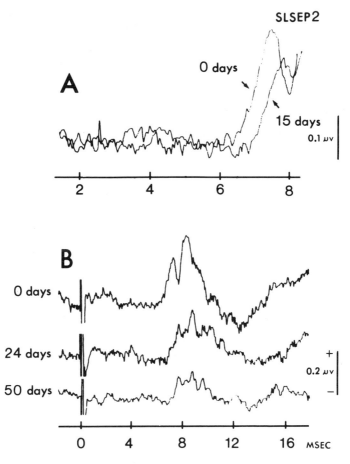

FIG. 8. A: Effects of acrylamide intoxication on onset and waveshape of the short-latency somatosensory evoked potential recorded overlying the cortical brainstem. **B:** Recordings at the
same site over long exposures to acrylamide.

Recent advances in computer-averaged electrophysiologic procedures permit the
noninvasive recording of activity within somatosensory fiber tracts of higher levels
of the CNS in man and experimental animals (5,7) (Fig. 7). Somatosensory evoked
potentials have been used to trace the onset of acrylamide-induced distal axonopathy in the primate (4). Initial dysfunction appears at the distal extreme of the
gracile component of the dorsal column system. The change consists of an increase
of the onset and peak of the short-latency components overlying this site following
stimulation of the lower limb (Fig. 8). The electrophysiologic findings in the CNS
precede any behavioral alteration or change in the peripheral conduction velocity
and appear coincident with the earliest detectable morphologic change in the gracile
nucleus.

Although evoked potentials may provide a sensitive index of neurotoxic insult, they are relatively expensive, time-consuming, and require sophisticated equipment and technical support. They are therefore not suitable as a screening measure for the evaluation of a large at-risk population. An effective screening program should target a specific function vulnerable to the neurotoxin in question. Dysfunction in the pacinian corpuscles and a consequent loss of vibration sensitivity are early and consistent features of central-peripheral distal axonopathies. The Optacon Tactile Tester stimulates fingers or toes with 144 individual metal rods that vibrate at 230 Hz and is compatible with the two-alternative forced-choice psychophysical paradigm. This device has been used in field studies of chemical workers and has proved sensitive to subclinical toxic axonopathies (3). A new device, the Pfizer Thermal Tester, has been developed to measure temperature sensitivity and thereby assess the integrity of small myelinated and unmyelinated fibers in the PNS (2). The combined use of these psychophysical measures may prove a reliable and rapid screening battery for many toxic neuropathies.

ACKNOWLEDGMENT

The authors thank Ms. Pat Vacchelli for secretarial assistance and Monica Bischoff and Nancy Brennan for preparing the illustrations. This work was supported by USPHS grants OH00535 and OH00851.

REFERENCES

1. Arezzo, J. C., Legatt, A. D., and Vaughan, H. G., Jr. (1981): Topography and intracranial sources of somatosensory evoked potentials in the monkey. II. Cortical components. *Electroencephalogr. Clin. Neurophysiol.*, 51:1–18.
2. Arezzo, J. C., Schaumburg, H. H., and Laudadio, C. (1983): The Pfizer Thermal Tester: A new portable device for measuring temperature sensation. *Ann. Neurol.*, 14:122.
3. Arezzo, J. C., Schaumburg, H. H., and Peterson, C. (1983): Rapid screening for peripheral neuropathy: A field study with the Optacon. *Neurology*, 33:626–629.
4. Arezzo, J. C., Schaumburg, H. H., Vaughan, H. G., Spencer, P. S., and Barna, J. (1982): Hind limb somatosensory evoked potentials in the monkey: The effects of distal axonopathy. *Ann. Neurol.*, 12:24–32.
5. Arezzo, J. C., Vaughan, H. G., Jr., and Legatt, A. D. (1979): Topography and intracranial sources of somatosensory evoked potentials in the monkey. I. Early components. *Electroencephalogr. Clin. Neurophysiol.*, 46:155–172.
6. Cho, E.-S., Spencer, P. S., and Jortner, B. S. (1980): Doxorubicin. In: *Experimental and Clinical Neurotoxicology*, edited by P. S. Spencer and H. H. Schaumburg, pp. 430–439. Williams and Wilkins, Baltimore.
7. Cracco, R. Q., and Cracco, J. B. (1976): Somatosensory evoked potential in man: Far field potentials. *Electroencephalogr. Clin. Neurophysiol.*, 41:460–466.
8. Lemon, R. N. (1979): Short-latency peripheral inputs to the motor cortex in conscious monkeys. *Brain Res.*, 161:150–155.
9. Spencer, P. S., Foster, G. V., Sterman, A. B., and Horoupian, D. (1980): Acetyl ethyl tetramethyl tetralin. In: *Experimental and Clinical Neurotoxicology*, edited by P. S. Spencer and H. H. Schaumburg, pp. 296–308. Williams and Wilkins, Baltimore.
10. Schaumburg, H. H., Wisniewski, H., and Spencer, P. S. (1974): Ultrastructural studies of the dying-back process. I. Peripheral nerve terminal and axon degeneration in systemic acrylamide intoxication. *J. Neuropathol. Exp. Neurol.*, 33:260–284.

11. Spencer, P. S., and Schaumburg, H. H. (1973): An ultrastructural study of the normal feline Pacinian corpuscle. *J. Neurocytol.*, 2:217–235.
12. Spencer, P. S., and Schaumburg, H. H. (1977): Central and peripheral distal axonopathy—The pathology of dying-back polyneuropathies. In: *Progress in Neuropathology, Vol. 3*, edited by H. M. Zimmerman, pp. 253–295. Grune and Stratton, New York.
13. Spencer, P. S., and Schaumburg, H. H. (1978): Distal axonopathy—One common type of neurotoxic lesion. *Environ. Health Perspect.*, 26:97–105.
14. Spencer, P. S., and Schaumburg, H. H. (1980): Classification of neurotoxic disease: A morphological approach. In: *Experimental and Clinical Neurotoxicology*, edited by P. S. Spencer and H. H. Schaumburg, pp. 92–99. Williams and Wilkins, Baltimore.
15. Sterman, A. B., Schaumburg, H. H., and Asbury, A. K. (1979): The acute sensory neuronopathy syndrome: A distinct clinical entity. *Ann. Neurol.*, 7:354–358.
16. Towfighi, J. (1980): Hexachlorophene. In: *Experimental and Clinical Neurotoxicology*, edited by P. S. Spencer and H. H. Schaumburg, pp. 440–455. Williams and Wilkins, Baltimore.

Toxicology of the Eye, Ear, and Other Special Senses, edited by A. W. Hayes. Raven Press, New York © 1985.

Basic Patterns of the Development of the Eye

Richard M. Hoar

Hoffmann-La Roche Inc., Nutley, New Jersey 07110

To an individual struggling to understand some basic mechanisms associated with normal embryology, the development of the eye is well worth study. Here induction has been clearly established as an essential mechanism, and one can discover examples of both primary and secondary inductive forces. Here, too, one finds examples of early developmental steps or events whose persistence (or absence) results in either congenital abnormalities or future disease states. And in this system one encounters examples of those unexplained spontaneous events that are so common in an embryologist's lexicon. An examination of the development of the eye should serve to remind us that embryogenesis is a continuum and, although discursive presentations such as this tend to emphasize the pieces rather than the puzzle, one should not lose sight of the whole when discussing its parts, because each event we shall discuss is part of an interdependent continuum that can be totally disrupted by the failure of any one of its components either to appear on time or to develop normally. Finally, the development of the eye serves to remind us that there are many instances in normal embryology in which development continues after birth and can be significantly altered by events in postnatal life. The presentation that follows is intended only as an outline of the development of the human eye. For those who wish to pursue the subject, a list of references has been supplied to assist you, and a figure of comparative development has been provided to remind you how rapidly these events occur in rodents and the chick as compared to man.

Now let us turn our attention specifically to the development of the eye. We see the optic primordium first in man on about day 22 as bilateral evaginations of the neuroectoderm of the forebrain (prosencephalon), which still remains open as bilateral neural folds. These evaginations, the optic peduncles, continue to proliferate laterally as the forebrain closes so that at about the 27th day they have become large single-layered vesicles, the primary optic vesicles, which are continuous with the third ventricle. As they reach the surface ectoderm these hollow balls of neuroectoderm, connected to the brain through hollow optic stalks, induce the formation of lens primordia, the lens placodes. This is the classic example generally offered as evidence for primary induction in normal development for, unless the optic vesicle reaches the surface ectoderm, no lens vesicle will develop. A groove appears on the inferior surface of each optic stalk and optic vesicle at about 29 days. This retinal (choroid or optic) fissure incorporates both mesenchyme and the hyaloid artery and vein by 33 days, vascularizing the optic stalk and the optic vesicle, which itself is undergoing further structural modifications. The hollow ball (vesicle) has become indented, creating the appearance of a cup with two layers, an internal and external retinal layer, separated by an intraretinal space that is still continuous through the optic stalk with the third ventricle.

The differentiation of this secondary optic vesicle continues with the fusion of the retinal layers and the disappearance of the intraretinal space except for anterior and posterior cul-de-sacs located at the ora serrata and the intraocular portion of the optic nerve, respectively. The external retinal layer becomes the pigmented layer of the retina by the 6th week and the internal layer differentiates into the neural layer, modification of which becomes obvious by 40 days and continues through the 7th month; one can visualize the definitive retinal pattern at approximately 175 days. The changes that occur in the neural layer are similar to those seen as the brain itself develops. At about 40 days, an internal germinal epithelial or ependymal layer may be found next to the pigmented layer, still separated from it by an occasional remnant of the intraretinal space. By 130 days, the ependymal layer gives rise to an external neuroblastic layer, an internal neuroblastic layer, and a ganglionic cell layer. By about 175 days, the internal neuroblastic layer has differentiated into the interneuron or bipolar cellular layer. Rudimentary neurosensory rods and cones appear during the 12th week and continue development after birth. Thus, because of the invagination of the primary optic vesicle to form the optic cup, the neural layer of the retina is inverted and the light-sensitive rods and cones are located adjacent to the pigmented epithelium so that light must cross the neural retina to reach the receptors.

In humans, from the 35th to the 210th day of gestation, the optic stalk has undergone a parallel modification creating an external layer continuous with the external retinal layer, thus providing the axons from the neural retina a pathway for easy access to the brain. By about the 9th week, the hyaloid vessels are incorporated within the optic stalk, and as it fills with axons the retinal fissure fuses (6th week), continuity with the intraretinal space and the third ventricle disappears, and the hyaloid vessels become the central retinal vessels.

By turning our attention now to the anterior region of the secondary optic vesicle, we can consider the development of the iris, ciliary bodies, lens, vitreous body, and aqueous chamber of the eye. As the optic vesicle doubles back on itself (invaginates) forming the optic cup and an inner and outer retinal layer, the point where the two layers meet anteriorly tends to extend over the developing lens to form a pupillary opening. These two layers in front of the lens will become the iris, a process that commences about the 7th week. The internal retinal layer (the neural layer) remains thin in this location and the external layer provides a pigmented epithelium. I wonder what determines the failure of the neural retina in this area to thicken and undergo cell division as it did on the posterior surface of the cup? Could it be the presence of the lens?

The ciliary bodies appear on the inner surface of the developing iris during the 9th week and begin secreting aqueous humor. It should be noted that this system develops from neuroectoderm and functions in a manner similar to that of the choroid plexus.

The lens itself may now be seen as a lens vesicle (hollow ball), having lost its connection to the surface ectoderm during the 6th week. The inner cells of the lens vesicle multiply and extend primary lens fibers toward the opposite external cells, gradually occluding the lumen of the lens vesicle. By the 7th week, the fibers extend between the walls of the vesicle, filling it and forming the nucleus of the lens. New fibers arise throughout life from cells positioned in the equatorial plane. The equatorial plane is located near the origin of the aqueous humor, which will become its principal source of nutrients after the hyaloid vessels disappear. Loose bundles of fibers derived from the vitreous framework appear between the ciliary body and the lens forming the suspensory ligament (zonule of Zinn) of the lens.

Posterior to the lens, in an area surrounded by the developing retina, the lenti-retinal space, the primary vitreous body is developing from mesenchyme that infiltrated through the retinal fissure. The retinal fissure begins to close at about 37 days, creating a circular optic cup with no inferior gap, and completely encloses the primary vitreous body by about 47 days. The primary vitreous body and the rapidly developing lens are both supplied by the hyaloid artery. However, the intravesicular vessels degenerate and the mesenchyme of the primary vitreous body becomes an acellular jelly, the secondary vitreous body, which fills the optic cup behind the lens—a process that is completed about the 9th week. The hyaloid vessels within the optic stalk do not degenerate, but remain as the central retinal artery and vein.

The aqueous chamber of the eye develops during the 7th week between the cornea and iris (anterior chamber) and between the iris and the lens (posterior chamber) under the influence of the lens. The anterior chamber develops as a space in the mesenchyme located between the developing lens and the overlying ectoderm. This space separates the mesenchyme into two layers, a thick outer layer that will become the cornea *(vide infra)* and a spidery combination of mesenchyme and developing choroid (the iridopupillary membrane) that covers the pupil but regresses and disappears before birth. The fluid medium of the two chambers, the aqueous humor, is produced by the ciliary body and is drained by a large vessel, the canal of Schlemm, located in the iridocorneoscleral angle, the drainage angle or angular sinus.

This complex structure, which has formed between the 3rd and 9th weeks of gestation, needs protective layers and muscles. Responding to the inductive forces of the pigmented outer layer of the optic cup during the 6th and 7th weeks, the surrounding mesenchyme forms a vascularized pigmented layer, the choroid (which is analogous to the pia-arachnoid layer of the brain), and a tough, white, collagenous sclera that surrounds the optic cup with tissue that is continuous with the dura mater of the brain. The cornea, which is continuous with the sclera, is created from mesenchyme *(vide supra)* that invades between the developing lens and the

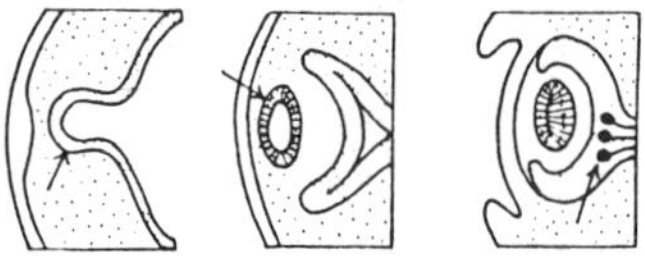

	Optic Vesicle Forming	Lens Separated	Optic Nerve Fibers Present
Man	24	35	48
Rat	10.5	12.5	14
Mouse	9.5	11.5	13
Chick	1.3	2.5	4

FIG. 1. Selected developmental stages of the ocular system accompanied by the age in days on which a particular event occurs in the rat, mouse, and human based on fertilization age and, in the chick, based on incubation age. (Modified from Monie, refs. 6 and 9.)

surface ectoderm and is covered with a multilayered epithelium anteriorly and a single-layered endothelium posteriorly. Under the influence of the lens, the cornea and the covering ectoderm (epithelium) become clear. The extrinsic ocular muscles and the ciliary muscles, which control convergence of the lens, are established *in situ* from mesenchyme between the 4th and 10th weeks. The dilator and constrictor muscles of the iris are of neuroectodermal origin, for they develop *in situ* from the pigmented layer of the iris, which was the external retinal layer.

The eyelids appear during the 6th week as folds of ectodermal tissue with a mesenchymal core. They grow until they meet and fuse during the 9th week, obliterating the palpebral opening, and they remain joined until about the 7th month. Upon fusion of the eyelids, a closed conjunctival sac is formed between the eyelids and the cornea. The lacrimal gland primordium begins to develop from the surface ectoderm in the upper lateral part (superior fornix) of the conjunctival sac during the 7th week. Although the morphogenesis of the eyelids and lacrimal apparatus is said to be independent of that of the eye, there is no question that the wetting action of the eyelid is absolutely essential to the integrity of the cornea and their independent development would appear to be more than fortuitously beneficial.

Having considered the development of the eye during its major period of organogenesis, between the 3rd and 9th weeks of gestation, one should remember that development of the eye continues into postnatal life. The fovea centralis of the retina is not differentiated until 4 months after birth. The cones, after appearing during the 12th week, remain poorly developed until about 4 months after birth. The dilator pupillae muscle continues its development until the 5th year of life, and the lens keeps adding fibers to its circumference throughout life at a pace that decreases with age.

I believe that a discussion of this vital system should include commentary on the origin of a few representative birth defects. Coloboma iridis is the result of failure of the retinal fissure to completely close during the 7th week. We now know why a gap in the iris may be indicative of damage to such structures as the ciliary bodies, the retina, or the optic nerve. A persistent iridopupillary membrane, on the other hand, need not be accompanied by a plethora of other defects, for its development appears to be an isolated event. Although the pigmented epithelium of the retina, the internal retinal layer, becomes firmly attached to the surrounding choroid layer, the retina itself may be separated from the pigmented layer along the lines of that fusion plane which was the intraretinal space. This separation may be assisted by the presence of a persistent hyaloid artery or vitreoretinal adhesions.

This chapter has only introduced the reader to the intricacies of the developing eye. However, it is hoped that sufficient stimulus has been provided so that, with the assistance of the general references (1–11) that have been appended, you will continue to investigate its complexities. To further your efforts, a figure of ocular development has been provided (Fig. 1) comparing the approximate timing of a particular event in the rat, mouse, and human, giving the age in days based on fertilization age, and in the chick according to its incubation age, also in days.

REFERENCES

1. Duke-Elder, S., and Cook, C. (1963): Embryology. In: *System of Ophthalmology, Vol. 3*, edited by S. Duke-Elder. The C. V. Mosby Company, St. Louis.
2. Fine, B. S., and Yanoff, M. (1979): *Ocular Histology, a Text and Atlas*. Harper and Row, Hagerstown, Maryland.
3. Hoar, R. M., and Monie, I. W. (1981): Comparative development of specific organ systems. In: *Developmental Toxicology*, edited by C. A. Kimmel and J. Buelke-Sam, pp. 13–34. Raven Press, New York.
4. Langman, J. (1974): *Medical Embryology*. 3rd Edition. Williams and Wilkins, Baltimore.
5. Mann, I. (1950): *The Development of the Human Eye*. Grune and Stratton, Inc., New York.
6. Monie, I. W. (1962): Comparative development of rat, chick and human embryos. In: *Teratologic Workshop Manual (Supplement)*. Pharmaceutical Manufacturers Association, Berkeley, California.
7. Moore, K. L. (1973): *The Developing Human*. W. B. Saunders Company, Philadelphia.
8. O'Rahilly, R. (1966): The early development of the eye in staged human embryos. *Contrib. Embryol.*, 38:1.
9. Otis, E. M., and Brent, R. (1954): Equivalent ages in mouse and human embryos. *Anat. Rec.*, 120:33.
10. Shepard, T. H. (1983): *Catalogue of Teratogenic Agents*. 4th Edition. Johns Hopkins University Press, Baltimore and London.
11. Tuchmann-Duplessis, H., Auroux, M., and Haegel, P. (1974): *Illustrated Human Embryology, Vol. 3: Nervous System and Endocrine Glands*. Springer-Verlag, New York.

Toxicology of the Eye, Ear, and Other Special Senses, edited by A.W. Hayes. Raven Press, New York © 1985.

Clinical and Laboratory Assessment of Visual Dysfunction

R. Heywood

Huntingdon Research Centre, plc, Huntingdon, Cambs, PE18 6ES, England

Chemical damage to the eye, with its subsequent effects on vision, is one of the sensitive areas of current toxicology.

Because of the problem of adverse reactions, it is now required by the regulatory authorities in most countries that new chemicals be tested for safety before their general release. Animal studies are essentially comparative, in that spontaneous and induced pathologic manifestations are compared in control and treated animals, respectively. The purpose is to identify variations from normal and to define underlying disturbances of physiological mechanisms. The conventional procedure for toxicity studies is to have a control group compared with three groups of animals given different dose levels of a compound, in order to identify target organ systems and to define levels at which there is no observable effect. The regulatory authorities stipulate that these studies must be carried out in a rodent and a nonrodent species. The purpose of this paper is to outline the methods for assessing ocular damage in the commonly used laboratory species following systemic administration of chemicals, with particular reference to underlying mechanisms of toxicity, and to draw attention to the limitations in both the use and understanding of these approaches to safety evaluation.

EXAMINATION OF THE EYE

Ocular toxicity can be monitored by using a variety of techniques; those applicable to animals are listed in Table 1. Because toxicological studies concern groups of animals, the techniques adopted must be simple and applicable to the unanesthetized animal. Examination of the eye may be by direct or indirect ophthalmoscopy; the latter is preferable, because the greater degree of illumination provided allows one to examine the cornea, lens, vitreous, and retina more rapidly than does the direct ophthalmoscope. The modern binocular instrument allows stereoscopic vision, facilitating the recognition of lesions on the fundus and within the vitreous. Large areas can be seen in one field and the peripheral fundus can be examined with comparative ease. It is easy to compare the two eyes quickly. Slit-lamp biomicroscopy is not recommended in the routine ophthalmoscopic examination. Tear flow can be measured by using commercially available Schirmer tear-test

TABLE 1. *Examination for ocular toxicity: techniques applicable to animals*

General examination
Examination with the ophthalmoscope
  Direct
  Indirect
Biomicroscopy
Schirmer test
Ocular pressure
Functional examination
Electrodiagnosis—ERG
Biochemistry
Pathological examination
  Light microscopy
  Electron microscopy

papers. Intraocular pressure can be measured by using either the Schiötz tonometer or, preferably, an applanation tonometer.

Functional examination is limited to the testing of the simple reflexes—the fixating, corneal, blink, and pupillary light reflexes. The fixating and blink reflexes are dependent on the afferent pathways of the optic nerve, optic tract, lateral geniculate body, optic radiation, and visual cortex. The efferent pathway is via the superior colliculus, the third, fourth, and sixth cranial nerves, and the cervical nerves. Constriction of the pupil is dependent on the optic nerve, optic tract, pretectal region with the efferent pathway, the third parasympathetic division, and the ciliary ganglion and nerve. The consensual response is dependent on decussations in the optic chiasma.

Physiologic measurement of retinal integrity can be made by recording electroretinograms (ERGs). The ERG represents the summated transient electrical activity evoked in response to a light stimulus of a large number of retinal cells. The wave pattern is illustrated in Fig. 1. It is now generally accepted that the outer layers of the retina give rise to the initial negative deflection, or "a" wave, while the activity of the inner layers of the retina is represented by the subsequent positive deflection, or "b" wave. The later positive potential, or "c" wave, is thought to originate in the pigment epithelium. The patterns of response of the rod and cone systems are known to differ, the cones having a higher stimulus threshold than the rods. The validity of the results obtained from an electroretinographic examination relies heavily on the minimization of all artifacts and on the standardization of the recording technique. Subtle changes in the ERGs recorded during or after treatment of experimental animals with novel compounds must be interpreted with caution, and assessed in conjunction with other clinical and ultrastructural histopathological findings. Without close correlation with behavioral or morphologic evidence, changes in the ERG are not necessarily attributable to disturbance of the visual function. The value of the electroretinographic examination in predictive chemical safety evaluations lies in the provision of supplementary evidence to confirm or refute ophthalmologic assessments based on conventional clinical and pathologic data.

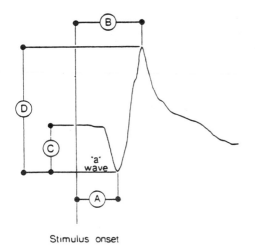

FIG. 1. Measurements taken from recorded electroretinogram: A ("a" wave), B ("b" wave): implicit times; C ("a" wave), D ("b" wave): amplitudes.

Stimulus onset

Considerable problems are encountered in preparing eyes for morphologic examination. Immediately after the animal has been killed, the eyes should be dissected from the orbit by the technique of Saunders and Jubb (32) and placed in a fixative. It is essential to use a fixative that will rapidly penetrate the sclera: Zenkers-acetic imposes critical timing but gives good results for the retina; Bouin's fluid is considered better for fixing the lens; however, the fixative most appropriate for routine toxicologic laboratories is Davidson's fluid. Formalin fixation inevitably causes separation of the retinal layers in the rat, and it is difficult to avoid inducing artifacts in the taking and fixing of eyes. After fixation the calottes are removed and the eye embedded in fibro-wax. It is useful if the eye can be correctly orientated before sectioning; this can sometimes be done by reference to the ocular muscle and/or by marking the cornea before fixation. Sagittal sections are cut at 5 μm and stained with hematoxylin and eosin. For electron microscopy the eyes are fixed in sodium cacodylate-buffered glutaraldehyde for 5 min. The cornea is then removed and the globe returned to the glutaraldehyde for a further 5 min, after which the iris is removed and the eye allowed to fix for a further 10 min. The lens and vitreous are then removed from the cup, which is allowed to fix for a further 45 min. The retina is subsequently postfixed in 2% osmium in cacodylate buffer for 1 hr before being dehydrated in alcohol and embedded in epoxy resin.

It is necessary to know the range of normal and spontaneous pathologic variations common to the test species. In the dog, rat, and primate, many spontaneous abnormalities occur congenitally, or as a result of trauma, infection, or developmental and aging processes.

MANIFESTATIONS OF OCULAR TOXICITY IN THE LABORATORY ANIMAL

Adverse drug reactions involving the eye are best classified according to the structures involved. The major reactions are summarized in Table 2.

TABLE 2. *Adverse drug reactions: eye*

Eyelids and periorbital tissue	Relaxation of eyelids Edema
Disorders of lacrimation	Decreased Increased
Conjunctiva	Conjunctivitis
Cornea	Corneal opacity Corneal edema
Pupil	Miosis Mydriasis
Iris	Iritis
Lens	Cataract
Retina	Retinopathy Hemorrhage Edema Retinal vessel occlusion Deposition
Optic nerve	Papilledema Optic neuropathy
Disorders of ocular movements	Nystagmus

Eyelids and Periorbital Tissue

Ptosis of the eyelids, although a common sign in acutely intoxicated rats, is rarely observed following chronic administration of compounds. It is a sign of paralysis of the third cranial nerve, which governs the muscle that elevates the upper lid.

The dog has a third eyelid, which is extensive and can cover the whole anterior aspect of the eye; compounds affecting the autonomic system can cause relaxation of this third eyelid.

Edema of the eyelids is occasionally seen, often associated with the administration of nonsteroidal antiinflammatory agents. An example is paracetamol intoxication in the dog, which induces palpebral edema at the dosage level of 450 mg/kg/day, with an associated reduction in the secretory activity of the meibomian glands.

Disorders of Lacrimation

If lacrimal secretion is affected, it is usually diminished. Keratoconjunctivitis sicca can readily be induced in dogs with a variety of compounds, including phenazopyridine hydrochloride (34) and some sulfonamides (35), and all anticholinergic compounds at high enough doses induce this condition, particularly in the dog. Secretion of lacrimal fluid is not exclusively parasympathetic in origin; stimulation of the sympathetic system also plays a part, and this accounts for the occasional cases of dry-eye seen in dogs given high doses of β-adrenergic receptor blocking agents. Clonidine has recently been found to induce keratoconjunctivitis sicca in the rat (41). The diagnosis of keratitis sicca is made on clinical examination, supported by evidence of reduced tear secretion. Schirmer tear test values of less than 9 mm/min, accompanied by ocular irritation, are considered suggestive of keratoconjunctivitis sicca in the dog. Schirmer tear test values of 4 to 6 mm/min are normal for the rat, and in the monkey one would expect the normal value to be around 18 mm of wetting/min. Excessive lacrimation has not been recorded in laboratory animals; however, the testing of lacrimogenic gases would be expected to increase tear flow.

In rats, there is a condition in which there is secretion of red tears (chromodacryorrhea), which is associated with stress factors or with overgrowth of the incisor teeth. Harkness and Ridgway (13) showed that injections of acetylcholine increased almost instantaneously the flow of a dull red secretion, the red color being caused by porphyrins.

Conjunctiva

Conjunctivitis as a clinical entity is rarely found in animal safety studies, and hypersensitivity reactions involving the conjunctiva have not been seen following systemic administration of chemicals. Practolol did not cause any conjunctival problems when administered to rats, mice, rabbits, guinea pigs, hamsters, dogs, and marmosets (28).

Cornea

For a systemically administered compound to affect the cornea, it must pass the blood-aqueous humor barrier, be secreted in the tears, or alter the composition of the tears. The cornea is a clear avascular structure maintained in its state of turgescence by being bathed externally by the tears and other secretions, and internally by the aqueous humor.

The simplest form of damage is the induction of corneal vacuoles. Vacuoles can be formed in the corneal epithelium; although the etiology of these vacuoles is obscure, it is suggested that they are formed by loosening of epithelial cells from the stroma. The vacuoles present in the corneal epithelium as shiny bubbles, but their positions within the cornea change on successive examinations. Vacuoles have been induced in rats with high dosages of imipramine and similar compounds. Corneal vacuoles are a recognized clinical entity in man, having been recorded following the administration of nicothiazine, thiacetazone, and n-butanol vapor (11). Any compound that destroys the integrity of either the epithelium or the endothelium will alter the state of hydration of the cornea. Epithelial erosions are the simplest form for the damage to take, but with continued insult, superficial lesions rapidly progress to keratitis of varying severity. Epithelial damage is thought to be caused by the direct action of a compound or its metabolites, since they are being excreted in the tears. Edema surrounds sites of local keratitis, whereas vascularization is always associated with keratitic pathologic processes. Whether the edema is the result of, or related to the cause of, vascularization is not known.

A number of compounds can induce this type of damage, including sulfonyl ureas, mimosine, tricyclic antidepressants, progesterones, and various vitamin deficiencies. Some compounds can reach concentrations within the aqueous humor sufficient to damage the corneal endothelium. If damage does occur, the stromal swelling becomes apparent in the whole cornea; the eye appears white and bulges from the orbit.

Corneal opacities can be induced in laboratory animals by a variety of compounds: in the rat, invariably by morphine (5) or the narcotic analgesics (29). Lipoidal opacities induced by nitroaniline have been described in the dog (4). Corneal opacities are not induced in laboratory animals, as in man, with antimalarial drugs such as chloroquine, hydroxychloroquine, and mepacrine.

Exacerbation of traumatic lesions and reactivation of old infections can be induced in laboratory animals following the administration of corticosteroids.

Toxicity involving the cornea is best diagnosed by clinical examination supported by histopathologic examination of the cornea.

Uveal Tract

A side effect of many chemicals is the disturbance of the refractive power of the eye and of the ability of the eye to accommodate.

The common response of the pupil is dilatation or constriction. Dilatation of the pupil is induced by the systemic administration of anticholinergic compounds and parasympatholytic agents; constriction is by direct cholinergic or parasympathomimetic action. The effects on the pupil can be modified by central nervous system effects.

The high vascularity of the uveal tract should make this a potential site for chemical immunologic reactions. However, this has not been the case and, in my experience, one compound only—an antiviral agent—caused sensitization of the uveal tract in a subhuman primate species, with resultant uveitis.

Lens

The lens arises from ectoderm. It is a biconvex transparent body, separating the aqueous and vitreous chambers. It has no blood supply and relies on the aqueous, and to a lesser extent the vitreous, for its supply of nutrients. The lens continues to grow through life by layering new fibers over the old fibers, so that the old cells become compressed into the center. The lens undergoes a progression of age-related changes and may also develop opacities. The characteristic response to injury is degeneration.

For a compound to be cataractogenic, it must traverse the blood-aqueous barrier to enter the anterior chamber. Toxic levels can be achieved only by high daily dosage, slow excretion, or prolonged administration. The selective entrance of drugs into the aqueous is dependent on molecular size and lipid solubility. Large molecules are held back by the capillary membrane, whereas lipid-soluble substances rapidly traverse the blood-aqueous barrier and reach equilibrium.

Chemically induced lenticular lesions are cataracts and can be classified into two major groups—transient lens opacities and permanent cataracts.

Transient Lens Opacities

Opacities of a transient nature, in which the lens returns to normal within a few hours, have been produced in young rats following the administration of substitute phenothiazines, catecholamines, and morphine-like analgesics. They have also been produced in young beagle dogs following the administration of some tranquilizers, some diuretics, and diisophenol. These opacities are usually associated with the anterior capsule, where they appear as crescents around the periphery of the lens or as opacification of the anterior subcapsular fibers (Fig. 2).

These acute reversible lens opacities are ascribed, in the main, to osmotic changes. The normal state of hydration in the lens is maintained by the integrity of the lens membranes and the cation pump, which extrudes sodium and concentrates potassium ions. The aqueous humor has a high level of sodium and a low level of potassium ions, whereas the cations in the lens have the opposite composition—high potassium and low sodium. Maintaining the pump-leak balance is crucial to preserving the viability of the lens. Osmotic change is a common feature of many cataracts, and if the pump-leak equilibrium is not rapidly restored permanent opacification results.

Acute reversible lens opacities have been seen in which osmotic change was not involved. The feature of these other forms of acute lens opacification was vacuolation within and just below the lens epithelium. It is postulated that here the compound within the aqueous humor interferes with the metabolism of the lens epithelium, and provided the lens epithelium is not disrupted, reversal is possible.

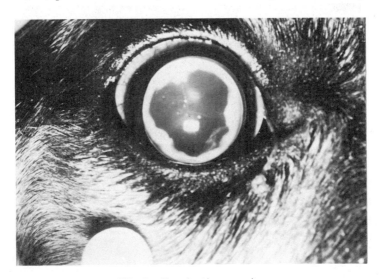

FIG. 2. Transient lens opacity.

Permanent Cataracts

The clinical development of permanent chemically induced cataracts follows distinct courses. There is always a latent period between the administration of a compound and the onset of lenticular change, and this can vary from a few days to several months. Many cataracts start at the equator of the lens. The first sign is the appearance of vacuoles and striation around the equator of the lens. The lens at the equator becomes opaque and appears to have a surrounding halo. Opacification of the superficial lens fibers continues and extends under the anterior or, more frequently, the posterior capsule of the lens. Initially only those lens fibers immediately below the capsule are involved. The most common form of chemically induced cataract is that which starts at the posterior pole of the lens. In the dog these cataracts appear to be roughly triangular at the posterior pole, involving only subcapsular fibers (Fig. 3). In the rat chemically induced cataracts show a variety of morphologic patterns, but often they first show as triangular opacities at the posterior pole (Fig. 4). The most likely explanation of the greater involvement of the posterior cortex of the lens in toxic cataracts is that posteriorly the capsule is thinner and epithelial cells are absent, allowing the toxic agent to penetrate into the superficial fibers more readily. At the posterior pole the lens is at its greatest stress with respect to nutrients and oxygen. The only other manifestation of lenticular toxicity that has been shown is that of changes in refraction. Changes in the transparency as well as in the refraction of the lens nucleus have been recorded following the administration of dimethyl sulfoxide (DMSO) (31) and with parachlorophenylalanine (10).

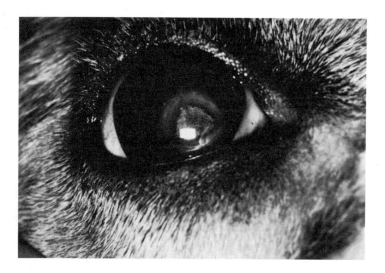

FIG. 3. Triangular posterior polar subcapsular opacity.

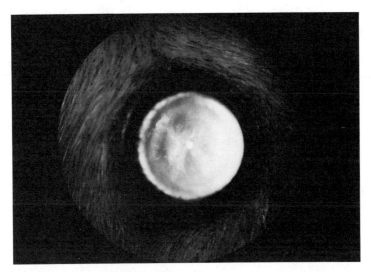

FIG. 4. Beginning of posterior polar triangular cataract in the rat.

Cataracts are best diagnosed by clinical examination; processing of the lens for histopathologic examination is of very limited value.

Chemicals with widely differing structures and pharmacologic activity have been reported to cause cataracts in laboratory animals; these agents have been reviewed by Gehring (9). Such compounds defy easy classification because the mechanisms of their cataractogenicity are poorly understood.

Cataracts can be induced by feeding high levels of galactose and xylose to rats. Animals that become diabetic by the administration of alloxan or streptozotocin, or high dose levels of progestational agents, develop cataracts. Here the common mechanism is the formation of sugar alcohols that accumulate and, because they are not easily metabolized, cause hypertonicity and osmotic swelling. Those alkylating agents that are cytotoxic induce cataracts by interfering with cell proliferation. Triparanol, a drug once used in the treatment of hypercholesterolemia, induces cataracts in the rat and the dog; these opacities appear as peripheral striate opacities, and sudanophilic material has been identified within the lens fibers. It is possible that this type of cataract is a manifestation of phospholipidosis. Cataracts induced by other compounds, such as the sulfonylurea drugs, the chelating agent desferrioxamine, sulfonamides, the steroids such as methallibure and clomiphene citrate, and chemicals such as diquat, heptachlor, and mirex, are the result of unknown mechanisms. Many of the agents inducing cataracts may do so by specific interference with enzyme systems. In experimental animals there is evidence that multiple cataractogenic factors have additive or even synergistic effects. The toxic effects of various substances on the lens are quantitatively very different in different species.

Retina

The response of the ocular fundus to chemical insult can be classified into five main categories: retinopathy, hemorrhage, edema, retinal vessel occlusion, and deposits.

Retinopathy

Drug-induced retinopathies have been reviewed by Meier-Ruge (24,25), with the main discussion directed toward the antimalarial chloroquine and the psychotropic phenothiazine derivatives. Of the three categories of phenothiazines, only the piperidines induce retinal lesions. Of these compounds, thioridazine has been most extensively studied. Retinal lesions can be readily induced with these compounds in the cat and dog; on clinical examination the retina of the tapetum has a coarse spotted appearance (Fig. 5). The lesions first occur in the primary visual cells, with secondary changes in the pigment epithelium. Meier-Ruge (25) has shown by histochemical techniques that there is a massive loss of enzyme activity in the ellipsoids of the rods. He is also of the opinion that the absorbent binding to melanin is of importance.

The binding capacity of the pigment tissues of the eye has been demonstrated for many compounds besides chloroquine and the phenothiazines. The beta-blockers, rifampicin, many antiprotozoals, tetracyclines, glycosides, and most polycyclic compounds bind to melanin. Compound uptake apparently increases with time, and once bound to melanin it can be retained for long periods. With the majority of compounds there is no resultant retinal toxicity, presumably because the compound is bound in an inactive form. In some cases, as with some phenothiazines and

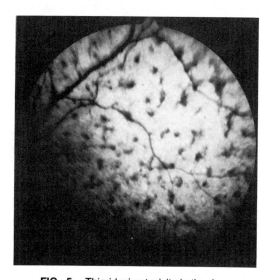

FIG. 5. Thioridazine toxicity in the dog.

chloroquine, once the binding capacity has been exceeded direct damage may result.

Experimental chloroquine retinopathy has caused considerable controversy over the mechanisms of the toxicity. It is certain that chloroquine binds to the pigmented tissues of the eye (22,25,26,30), but it is doubtful whether the pigment binding is of relevance to the primary retinopathy. From work carried out in the albino rat and pigmented strains, rabbits, beagle dogs, cats, and rhesus monkeys, the initial reaction of the retina is the formation of membranous cytoplasmic bodies (myelinoid bodies), and these myelinoid bodies can be induced within 1 week of starting treatment. Rosenthal et al. (30) clearly demonstrated that degenerative changes in the eye of the monkey occur in the nucleus and cell body of both the rods and cones and that the pigment epithelial damage is a later manifestation of chloroquine toxicity. In this experiment in the rhesus monkey, very extensive damage was found to have occurred in the retina, although there was no clinical or functional evidence of change.

The administration of amphophilic compounds to the rat results in the formation of myelinoid bodies in many cell types. These myelinoid bodies are uni- or multicentric. They are particles limited by a single membrane and containing osmiophilic membranes in concentric arrangement. The formation of myelinoid bodies is a manifestation of chemically induced lysosomal storage disease. Generalized phospholipidosis has been induced by a variety of chemical agents, which include antihistamines, hypolipidemics, antiinflammatories, antidepressants, anorectics, and coronary vasodilators (17,18). In chemical safety evaluation studies, it has been the drug-induced pulmonary lipidosis with the accumulation of foamy macrophages that has promoted interest. Drenckhahn and Lullmann-Rauch (3) have focused attention on drug-induced retinal lipidosis, which has been caused by several compounds. Myelinoid bodies have been found in the inner retinal cell types and the pigment epithelium. Different compounds have given different distributions; some compounds, like triparanol, have shown a predilection for pigment epithelial cells, whereas chloroquine affects mainly the ganglion cells. Some compounds that have been shown to produce a marked generalized phospholipidosis involving lungs, liver, endocrine tissues, peripheral and central nerve cells, and epididymal tissue have induced only a mild degree of lipidosis in the retina. It seems that the accumulation of myelinoid bodies within the cell does not lead to cell death, and there is some evidence that, even with the continued administration of compounds, the cells recover from the initial shock and the accumulated myelinoid is not progressive. Myelinoid bodies tend to disappear after cessation of treatment. The use of electron microscopy is essential to look for these myelinoid bodies (Fig. 6). Myelin figures can be produced in tissues fixed in glutaraldehyde, if fixation is prolonged, and these figures could be mistaken for pathologic change.

Some chemicals cause a loss of tapetal color. The change first appears as patchy fading of the tapetal color, until eventually the entire tapetum has a bleached appearance. No histopathologic change can be detected by light microscopy, but electron microscopy shows the presence of ultrastructural changes. Tapetal cells

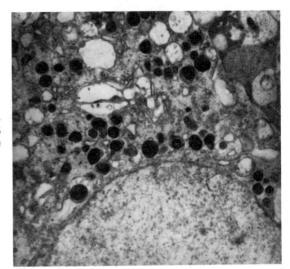

FIG. 6. Myelinoid bodies in ganglion cells of rat. (Chloroquine 5 daily doses, 100 mg/kg/day.) × 10,725.

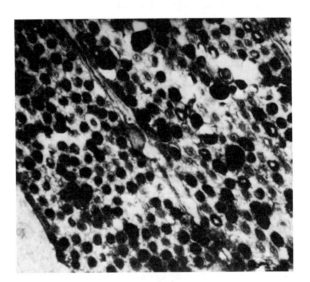

FIG. 7. Normal tapetal cells. × 15,150.

from normal dogs are characterized by the presence of parallel groups of uniformly dense intracytoplasmic rods; in animals with bleached tapeta, the parallel arrangement of the rods is disrupted, and these rods are surrounded by vacuoles that are not uniformly dense, but appear swollen with indistinct outlines (Figs. 7 and 8). No functional alteration can be detected by ERG other than slight prolongation of the implicit time of the wave forms evoked in response to low-intensity stimuli in the dark-adapted state. These changes are attributed to the chelating action of these compounds; ethambutol is one such compound (40).

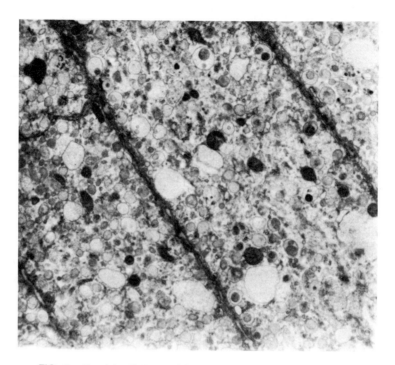

FIG. 8. Tapetal cells from animal with bleached tapetum. ×20,200.

Retinopathies have been induced in laboratory animals by a variety of compounds, such as monosodium glutamate and aspartate in neonate rodents, psychotropic agents such as cyproximide, methyl nitroso ureas, aminooxypropionic acid derivatives, and the hydroxypyridinethiones.

Hemorrhage

Compounds that cause hemorrhage do so by acting directly or indirectly on the clotting mechanisms. The most common examples are the coumarin anticoagulants such as dicoumarol. Butylated hydroxytoluene (BHT), a widely used antioxidant in food, induces vitamin K deficiency in the rat, although it is suggested that the mechanism of BHT-induced hemorrhage differs from that of dicoumarol-induced hemorrhage (37). The blood frequently penetrates the hyaloid membrane and appears in the vitreous as blobs or clots.

Edema

Edema of the retina has been seen on occasion in the dog, this condition being the most apparent over the tapetum lucidum. Plasma exudate between the epithelial layers, notably between the pigment epithelium and the other retinal layers, can appear as either circinate or linear lesions. The circinate areas of detachment give a watermarked appearance to the retina (Fig. 9). The linear lesion is always above the optic disc and appears to follow the line of the long posterior artery that travels along the horizontal meridian of the globe. Cellular infiltrates occur in inflammation of the retina, appearing as cotton-wool patches on the retina.

Vessel Occlusion

Changes in the size of retinal blood vessels are rarely recorded. In the dog drug-induced hypertension has been found not to alter the caliber of retinal vessels, but hypotension may cause attenuation of the retinal vessels, particularly those on the optic disc when the blood pressure is lowest. In the rat changes in the retinal vessels have been associated with compounds inducing hypertension. The normal blood pressure of the rat is 120 mm Hg systolic and 80 mm Hg diastolic; the retinal changes occur when the systolic pressure is greater than 220 mm Hg, and the diastolic greater than 140 mm Hg. The first change induced is irregular narrowing of one or more of the arteries, which may become more tortuous with the veins becoming markedly congested. In cases of profound anemia, the retinal vessels are threadlike and the retina has a pale, opaque appearance caused by cloudy swelling of the retinal ganglion cell layer.

Deposits

Occasional compounds, or their metabolites, have been seen to leak from damaged vessels, causing deposits to occur on the retina.

Optic Nerve

The response of the optic nerve is limited; it may show atrophy or it may increase in size (Fig. 10). The cases of atrophy show as a reduction of myelinated axons or

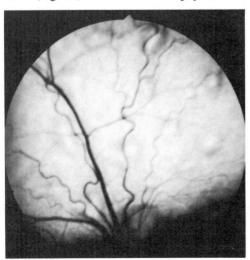

FIG. 9. Retinal detachment: dog.

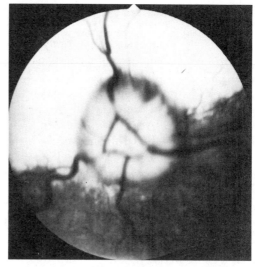

FIG. 10. Edema of the lens: dog.

demyelination of the optic nerve. In the dog an organophosphate pesticide, ethyl-thioemeton (19), and clioquinol (38) induce this type of change. Ethambutol has caused demyelination of the optic nerve, chiasm, and tract in the monkey (33) and the rat (21).

Edema of the disc is reported in monkeys with methyl alcohol poisoning (23) and trimethyl tin acetate (14). In the dog salicylanilide (2) causes vacuolation of the cerebral white matter and edema of the disc, and hexachlorophene (36) induces peripapillary exudations.

Changes in the optic nerve are readily diagnosed by the standard clinical and histopathologic methods, although impairment of the pupillary light reflex is frequently the first evidence of damage.

Disorders of Ocular Movement

Of the disorders of ocular movement, the one most readily diagnosed in laboratory animals is nystagmus, which is central in origin and usually horizontal. Many of the centrally active compounds, including the diazepams and the monoamine oxidase inhibitors, can induce nystagmus at high dosages, particularly in nonhuman primate species.

DISCUSSION

There is an overwhelming number of reports on ocular toxicity (1,8,11,12,27), which give the impression that the eye is a potential target organ of every chemical ever discovered. It is important that these adverse reactions are seen in perspective. Animal studies fall into two main categories—predictive evaluation of new compounds, and their incorporation into schemes designed to help lessen or clarify a recognized hazard. It is appropriate to ask, how predictive are the common laboratory animal species with respect to ocular toxicity?

In a survey of the toxicologic profiles of 50 compounds studied in rodent and nonrodent species, Heywood (15,16) found that in the dog and the monkey, 26% and 7% of the compounds, respectively, induced some form of ocular toxicity, whereas in the rodent, none of the compounds affected the eye. In a survey of the published toxicity of 37 compounds studied in the rat and the beagle dog, it was found that 5% of the compounds induced ocular toxicity in the dog and 3% in the rat. This considerable difference in the dog is most likely attributable to observer differences and to levels of recording. In a survey of 213 compounds, Falahee et al. (6) recorded a 1.4% incidence of ocular toxicity in both rat and dog. Correlations between rodent and nonrodent species were not established. A review of the literature shows some correlations for ocular toxicity between rodent and nonrodent species—for example, triparanol, some sulfonamides, chloroquine, iminodipropionitrile—but such correlations are rare. The toxic effects of various substances on the eye are quantitatively very different in the different species; this is probably attributable to differences in metabolism, particularly at the cellular level.

Venning (39) has surveyed the major adverse drug reactions that have been recorded since thalidomide, and from this survey the adverse reactions of the sense organs were abstracted (Table 3). It can be seen that practolol and clioquinol were rated as having caused major problems, yet neither was predicted by animal toxicity studies. If we compare known adverse drug reactions involving the eye in man with toxic findings in animals, again the correlations are shown to be poor (Table 4).

Some findings in animals have not been confirmed by human clinical experience. In aging monkeys hyperfluorescent spots around the macula have been described, both in controls and particularly in those animals undergoing long-term administration of progestogens. Fine and Kwapien (7) have shown that these lesions consist almost exclusively of lipoid degeneration of the pigment epithelial cells. The significance of this finding in relation to women using oral contraceptives is not known; however, there is no clinical evidence to establish adverse effects of oral contraceptives on the retina.

Many compounds affect physiologic processes that may involve the visual system and that cannot be predicted from animal experimentation. Of 56 compounds investigated by Laroche and Laroche (20), 34 were found to decrease color dis-

TABLE 3. *Adverse reactions of sense organs to drugs*

Adverse reactions	Drug	Incidence rating by 20 physicians
Oculomucocutaneous syndrome	Practolol	19
SMON	Clioquinol	10
Retinopathy	Chloroquine	3
Deafness	Streptomycin	2
Deafness	Neomycin	1
Cataract	Triparanol	1

SMON, subacute myelooptic neuropathy.

TABLE 4. *Adverse drug reactions in animals and humans*

Compound	Human	Animal
Iodochloro-hydroxyquine	SMON	Dog—optic neuritis
Aminoquinolines	Corneal deposits	Rat—lipidosis
	Toxic maculopathy	
Thioridazine	Retinal pigmentary	Dog—retinal pigmentary
	degeneration	degeneration
Cordarone (amiodarone)	Corneal deposits	NAD[a]
Practolol	Ocular mucocutaneous	NAD
	syndrome	
Adrenal corticosteroids	Cataract	NAD

[a]NAD = Nothing abnormal detected.

crimination significantly; 18 of the 56 compounds were antibiotics and nine caused some impairment of vision. The classic example is that of digitalis, for 10 to 25% of patients on digitalis experience some visual symptoms of toxicity (1).

The eye may show side effects from a wide variety of drugs used in clinical medicine. Some of these side effects, although undesirable, must be accepted as unavoidable. Most of the ocular side effects are caused by overdosage or indirect consequences of the drug's prime reaction, or by an individual idiosyncrasy. The eye is an emotive target organ in safety evaluation studies; however, this should not affect judgment when evaluating animal safety data. Mechanisms of ocular toxicity are poorly understood, and the limitations of animal studies in predicting side effects in man must be appreciated.

REFERENCES

1. Bron, A. J. (1979): Mechanisms of ocular toxicity. In: *Drug Toxicity*, edited by J. W. Gorrod, pp. 229–253. Taylor & Francis, London.
2. Brown, W. R., Rubin, L., Hite, M., and Zwickey, R. E. (1971): Experimental papilledema induced by a salicylanilide. *Toxicol. Appl. Pharmacol.*, 27:532.
3. Drenckhahn, D., and Lullmann-Rauch, R. (1978): Drug-induced retinal lipidosis. *Exp. Mol. Pathol. (Suppl.)*, 8:360–371.
4. Earl, F. L., Curtis, J. M., Bernstein, H. N., and Smalley, H. E. (1971): Ocular effects in dogs and pigs treated with Dichloron. *Food Cosmet. Toxicol.*, 9:819.
5. Fabian, R. J., Bond, J. M., and Drobeck, H. P. (1967): Induced corneal opacities in the rat. *Br. J. Ophthalmol.*, 51:124.
6. Falahee, K. J., Rose, C. S., and Seifried, H. E. (1983): In: *Alternatives in Toxicity Testing*, edited by A. M. Goldberg. *Vol. 1*, pp. 139–162.
7. Fine, B. S., and Kwapien, R. P. (1978): Pigment epithelial windows and drugs. *Invest. Ophthalmol.*, 17:1059.
8. Frauenfelder, F. T. (1976): *Drug-Induced Ocular Side-Effects and Drug Interactions*. Lea and Febiger, Philadelphia.
9. Gehring, P. J. (1971): The cataractogenic activity of chemical agents. *Crit. Rev. Toxicol.*, 1:93.
10. Gralla, E. J., and Rubin, L. F. (1970): Ocular studies with *para*-chlorophenylalanine in rats and monkeys. *Arch. Ophthalmol.*, 83:734.
11. Grant, W. M. (1974): *Toxicology of the Eye*. Charles C. Thomas, Springfield, IL.
12. Green, H., and Spencer, J. (1969): *Drugs with Possible Ocular Side-Effects*. Barrie & Rockliff, London.

13. Harkness, J. E., and Ridgway, M. D. (1980): Chromodacryorrhea in laboratory rats. *Lab. Anim. Sci.*, 30:841.
14. Hedges, T. R., and Zaren, H. A. (1969): Experimental papilledema. *Neurology*, 19:359.
15. Heywood, R. (1981): Target organ toxicity. *Toxicol. Lett.*, 8:349.
16. Heywood, R. (1983): Target organ toxicity. II. *Toxicol. Lett.*, 18:83.
17. Hruban, Z. (1976): Pulmonary changes induced by amphophilic drugs. *Environ. Health. Perspect.*, 16:111.
18. Hruban, Z., Slesers, A., and Hopkins, E. (1972): Drug-induced and naturally-occurring myelinoid bodies. *Lab. Invest.*, 27:62.
19. Ishikawa, S., and Mukono, K. (1977): Histopathological study of canine optic nerve and retina treated by organophosphate pesticide. *Invest. Ophthalmol.*, 16:877.
20. Laroche, J., and Laroche, C. (1972): Modifications de la vision des couleurs appostées par l'usage, à dose thérapeutique normale, de quelques médicaments. *Ann. Pharm. Fr.*, 30:433.
21. Lessell, S. (1976): Histopathology of experimental ethambutol intoxication. *Am. J. Med. Sci.*, 272:765.
22. Lindquist, N. G., and Ullberg, S. (1972): Melanin affinity of chloroquine and chlorpromazine. *Acta Pharmacol. Toxicol.*, 31(Suppl. II).
23. Martin-Amat, G., Tephly, T. R., McMartin, K. E., Makar, A. B., Hayreh, M. S., Hayreh, S. A., Baumback, G., and Cancilla, P. (1977): Methyl alcohol poisoning. *Arch. Ophthalmol.*, 95:1847.
24. Meier-Ruge, W. (1967): *Medikamentose Retinopathies*. Thieme, Stuttgart.
25. Meier-Ruge, W. (1972): Drug-induced retinopathy. *Crit. Rev. Toxicol.*, 1:325.
26. Potts, A. M. (1964): Further studies concerning the accumulation of polycyclic compounds in uveal melanin. *Invest. Ophthalmol.*, 3:405.
27. Potts, A. M., and Gonason, L. M. (1980): Toxic responses of the eye. In: *Toxicology*, edited by J. Doull, C. D. Klaassen, and M. O. Amdur, pp. 275–310. Macmillan, New York.
28. Reeves, P. R., McCormick, D. J., and Jepson, H. T. (1979): Practolol metabolism in various small animal species. *Xenobiotica*, 9:453.
29. Roerig, D. L., Hasegawa, A. T., Harris, G. J., Lynch, K. L., and Wang, R. I. H. (1980): Occurrence of corneal opacities in rats after acute administration of 1-α-acetylmethadol. *Toxicol. Appl. Pharmacol.*, 56:155.
30. Rosenthal, A. R., Kolb, H., Bergsma, D., Huxsoll, D., and Hopkins, J. L. (1978): Chloroquine retinopathy in the rhesus monkey. *Invest. Ophthalmol.*, 17:1158.
31. Rubin, L. F., and Mattis, P. A. (1966): Dimethyl sulphoxide. *Science*, 153:83.
32. Saunders, L. Z., and Jubb, K. U. (1961): Notes on techniques for post-mortem examination of the eye. *Can. Vet. J.*, 2:123.
33. Schmidt, I. G. (1966): Central nervous system effects of ethambutol in the monkey. *Ann. N.Y. Acad. Sci.*, 135:759.
34. Slatter, D. H. (1973): Keratoconjunctivitis sicca in the dog produced by oral phenazopyridine hydrochloride. *J. Sm. Anim. Pract.*, 14:749.
35. Slatter, D. H., and Blogg, J. R. (1978): Keratoconjunctivitis sicca in dogs. *Aust. Vet. J.*, 54:444.
36. Staben, P. (1980): The effect of hexachlorophene on the optic nerve and visual faculty in beagle dogs after prolonged dermal application. *Toxicol. Lett.*, 5:77.
37. Suzuki, H., Nakao, T., and Hiraga, K. (1979): Vitamin K deficiency in male rats fed diets containing butylated hydroxytoluene (BHT). *Toxicol. Appl. Pharmacol.*, 50:261.
38. Tateishi, J., Kurodas Slato, A., and Otsuki, S. (1972): Clioquinol toxicity. *Lancet*, 1:1289.
39. Venning, G. R. (1983): Identification of adverse reactions to new drugs. (4 parts). *Br. Med. J.*, 286: I. What have been the important adverse reactions since thalidomide? p. 199. II. How were 18 important adverse reactions discovered, and with what delays? p. 289. II. (cont.) How were 18 important adverse reactions discovered and with what delays? p. 365. III. Alerting processes and early warning systems. p. 458. IV. Verification of suspected adverse reactions. p. 544.
40. Vogel, A. W., and Kaiser, J. A. (1963): Ethambutol-induced transient change and reconstruction of the tapetum lucidum colour in the dog. *Exp. Mol. Pathol. (Suppl.)*, 2:136–149.
41. Weisse, I., Hoefke, W., Greenberg, S., Gaida, W., Stoltzer, H., and Kreuger, H. (1978): Ophthalmological and pharmacological studies after administration of clonidine in rats. *Arch. Toxicol.*, 41:89.

Toxicology of the Eye, Ear, and Other Special Senses, edited by A. W. Hayes. Raven Press, New York © 1985.

Psychophysical Assessment of Sensory Dysfunction in Nonhuman Subjects

*Patricia M. Blough and **John S. Young

*Department of Psychology, Brown University, Providence, Rhode Island 02912; and
**Environmental Stress Program Center, Naval Medical Research Institute, National Naval Medical Center, Bethesda, Maryland 20814

Psychophysical methodology provides a variety of tools for measuring the sensory capabilities of organisms. These techniques permit us to specify stimulus events and to establish the relationships between stimulus and behavioral changes. Thus psychophysics provides us with the ability to describe the functional consequences of sensory input. For the toxicologist, the potential of these procedures expands because of their applicability to nonhuman subjects. In this chapter we focus on animal psychophysical methodology.

In choosing and applying psychophysical techniques, there are several important requirements. We must achieve good control by the stimulus of interest, and we must separate sensory from nonsensory influences. When subjects are animals, we must bypass verbal instructions in establishing the stimulus-behavior relationship. For toxicologic research especially, we must consider efficiency.

STIMULUS CONTROL

Good stimulus control is seen when there is a smooth relationship between the stimulus and response, when the subject remains attentive, and when control is restricted to the dimension of interest.

Establishment of the Psychophysical Relation

A fundamental relationship in psychophysics is the psychometric function. It describes the variation in a response measure with the variation of a stimulus along a clearly defined continuum. Figure 1 illustrates functions that indicate good control. In particular, the measure is increasing and monotonic, suggesting a clear dependence of the response on the stimulus value. The strong stimulus-response association at high stimulus intensities indicates that attention was good. It is also important that the response measure approaches chance values at low stimulus intensities; thus there did not appear to be extrastimulus cues affecting the behavior.

One reason for the establishment of a complete psychometric function is that drugs and toxins seem to have their clearest effects when external control of

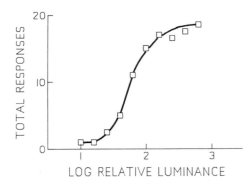

TOTAL RESPONSES

LOG RELATIVE LUMINANCE

FIG. 1. Number of responses to lights of varying luminance. There were 20 opportunities to respond to each of the 10 values. The pigeons were rewarded for responding to the lighted keys, but not to dark ones. Thus failures to respond reflect the birds' inability to detect the light, and the function provides an index of the absolute threshold. (Reproduced from Blough and Young, ref. 3, by permission.)

behavior is weak (19). For example, Evans (7) has shown that scopolamine interacts with stimulus discriminability in its effects on performance. To describe the early or subtle effects of toxins, it may be most useful to consider stimuli in the range where discrimination is poor; these would be values in the intermediate portion of the psychometric function. Establishment of the remainder of the function is important for assessing stimulus control.

Problems for Specific Sensory Systems

Establishment of a psychometric function requires physical manipulation of a stimulus source. It is necessary to consider both the equipment and the sensory modality under investigation if control is to be restricted to the dimension of interest. For example, the stimuli used in obtaining Fig. 1 varied in luminance alone, because neutral density filters controlled the energy of the light. Neutral density filters attenuate all wavelengths equally; had changes in electrical resistance been used to vary energy, the stimulus continuum would have represented a mixture of wavelength and intensity changes.

Analogously, in studying audition, we cannot assume that supplying a constant signal voltage to an earphone or loudspeaker will provide a constant sound intensity at different stimulus frequencies. Virtually no speakers are equally sensitive to all frequencies, and even "identical" speakers may differ considerably. These are just two examples of the complex problem of controlling stimuli; for vision, technical details are discussed by Boynton (4), among others; in audition, a good source is Vernon, Katz, and Meikle (34).

Another consideration, pertaining specifically to vision, concerns the duplexity of the visual system. Subjects working in well-lighted conditions probably use photopic or daylight vision, mediated by the retina's cones and good for tasks requiring acuity or color vision. Subjects who are adapted to darkness use the scotopic visual system, mediated by rods, and especially sensitive to dim light. There are other procedures for separating the two systems; for example, the photopic system is relatively more sensitive to long wavelengths and to lights flickering at high speeds. Recent research of Merigan (21) has elucidated the effects of methylmercury by varying both adaptation conditions and frequency of a temporally modulated light. His findings, suggesting that the photopic visual system is involved, help to clarify the constriction of the visual field seen after mercury poisoning.

ANIMAL METHODS

With human subjects, verbal instructions direct the subject's attention to the proper stimulus dimension and the appropriate mode of response. With nonhuman animals, verbal instructions are replaced by careful training or special attention to stimulus-elicited responses.

Training Methods

Through operant or classical conditioning, animals can learn to discriminate among stimuli by associating different responses with different stimulus cues. The animal psychophysicist starts with an easy discrimination and then varies the stimuli along the desired dimension in order to find a "threshold" or point at which the discrimination breaks down. A simple operant conditioning procedure provided the data in Fig. 1. Hungry pigeons were rewarded with food for pecking a disc illuminated with light; when the disc was dark, pecks were not rewarded. Thus the function in Fig. 1 describes the pigeons' ability to discriminate the presence of light when its intensity varied. Data such as these permit the assessment of the pigeons' absolute threshold for light. Later sections will refer to variations that improve precision and efficiency in sensory measurement. Reviews published elsewhere (2,28) examine in more detail the use of operant methods in animal psychophysics.

Reflex Modification

A disadvantage of conditioning methods is the need for extensive training. Thus operant techniques are more appropriate for research that uses repeated measures on a small number of subjects. In toxicologic research, where irreversible treatments may be combined with a need for a complete dose-response relationship, it is often necessary to use many subjects. Thus more efficient pretreatment procedures may be desirable.

One alternative to training procedures is to study reflexes elicited by stimuli in the modality of interest. For example, light elicits a pupillary reflex and sound elicits a pinna-flick (Preyer reflex) in rodents. Unfortunately, such procedures lack sensitivity. Preyer reflex thresholds, for instance, can be 80 dB (8 orders of magnitude) less sensitive than operant detection thresholds (22,24).

A promising elaboration of simple reflex procedures is based on the phenomenon known as reflex modification (RM). In essence, a low-intensity prestimulus, when presented 20 to 500 msec before a startle-eliciting event, reduces the amplitude of the startle response. While this phenomenon was first described over a century ago, it has recently received considerable attention [see Hoffman and Ison (11) and Ison and Hoffman (16) for reviews]. Reflex modification has been seen with a variety of reflexes (e.g., 32,33), but perhaps has been studied most frequently in connection with the acoustically elicited startle in the rat. The prestimulus may be auditory (12, 13), visual (5,15), or cutaneous (23,26). It need not be the onset of a stimulus; termination of (30) or gaps in (14,18) an ongoing event or changes in the frequency distribution of a continuous noise (31) also inhibit startle. Recent research with humans has shown that an effective prestimulus can be the onset of binocular disparity in a random dot display (33).

From the perspective of the animal psychophysicist, RM is of interest because the amount of inhibition varies with the strength of the prestimulus. Further, at least in audition, the intensity of the prestimulus just required for inhibition is quite close to the absolute detection threshold (25). By eliminating the period of training required by operant psychophysics, RM is proving useful in work with species that do not seem to learn well. An early application of RM was to estimate the auditory capacities of the frog (35); current research has successfully extended these results with more sophisticated equipment (20a).

Reflex modification has proven effective in studies of sensory system toxicity (26; also 36). In examining auditory and cutaneous sensitivity, Russo (26) employed pairs of startle trials. Each pair compared the elicited startle with and without a prestimulus. The criterion of inhibition was that the prestimulus trial produces a smaller amplitude response than the paired trial without the prestimulus. Russo adjusted stimulus intensity to track the threshold of startle inhibition. Thresholds for 1/3-octave noisebands and electrocutaneous stimuli were determined in this fashion and were similar to those obtained in operant discrimination studies. The method also detected temporary threshold shifts induced by noise (auditory) and lidocaine injection (tactile).

More recent research has employed an automated startle inhibition procedure for obtaining pure-tone audiometric functions (8,36). By using a predetermined set of stimulus intensities (Method of Constant Stimuli), it is possible to study several subjects simultaneously with a single stimulus generation system. Figure 2 compares pure tone audiograms obtained with this procedure with examples of equivalent operant data. The functions are quite similar, with RM thresholds within 12 to 15 dB of operant determinations, a difference that may be explained by stimulus duration differences. Figure 3 shows the influence of neomycin and saline injections on these thresholds. The characteristic pattern of neomycin-induced high-frequency hearing loss is evident.

The RM procedure does have several limitations as a psychophysical technique. Most important is its limited dynamic range, since stimuli of low intensity will produce large decrements of startle amplitude. Further, the method requires extreme care in the control of the testing environment. Extraneous stimuli in any modality can inhibit the reflex, making it impossible to partial out the effects of the stimulus under investigation.

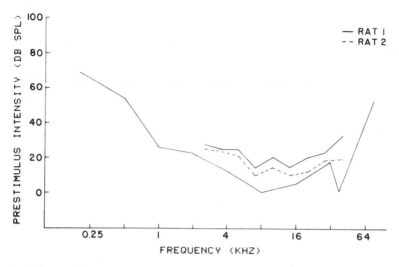

FIG. 2. Reflex modification (RM) audiograms for two groups of rats, with an audiogram determined in an operant conditioning study (17). The first *upper solid line* represents mean RM thresholds for 4 rats; the *dashed line*, 3 additional rats. The operant determination represents data from 3 rats. The slightly decreased sensitivity of the RM procedure may result from the use of brief (20 msec) prestimuli, in contrast to the operant procedure, in which tones were of long duration (up to 10 sec). (Reproduced from Young and Fechter, ref. 36, by permission of the American Institute of Physics.)

ISOLATION OF SENSORY EFFECTS

It is well known that toxic agents affect many aspects of behavior. The assessment of strictly sensory effects requires special precautions to preclude confounding behavioral deficits. Research of Hayes (10) illustrates this problem. These experiments attempted to separate the sensory effects of certain drugs from their effects on the subjects' attention. A drug that leads to an attentional deficit should affect performance in all phases of a discrimination task, regardless of its difficulty. If the effect is strictly sensory, however, we would expect to see the deterioration limited to more difficult discrimination.

Hayes's (10) research used a more sophisticated application of the operant method seen in our earlier example. Pigeons were trained to discriminate among wavelengths of light. In this case, however, there were two response keys available. The birds were rewarded for pecking the one on the left if the wavelength was shorter than 572 nm; for longer wavelengths, they were rewarded for pecking the right-hand key. The functions in Fig. 4 illustrate an attentional deficit induced by pentobarbital. The slopes of these curves describe wavelength sensitivity; steeper slopes indicate better discriminability or smaller differential thresholds. In contrast, the asymptotes of these curves provide a measure of attention. If attention were perfect, the left asymptote would be at zero and the right at 100% correct; that is, the pigeon would never peck the right key when the wavelength was very short, and it would always do so when the wavelength was very long. Hayes's findings

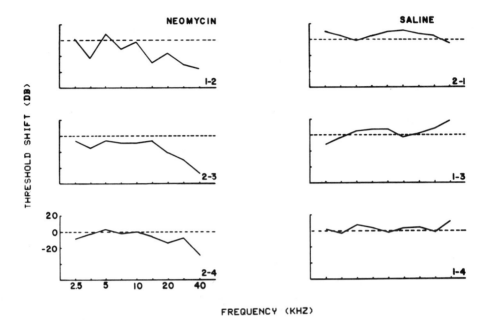

FIG. 3. Shifts in reflex modification (RM) thresholds (changes in threshold from preexposure test to postexposure test) at nine frequencies for 3 rats injected with neomycin sulfate dissolved in normal saline (100 mg/kg/day for 5 days) and 3 rats injected with equivalent volumes of saline. Negative shifts represent decreased auditory sensitivity. The neomycin-treated animals showed a characteristic pattern of high-frequency loss. (Reproduced from Young and Fechter, ref. 36, by permission.)

indicate that pentobarbital affects both the slopes and the asymptotes of these psychometric functions. Thus the drug effect on a sensory system was confounded by its effect on an attentional system.

A related problem concerns the separation of response bias from stimulus sensitivity. Suppose, for example, that a certain toxin led to an increased activity level that, for a pigeon, was reflected in an increased likelihood of the pecking response. Had the procedure been the go/no-go method illustrated in Fig. 1, the effect would have been an increase in response probability to all luminances and an apparent, but misleading, increase in sensitivity. In fact, drugs may have a selective effect on bias (6). The theory of signal detection (9) provides techniques for coping with this problem. Blough and Blough (2) discuss their application to animal psychophysics. When the two-response method used by Hayes (10) is employed, it is possible to evaluate effects on bias as well as those on attention.

Other data, mainly from behavioral pharmacology, suggest that psychophysical tools should be selected with caution. For example, rate measures (number of responses over an extended trial) are prevalent in the operant discrimination literature. Yet a considerable body of data suggests that drugs have complicated effects on response rate (e.g., 20). In some cases, a particular agent may raise an initially

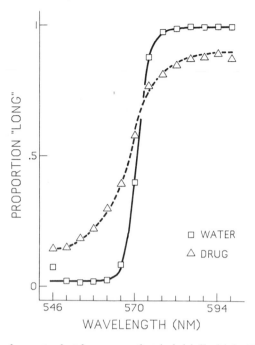

FIG. 4. Psychometric functions obtained following injections of water or pentobarbital in pigeons. Two responses were available. The one shown was correct only when the stimulus wavelength was greater than 572 nm. The drug appeared to reduce attention, since treatment led to more errors on easy as well as hard discriminations. (Reproduced from Blough and Young, ref. 3, by permission.)

low rate, but lower one that is initially high. Thus rate measures are unsuitable for the assessment of sensory effects. The experiments illustrated in Figs. 1 and 4 used trialwise procedures. Each trial began with the presentation of the stimulus and lasted only briefly. The resulting measure, the probability of a particular response during a brief trial, is a more reliable index than the traditional rate measure.

Researchers using RM must also be alert for sources of error. Fortunately, at least in humans, attention to the prestimulus does not appear to be necessary for the inhibitory effect to occur; this finding, along with others, suggests that RM is relatively independent of high-level neural processes (27). Thus it may be less subject to complex biases seen in conditioning procedures.

In the RM assessment of toxins, it is important to consider effects of the poison on other sensory modalities and on nonsensory systems. One way to test for such effects is to evaluate two or more modalities simultaneously. If a toxin has effects specific to a particular sensory system, the unaffected modality will show normal RM functions. In fact, however, some toxins may indeed have effects that are specifically sensory, but that affect more than one modality.

Nonsensory toxic effects may affect the amplitude of the reflex in cases where the sensory system remains intact. A useful control is to monitor the amplitude of the reflex in the absence of the prestimulus and to evaluate sensory effects on the basis of such control trials. Figures 5 and 6 illustrate robust RM effects in the face of nonsensory toxicity. These data are from a study (8) in which rats were given triethyltin bromide in their drinking water. This potent neuromuscular toxin produced severe hindlimb paralysis, which was presaged by marked decreases in

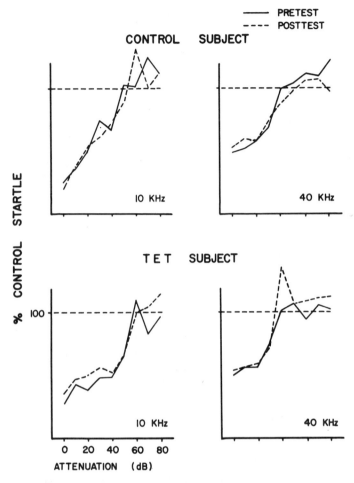

FIG. 5. Representative reflex modification (RM) psychometric functions from 2 subjects, obtained before *(solid line)* and after *(dashed line)* exposure to saline (control subjects) or to triethyltin (TET). Response amplitudes on trials with prestimuli attenuated to various degrees are plotted as a percentage of mean response amplitude on interspersed trials on which no prestimuli were presented. Despite a substantial reduction in control trial reflex amplitude in the TET-exposed subjects, these inhibition functions are essentially unchanged. (Reproduced from Fechter and Young, ref. 8, by permission of Academic Press.)

(uninhibited) startle amplitude. Despite these baseline shifts of 80% and more, psychometric functions relating relative startle decrement to prestimulus intensity were essentially normal, as were thresholds of startle inhibition. Thus sensory modification of startle is to a large extent independent of other factors that influence the startle response.

IMPROVING EFFICIENCY

Operant training for psychophysical tasks is notoriously time-consuming. Animals typically improve over time, and stable pretreatment performance may not be

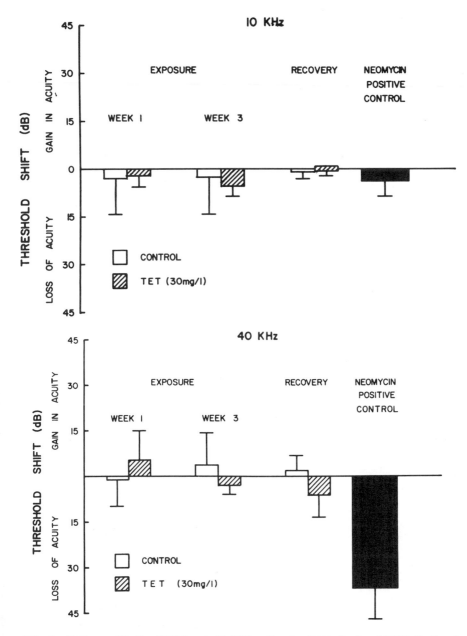

FIG. 6. Reflex modification (RM) threshold shift functions for 10 kHz **(top)** and 40 kHz **(bottom)** prestimuli, after 1 and 3 weeks of exposure to triethyltin (TET), and 3 weeks after the termination of TET exposure. Data from neomycin-exposed subjects are also shown for comparison. Despite its effects on control-trial startle amplitudes, TET did not alter thresholds of reflex inhibition. (Reproduced from Fechter and Young, ref. 8, by permission of Academic Press.)

reached for several weeks. An additional problem concerns limitations on the amount of data that can be obtained in a single session. In typical operant studies, this constraint is imposed by the amount of food or water reward that can be consumed without satiating the subject. For certain toxins, it may be desirable to administer the toxin only once and to maximize the amount of data collected immediately afterward. One way to improve the efficiency of single sessions is to reduce the probability or the amount of reward. When these values are low, satiation occurs less quickly, and a session can consist of more trials. Well-trained pigeons will maintain good stimulus control when correct responses are reinforced as rarely as once in 16 occurrences. Thus the lengthy training required for operant psychophysical training can pay off with quickly obtained, reliable posttreatment data.

Another method of improving efficiency during the posttreatment stage is to maximize presentations of test stimuli in the region of the threshold. A useful set of methods, known as "tracking" (1), uses feedback from the subject to determine stimulus values. The stimulus initially diminishes in strength until the response measure indicates that the subject no longer detects it. Strength is then increased until a criterion for detection is reached; again strength is decreased, and so forth. Figure 7 provides an illustration. Stebbins (29) has modified this tracking method and applied it in his extensive research in studies of ototoxicity. While tracking is most frequently described in the literature relating to operant techniques, it is also feasible when RM is used, as in Russo's study (26). The principal drawbacks of the procedure are its cost in stimulus-generating equipment and the fact that it does not yield a complete psychometric function.

Reflex-modification psychophysical procedures are inherently efficient, because no training time is necessary. The audiometric determinations made by Young and Fechter (36), employing nine stimulus frequencies and a large number of intensities, required only 14 10–hr sessions. Fechter and Young (8) obtained satisfactory functions for two frequencies with a series of seven 3-hr tests. The limiting factor in these determinations is the need for a fairly long intertrial interval; these periods guard against the possibility of threshold shifts induced by startle-eliciting stimuli.

CONCLUSION

Animal psychophysics can supply valuable information regarding sensory system toxicity. Although traditional learning procedures have proven precise, the lengthy

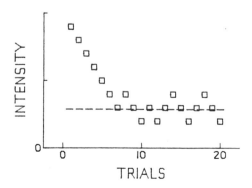

FIG. 7. Schematic representation of a modified tracking procedure. The subject's behavior on each trial determines stimulus intensity for the following trial. A correct detection decreases intensity; when the subject fails to detect the stimulus, its intensity is increased. The *dashed line* indicates an intensity that might be taken as absolute threshold. (Reproduced from Blough and Young, ref. 3.)

training required may render them inappropriate for some toxicologic research. Thus in addition to reviewing operant techniques, we have described recent applications of reflex modification. Properly used, either method can reveal the needed information about the normal and toxin-impaired capacities of nonhuman subjects.

ACKNOWLEDGMENT

We thank Laurence D. Fechter for his helpful comments during the preparation of this manuscript.

REFERENCES

1. Blough, D. S. (1958): A method for obtaining psychophysical thresholds from the pigeon. *J. Exp. Anal. Behav.*, 2:31–43.
2. Blough, D. S., and Blough, P. M. (1977): Animal psychophysics. In: *Handbook of Operant Behavior*, edited by W. K. Honig and J. E. R. Staddon, pp. 514–539. Prentice-Hall, Englewood Cliffs, N.J.
3. Blough, P. M., and Young, J. S. (1982): Psychophysical assessment of visual dysfunction. *Environ. Health Perspect.*, 44:47–53.
4. Boynton, R. M. (1966): Vision. In: *Experimental Methods and Instrumentation in Psychology*, edited by J. B. Sidowski, pp. 273–330. McGraw-Hill, New York.
5. Buckland, G., Buckland, J., Jamieson, C., and Ison, J. R. (1969): Inhibition of the startle response to acoustic stimulation produced by visual prestimulation. *J. Comp. Physiol. Psychol.*, 67:493–496.
6. Dykstra, L. A., and Appel, J. B. (1974): Effects of LSD on auditory perception: A signal detection analysis. *Psychopharmacologia*, 34:289–307.
7. Evans, H. L. (1975): Scopolamine effects on visual discrimination: Modification related to stimulus control. *J. Pharm. Exp. Ther.*, 195:105–113.
8. Fechter, L. D., and Young, J. S. (1983): Discrimination of auditory from nonauditory toxicity by reflex modulation audiometry: Effects of triethyltin. *Toxicol. Appl. Pharmacol.*, 70:216–227.
9. Green, D. M., and Swets, J. A., editors (1966): *Signal Detection Theory and Psychophysics*. Wiley, New York.
10. Hayes, W. F. (1980): Drug effects on wavelength discrimination in pigeons. Ph.D. Dissertation, Brown University.
11. Hoffman, H., and Ison, J. R. (1980): Reflex modification in the domain of startle: I. Some empirical findings and their implications for how the nervous system processes sensory input. *Psychol. Rev.*, 87:175–189.
12. Hoffman, H., and Searle, J. L. (1965): Acoustic variables in the modification of startle reaction in the rat. *J. Comp. Physiol. Psychol.*, 60:53–58.
13. Hoffman, H., and Searle, J. L. (1968): Acoustic and temporal factors in the evocation of startle. *J. Acoust. Soc. Am.*, 43:269–282.
14. Ison, J. R. (1982): Temporal acuity in auditory function in the rat: Reflex inhibition by brief gaps in noise. *J. Comp. Physiol. Psychol.*, 96:945–954.
15. Ison, J. R., and Hammond, G. R. (1971): Modification of the startle reflex in the rat by changes in the auditory and visual environments. *J. Comp. Physiol. Psychol.*, 75:435–452.
16. Ison, J. R., and Hoffman, H. S. (1983): Reflex modification in the domain of startle: II. The anomalous history of a robust and ubiquitous phenomenon. *Psychol. Bull.*, 94:3–17.
17. Kelley, J. B., and Masterton, B. (1977): Auditory sensitivity of the albino rat. *J. Comp. Physiol. Psychol.*, 91:930–936.
18. Kellogg, C., Ison, J. R., and Miller, R. K. (1983): Prenatal diazepam exposure: Effects on auditory temporal resolution in rats. *Psychopharmacology*, 79:332–337.
19. Laties, V. G. (1975): The role of discriminative stimuli in modulating drug action. *Fed. Proc.*, 43:1880–1888.
20. McKearney, J. W. (1970): Rate-dependent effects of drugs: Modification by discriminative stimuli of the effects of amobarbital on schedule controlled behavior. *J. Exp. Anal. Behav.*, 14:167–175.
20a. Megela-Simmons, A., Moss, C. F., and Daniel, K. M.: Behavioral audiograms of the bullfrog (*Rana catesbiana*) and the green treefrog (*Hyla cineria*). *J. Acoust. Soc. Am.* (in press).
21. Merigan, W. H. (1980): Visual fields and flicker thresholds in methylmercury-poisoned monkeys.

In: *Neurotoxicity of the Visual System*, edited by W. H. Merigan and B. Weiss, pp. 149–163. Raven Press, New York.

22. Neidl, M. J., Liddell, M. R., Montenaro, M. J., Hawkins, J. E., Jr., and Drobeck, H. P. (1981): The ototoxicity of hydroxygentamicin, a new aminoglycoside antibiotic, in guinea pigs. *Fundam. Appl. Toxicol.*, 1:395–402.

23. Pinckney, L. A. (1976): Inhibition of the startle reflex in the rat by prior tactile stimulation. *Anim. Learn. Behav.*, 4:467–472.

24. Prosen, C. A., Peterson, M. R., Moody, D. B., and Stebbins, W. C. (1978): Auditory thresholds and kanamycin-induced hearing loss in the guinea pig assessed by a positive reinforcement procedure. *J. Acoust. Soc. Am.*, 63:559–566.

25. Reiter, L. A., and Ison, J. R. (1977): Inhibition of the human eyeblink reflex: An examination of the Wendt-Yerkes method for threshold detection. *J. Exp. Psychol. (Hum. Percept.)*, 3:325–336.

26. Russo, J. M. (1980): Sensation in the rat and mouse: Evaluation by reflex modification. *Diss. Abstr. Int.*, 41:392-B.

27. Silverstein, L. D., Graham, F. K., and Callaway, J. M. (1980): Preconditioning and excitability of the human orbicularis oculi reflex as a function of state. *Electroencephalogr. Clin. Neurophysiol.*, 48:406–417.

28. Stebbins, W. C., editor (1970): *Animal Psychophysics: The Design and Conduct of Sensory Experiments*. Appleton-Century-Crofts, New York.

29. Stebbins, W. C., and Rudy, M. C. (1978): Behavioral ototoxicology. *Environ. Health Perspect.*, 26:43–51.

30. Stitt, C. L., Hoffman, H., and Marsh, R. (1973): Modification of the rat's startle reaction by termination of antecedent acoustic signals. *J. Comp. Physiol. Psychol.*, 84:207–215.

31. Stitt, C. L., Hoffman, H., Marsh, R., and Boskoff, K. J. (1974): Modification of the rat's startle by an antecedent change in the environment. *J. Comp. Physiol. Psychol.*, 86:826–836.

32. Stitt, C. L., Hoffman, H., Marsh, R. R., and Schwartz, G. M. (1976): Modification of the pigeon's visual startle reaction by the sensory environment. *J. Comp. Physiol. Psychol.*, 90:601–619.

33. Uhlrich, D. J. (1983): Inhibition of the human blink reflex by visual form stimuli. Ph.D. Dissertation, Brown University.

34. Vernon, J. A., Katz, B., and Meikle, M. B. (1976): Sound measurement and calibration of instruments. In: *Handbook of Auditory and Vestibular Research Methods*, edited by C. A. Smith and J. A. Vernon, pp. 306–356. Charles C. Thomas, Springfield, IL.

35. Yerkes, R. M. (1905): The sense of hearing in frogs. *J. Comp. Neurol. Psychol.*, 15:279–304.

36. Young, J. S., and Fechter, L. D. (1983): Reflex inhibition procedures for animal audiometry: A technique for assessing ototoxicity. *J. Acoust. Soc. Am.*, 73:1686–1693.

Toxicology of the Eye, Ear, and Other Special Senses, edited by A. W. Hayes. Raven Press, New York © 1985.

Newer Laboratory Approaches for Assessing Visual Dysfunction

Paul G. Shinkman, Michael R. Isley, and Diane C. Rogers

Department of Psychology, University of North Carolina, Chapel Hill, North Carolina 27514

VISUAL CORTICAL RECEPTIVE FIELDS AND THEIR PROPERTIES

Over the past 20 years, a number of basic concepts have emerged concerning the organization of the mammalian visual system, particularly at the cellular level. A centrally important concept, which ultimately describes the fundamental building blocks of visual circuitry, is the receptive field (RF). Each neuron along the retinogeniculocortical pathway (as well as other visual pathways) is concerned with the analysis of a small subregion of the total visual field. At each level, the RFs are arranged in a systematic topographic (i.e., retinotopic) manner such that the entire visual world is laid out multiply across the occipital cortex with an overrepresentation of the central region. A specific stimulus presented within the boundaries of a cell's RF will evoke a maximal discharge of impulses from that cell. The particular stimulus pattern evoking the strongest response is said to embody the "stimulus trigger features" or RF properties of that cell. For example, a well-known stimulus requirement of cortical units is orientation or angular position of the optimal stimulus.

Although there is a significant primate literature, most of our knowledge of how RF properties code form, movement, and depth in the visual world has been obtained from the feline visual system using recently developed microelectrode recording and stimulating techniques. The domestic cat has been so widely used as a subject that its use in the vision laboratory has been characterized as "currently representing the primary source of neural building blocks from which the majority of models of human vision are constructed" (1, p. 423). In a series of pioneering studies on the feline visual system, Hubel and Wiesel (2,3) laid down the basic foundation for interpreting the specific RF properties of cortical visual neurons.

The two RF properties that have received the most attention are ocular dominance and orientation selectivity. In the normal mammalian visual cortex, the majority (80–85%) of cortical neurons receive excitatory input from each eye, i.e., they are binocular. The remaining small population of cells, categorized as monocular units, receive input from one eye or the other. Furthermore, for cells receiving a dual input, that input is not necessarily equal for the two eyes. A seven-class scheme or an ocular dominance (OD) index characterizing this relative ocular input to a particular cortical cell was proposed by Hubel and Wiesel (2). This nomenclature has been universally adopted among visual neurophysiologists, and probably represents the easiest RF property to determine. A typical OD histogram and definitions for the various categories appear in Fig. 1. For a normal adult cat, the distribution for a population of cortical cells is bell-shaped with some contralateral skewing.

Of all the specific stimulus trigger features of visual cortical RFs, perhaps the most fundamental requirement is orientation specificity. That is, the appropriate stimulus must assume some critical angular position within the boundary of the RF for maximal stimulation of that cortical unit, and any deviation (± 10–25°) from the optimal orientation results in dramatically decreasing or eliminating the neural response. Typically, angular selectivity is determined by moving an appropriate stimulus, usually a light or dark edge (e.g., a bar), through the RF at different orientations while measuring the response. The response profile of a single cortical cell as a function of stimulus orientation is referred to as the orientation tuning curve (OTC), depicted in Fig. 2 for a hypothesized RF. An OTC can be compiled by one of two RF plotting techniques. The first consists of simply listening to the

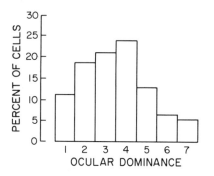

FIG. 1. Ocular dominance histogram showing the relative influence of the two eyes on a sample of cortical units in a normal adult cat. Each cell is assigned to one of seven categories: Monocular cells are driven exclusively by the contralateral eye *(1)* or the ipsilateral eye *(7)*, while binocular cells are driven equally by each eye *(4)*, more strongly by the contralateral eye *(2 or 3)*, or more strongly by the ipsilateral eye *(5, 6)*.

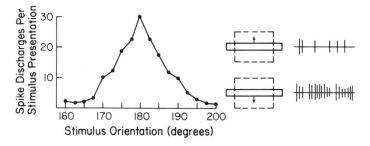

FIG. 2.a: Computer-determined orientation tuning curve for a cortical cell's receptive field, showing the response to a slit of light at several orientations. This cell is tightly tuned for a stimulus oriented near 180°. **b:** Schematic representation of directional selectivity for the same unit. Shown on the left is a slit of light moving through the receptive field in both directions, orthogonal to the optimal orientation. On the right are responses evoked by these stimuli.

amplified response of the unit over an audio monitor while simultaneously monitoring the activity on an oscilloscope (the manual/auditory feedback method popularized by Hubel and Wiesel) (2,3). The second approach, one advantage of which is to eliminate possible experimental bias, uses a computer or automatically controlled visual stimulation system. Measurements of orientation preference and the degree of selectivity made by these two methods generally stand in good agreement with each other (e.g., 4).

There exists an elegant layout of ocular dominance and orientation specificity within the cortex that has been convincingly demonstrated electrophysiologically and anatomically in both the cat and monkey striate cortex (e.g., 5–8). Two independent sets of vertical "columns" or cortical slabs, ocular dominance and orientation, represent the fundamental building blocks of visual cytoarchitectonics. Cells favoring the same eye or preferring approximately the same optimal stimulus orientation are grouped into functional slabs arranged perpendicularly to each other and the cortical surface and through the six layers of gray matter reveal systematic changes in both ocular dominance and orientation preference. Orientation changes occur in a clockwise or counterclockwise direction such that 180° is represented across about 1 mm of cortex before a reversal. All orientations are about equally represented, with neighboring columns varying by about 10 to 15°. Likewise, ocular dominance changes progressively; one eye is dominant, then the two become roughly equal, and finally the other eye becomes dominant in roughly the same cortical distance but independently of a 180° orientation sequence. One complete set of these columns, an orientation cycle or ocular dominance cycle, has been termed a hypercolumn.

Another RF feature characteristic of most normal cortical neurons is that a more vigorous response is elicited by a moving than a stationary stimulus. Furthermore, the majority of cortical units display a directional preference, responding more strongly to movement of the optimal stimulus in one direction than in the other direction. This, too, is illustrated in Fig. 2; the cell prefers the appropriate stimulus moving in a downward direction orthogonal to the optimal orientation. Other RF properties of cortical visual neurons include the spatial layout of excitatory and inhibitory subregions (shape) that compose an RF, preference for specific velocities of a moving stimulus, and interocular relationships such as RF locational or orientational disparities of binocular cells.

On the basis of the uniformity in RF properties, cortical units have been categorized by various investigators. The most commonly used system comes from the early studies of Hubel and Wiesel (2,3), who proposed the now classic simple, complex, and hypercomplex RF types. Extraction of stimulus features from the visual world, as conceived by these authors, is carried out by a hierarchical arrangement of these three basic RF types in visual cortex. In this model the properties of simple cells' RFs are determined by direct excitatory input from a number of lateral geniculate cells, while the RFs of complex cells are determined by input from several simple cells. Complex cells, in turn, provide the input to the RFs of hypercomplex cells. This strictly serial model, however, has been seriously challenged on both anatomic and electrophysiologic grounds (e.g., 9). The central visual circuitry, particularly from retina to cortex via the dorsal lateral geniculate nucleus, is composed of several functionally distinct, parallel-running subgroups of cells, two of which have been called the X- and Y-pathways. At the cortex, these separate systems are less easily identified, although several electrophysiologic studies point to a strong correlation between particular RF types and these parallel afferents. It is currently thought that the X-system influences mainly simple cells while the Y-system influences mainly complex cells. Important clues to understanding the functional roles of the X/Y dichotomy have been provided by differences in retinal distribution, spatial and temporal stimulus properties defined electrophysiologically, and cortical synaptology. The X-system is primarily concerned with detailed, central vision and binocular stereoscopic vision, while the Y-system subserves some functions of peripheral vision, such as the detection of motion, location, and possibly coarse outlines.

NEUROELECTRIC APPROACHES

Generally, more varied and advanced methods of assessment exist for the visual system than for other sensory systems. Like all sensory systems, its development is susceptible to environmental factors, including chemical agents; i.e., although genetics defines the potential, a high level of neuronal plasticity is present. Postnatal plasticity is greatest during early development, a time referred to as the critical period (CP), since normal visual experience during this time is crucial to normal development. Absences or abnormalities in visual experience are manifested as long-lasting functional and physiologic deficits. For example, occluding one eye (monocular deprivation or MD) of a kitten during the traditionally defined CP, 1 to 4 months of age, results in a loss of vision through that eye and a severe shift in ocular dominance in favor of the experienced eye (10). It is of particular interest to visual scientists to determine the extent to which RF properties as well as overall visual physiology are influenced by innate factors, passive maturational changes, and environmental contributions. That is, at each developmental stage, to what extent is the system susceptible to impairment or loss of function caused by various degrees of abnormal experience?

Because alterations in neural function following exposure to toxic substances, especially at long-term low-level exposures, are often quite subtle, and because it is necessary to determine threshold levels for toxins, it is desirable to have measures of nervous system function that are very sensitive. One suitable tool may be the neurophysiologic method of single-cell recordings. RF properties of single cells are finely tuned, and are highly sensitive and responsive to environmental manipulations during the CP. In particular, the properties of ocular dominance, orientation preference, and directional preference have demonstrated highly robust effects. For example, a number of innovative studies (e.g., 11,12) have found that if only one orientation (e.g., vertical) is experienced during the CP, most cortical cells will be tuned to that orientation. More importantly, behavioral measures mirror this: the animal appears to be blind to stimuli at nonexperienced orientations.

In most of these "environmental surgery" studies, animals have been exposed to a unique visual experience throughout the CP. However, some researchers, with the goal of determining the sensitivity of the system, have attempted to delineate the minimal amount of experience needed to alter RF properties. One interesting but controversial study (13) reported that as little as 1 hr of exposure to a highly redundant environment (vertical gratings) could significantly alter the normal orientation distribution in kitten cortex; i.e., disproportionately many cortical units were tuned to vertical orientations. Others have shown that ocular dominance can be dramatically shifted after only a few hours of monocular exposure during the peak of the CP (e.g., 14). On the other hand, important differences in the degree of susceptibility of certain RF properties to environmental insult are beginning to be unraveled. Velocity preferences, for example, appear to be more resistant to a "matching effect" than any other RF property (e.g., 15). Others contend that certain subclasses of orientation preferences are also quite resistant to environmental manipulations, pointing to a strong genetic determination (e.g., 16). In short, this sort of selective versus instructive question currently represents a major controversy among visual neurophysiologists. Since exposure to toxic substances can be restricted to either prenatal or postnatal periods, or be of a more chronic nature throughout adult life, knowledge of such developmental differences and their chronologies provides still another means for measuring the relative sensitivity of the visual system to neurotoxicity at the level of individual RF properties.

The effect of chemical agents on RF properties is a topic that has scarcely been broached, but indications are that this might be a highly sensitive and responsive measure, useful for revealing mechanisms of dysfunction. For instance, two observations made on cats during acute single-unit preparations are (a) administration of barbiturate anesthetic agents leads to a sharpening of orientation tuning of visual cortical units (17); and (b) improper regulation of oxygen, as measured by end-tidal CO_2 concentration, leads to a rapid and severe degradation of visual RF quality, e.g., high erratic base rate and poor responsiveness (e.g., 18). Another study, explicitly addressing changes in visual RF properties after neurotoxic exposure, reported that the widely used organophosphate pesticide, mevinphos, and related cholinergic drugs (e.g., agonists such as pilocarpine or antagonists such as atropine sulfate) abolish the highly tuned directional selectivity of single cells in the avian nucleus rotundus (19). A similar effect was reported after ethanol exposure. These effects may be the neuronal basis for visual behavioral impairment at certain levels of intoxication (e.g., decrease or loss of visual attention, orientation behavior, and peripheral vision).

Another neuroelectric technique, which has already been widely adapted for neurotoxin testing, is the visually evoked potential (VEP) (20). The VEP is a gross recording, obtained through scalp or depth electrodes, which simultaneously measures thousands of cells' responses to visual stimulation. The EP signal is generally localized to the small area of brain directly below the electrodes. Since the response is obscured in a single trace because of trial-to-trial variability, inherent noise, and background EEG, a reliable EP record is obtainable only through signal averaging techniques. A standard cortical VEP (VECP) record evoked from visual cortex by a light flash is diagrammed in Fig. 3. Like all EPs, the VECP is a complex waveform consisting of a series of positive (P1, P2, P3) and negative (N1, N2, N3) peaks, the amplitude and latency of which are determined by a number of factors: stimulus parameters, location and mode of recording, and age and physiology of the animal. Two phases comprise the VEP, and alterations in peak onset latency or amplitude (baseline-to-peak or peak-to-peak) of specific components may reveal CNS dysfunction. The early primary components (latency<50 msec), P1-N1 and N1-P2, are most sensitive to changed input parameters and are commonly thought to depend on retinogeniculate activity, while the late secondary components (50–200 msec latency), P2-N2, N2-P3, and P3-N3, which are believed related to diffuse activity of thalamic, mesencephalic, and cortical origins, are quite variable in waking brains and are suppressed by anesthetics.

This technique has advantages over single-unit records: (a) it can be quickly, easily, and repeatedly applied, and (b) it can be applied to humans as well as animal subjects. Its use as a research tool for determining mechanism of dysfunction, however, is restricted to a molar level. Clearly, it is of considerable theoretical and practical importance to establish correlations between specific parameters of gross evoked potentials, on the one hand, and the activity of various classes of single units, on the other. A number of studies have approached this question (e.g., 21), but a comprehensive picture has not yet emerged.

The ease with which the VEP can be measured has made it a prime candidate for clinical use, epidemiologic or experimental field studies, and longitudinal studies. It is currently used as a diagnostic tool for amblyopia in very young children and other nonverbal patients. Also, it has been proposed for use in evaluating neurotoxicity in individuals who have had prolonged occupational contact with possibly toxic substances. However, little toxicologic information is actually obtained from human subjects, since controlled administration of toxins cannot exceed threshold levels. For developmental or longitudinal studies, the VEP is well suited, since components emerge in a chronologically orderly sequence, and the waveform,

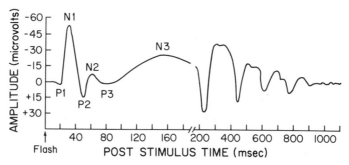

FIG. 3. Electrical activity in rat visual cortex following a light flash, showing the various components of the evoked potential and the subsequent 3- to 6-Hz afterdischarge. (After Fig. 1, ref. 20.)

which does not assume adult characteristics until a relatively late developmental stage, changes again during senescence (e.g., 22).

The VEP is currently being used to study effects of such common toxicants as CO, some heavy metals (e.g., lead, methylmercury), and some organophosphate compounds (e.g., mevinphos). For example, one study of the effects of methylmercury (23) reported that rats prenatally exposed to this heavy metal (their mothers ingested a single low dose) showed a visual dysfunction, as measured by the VEP, in adulthood. The early primary VECP components in these animals had an increased amplitude relative to controls, indicating a disruption of function in the retinogeniculate-striate system. Also, the P2 and N2 peaks had a shortened latency, which, in conjunction with other reports, suggests a greater susceptibility to damage by methylmercury for slowly conducting axons than for other axons.

A common feature of mammalian visually evoked cortical activity, which follows the VEP (120–200 msec latency) and persists for 2 sec or longer, is a rhythmic 3–6 Hz repetitive discharge known as the visually evoked response afterdischarge (VER AD) (see Fig. 3). It is generated and maintained by recurrent circuitry at the dorsal lateral geniculate nucleus (LGN) level and is modulated by a variety of limbic, brainstem, and thalamic systems (see refs. 24 and 25 for a review). This response, which has only recently been explored, is a sensitive measure of visual dysfunction caused by some substances when the VEP is insensitive. The VER AD is especially sensitive to drugs such as convulsants and anticonvulsants that have a predominantly thalamic level of action. Thus one promising use of the VER AD is as a model for the treatment of epilepsy.

NEUROCHEMICAL APPROACHES

Studies of chemically induced changes in single visual cortical neurons are quite limited, although the development of new neurochemical techniques has made this a major objective. Potentially fruitful approaches for assessing both acute and chronic administration of toxic substances to developing and adult visual cortical neurons have been provided by studies of specific functions of neurotransmitters in visual cortex. The value of this technology is that it permits relatively specific pharmacologic control of locally applied chemicals to sensory regions (e.g., visual cortex) of the brain and concurrent or subsequent electrophysiologic evaluation of specific, patterned cellular activity evoked by appropriate sensory stimuli. In particular, two techniques have been used in elucidating neurochemical mechanisms operating in the visual cortex of the cat. Importantly, both allow for within-animal controls (e.g., interhemispheric comparisons).

The first preparation, most suited to ascertain immediate or acute effects of exposure to toxic substances, is the microiontophoretic administration of substances of interest while simultaneously recording single-cell activity. Briefly, this technique involves penetrating the visual cortex with multi-barrel micropipettes. Typically, the center barrel is used as a recording/marking electrode for single units while the other barrels contain agents to be released at specific sites by passing a small ejecting current through the desired solution. For example, Sillito (26) and others (e.g., 27) have demonstrated in visual cortex that the action of γ-aminobutyric acid (GABA), an important inhibitory neurotransmitter in the mammalian brain, can be reversibly antagonized by iontophoretic application of the alkaloid bicuculline. The general effect of bicuculline on single cells is a disruption of response specificity for stimulus parameters such as orientation and direction of movement. In addition to the general disruption of RF properties, specific differences were noted for RF types such as simple versus complex. A corollary question, arising from these specific cortical effects following neurochemical manipulations, is the following: To what extent are specific differences manifested systematically throughout the central visual pathways following environmental insult, such as from toxic exposure, since functionally different systems (e.g., the X/Y dichotomy) are believed to be connected to these different cell types? Such an assessment would offer a means for measuring the relative sensitivity of the visual system to neurotoxicity at a more integrative level. The primary impetus for investigating these functional differences has already been provided by studies that have demonstrated that special critical period exposure for kittens can selectively disrupt normal function of the Y-system, while the same maneuver, in this case paralysis of one eye, performed on the adult cat degrades the X-system (e.g., 28).

Equally important questions concern changes in visual cortical RF properties following chronic administration of chemical agents, or low-level exposures during early postnatal development. Consequences in the latter case may not be fully manifested until late in life and may thus demand longitudinal analysis. A preparation that is quite adaptable for these maneuvers involves a continuous microperfusion technique using the newly developed Alzet osmotic minipump. Like the first technique, it too has yielded a means for coupling neurochemical and electrophysiologic approaches in the study of single neurons in the developing and adult visual cortices. This simple procedure involves subcutaneously implanting a minipump system with a connecting cannula that delivers the contents slowly and continuously over a specific cortical site. After the contents have been emptied, minipump replacement, if so desired, can be performed easily and quickly. Subsequently, electrophysiologic examination of single neurons is performed, using conventional procedures. Most recently, this preparation has been employed to investigate neurochemical mechanisms that possibly control the time course of the postnatal CP as manifested by the monocular deprivation effect in the feline visual system. Intraventricular injections (29) or local cortical microperfusions via an implanted osmotic minipump/cannula system (30) of the neurotoxin 6-hydroxydopamine (6-OHDA) prevent the loss of binocularity that normally follows monocular deprivation during the CP. These findings, along with subsequent studies, indicate that a normal balance of catecholamines plays a crucial role in promoting neuronal plasticity in the feline visual system. For example, concurrent microperfusion of the visual cortex with *l*-norepinephrine HCl blocked the 6-OHDA effect for monocularly deprived kittens, who then showed the expected shift in ocular dominance (31). Furthermore, the susceptibility to monocular deprivation of kittens well beyond the CP (13 weeks) and, to a lesser degree, of adult cats (2 years old) is restored by extended periods (2 weeks) of cortical microperfusion with norepinephrine (30).

BEHAVIORAL APPROACHES

Behavior is the most complex but also the most relevant level at which the effects of environmental manipulations can be examined. The assessment of visual behaviors, which has been extensive in the cat, has been approached in various ways. The first has involved observing and cataloguing naturally occurring visual behaviors in the normal adult organism. A second approach, related to the first, entails evaluating the development of such behaviors and various factors that affect them, especially during development. Commonly studied visual behaviors have traditionally included gross visuomotor responses such as the looming reflex, visual orienting, following and pursuit of visual targets, obstacle avoidance in an open field, triggered visual placing, coordinated jumping, and depth perception as tested on a visual cliff. Unfortunately, a good correspondence between visual deficits defined physiologically at the single-cell level and behaviorally via gross visuomotor performance may not occur. These behavioral tests are often not sensitive enough, and further, extensive visuomotor adaptation can mask real deficits or anomalies of visual function. Tests using refined and controlled psychophysical procedures have provided the necessary sensitive measures of visual function in normal and experimental animals. Attention will be confined to these procedures since they offer a method for pinpointing the nature and chronology of sensory deficits and, more importantly, a means for comparison of human and infrahuman results.

Two behavioral tests, a nose-key operant (4,32) and a modified Lashley jumping stand (33), require an animal to perform in a two-response forced-choice discrimination task. These tests have considerable appeal, since training is relatively fast and easy, allowing a variety of visual functions with known parameters for humans to be determined: acuity, orientation perception, depth perception, vernier alignment, and contrast sensitivity. With these techniques the functional significance of single-unit disruption can be directly addressed; i.e., does the quality of RF properties define visual capacities? Several studies have provided partial answers: A kitten monocularly deprived during the critical period has a mostly monocular cortex, as seen by single-unit studies (10). The behavioral manifestation, determined using a conditioned suppression paradigm, is that binocular visual functions (e.g., stereopsis) are absent or extremely attenuated (34). A second manipulation, which alters the cortical distribution of RF orientations, has been shown to affect perceptual performance as well. Kittens reared experiencing a restricted range of orientations (horizontal or vertical) develop biased visual cortices (i.e., most units are tuned to horizontal and vertical, respectively) and are visually more sensitive to the experienced orientations (4).

CONCLUSIONS

The relative sensitivity of visual cortical RF properties to environmental influences suggests a potential utility of RF analysis as a neurotoxicity screening tool.

New and improved laboratory techniques including neuroelectric, neurochemical, and behavioral approaches adaptable to this area of research were briefly reviewed. Their usefulness as screening tools remains to be fully demonstrated.

REFERENCES

1. Blake, R. (1979): The visual system of the cat. *Percept. Psychophys.*, 26:423–448.
2. Hubel, D. H., and Wiesel, T. N. (1962): Receptive fields, binocular interaction and functional architecture in the cat's visual cortex. *J. Physiol. (Lond.)*, 160:106–154.
3. Hubel, D. H., and Wiesel, T. N. (1965): Receptive fields and functional architecture in two nonstriate visual areas (18 and 19) of the cat. *J. Neurophysiol.*, 28:229–289.
4. Blasdel, G. G., Mitchell, D. E., Muir, D. W., and Pettigrew, J. D. (1977): A physiological and behavioural study in cats of the effect of early visual experience with contours of a single orientation. *J. Physiol. (Lond.)*, 265:615–636.
5. Hubel, D. H., and Wiesel, T. N. (1974): Sequence regularity and geometry of orientation columns in the monkey striate cortex. *J. Comp. Neurol.*, 158:267–293.
6. Hubel, D. H., Wiesel, T. N., and Stryker, M. P. (1977): Orientation columns in macaque monkey visual cortex demonstrated by the 2-deoxyglucose autoradiographic technique. *Nature*, 269:328–330.
7. LeVay, S., Stryker, M. P., and Shatz, C. J. (1978): Ocular dominance columns and their development in layer IV of the cat's visual cortex: A quantitative study. *J. Comp. Neurol.*, 179:223–244.
8. Albus, K. (1979): ^{14}C-Deoxyglucose mapping of orientation subunits in the cat's visual cortical areas. *Exp. Brain Res.*, 37:609–613.
9. Lennie, P. (1980): Parallel visual pathways: A review. *Vision Res.*, 20:561–594.
10. Hubel, D. H., and Wiesel, T. N. (1970): The period of susceptibility to the physiological effects of unilateral eye closure in kittens. *J. Physiol. (Lond.)*, 206:419–436.
11. Blakemore, C., and Cooper, G. F. (1970): Development of the brain depends on the visual environment. *Nature*, 228:477–478.
12. Hirsch, H. V. B., and Spinelli, D. N. (1970): Visual experience modifies distribution of horizontally and vertically oriented receptive fields in cats. *Science*, 168:869–871.
13. Blakemore, C., and Mitchell, D. E. (1973): Environmental modification of the visual cortex and the neural basis of learning and memory. *Nature*, 241:467–468.
14. Peck, C. K., and Blakemore, C. (1975): Modification of single neurons in the kitten's visual cortex after brief periods of monocular visual experience. *Exp. Brain Res.*, 22:57–68.
15. Tretter, F., Cynader, M., and Singer, W. (1975): Modification of direction selectivity of neurons in the visual cortex of kittens. *Brain Res.*, 84:143–149.
16. Stryker, M. P., and Sherk, H. (1975): Modification of cortical orientation selectivity in the cat by restricted visual experience: A reexamination. *Science*, 190:904–906.
17. Pettigrew, J. D. (1974): The effect of visual experience on the development of stimulus specificity by kitten cortical neurones. *J. Physiol. (Lond.)*, 237:49–74.
18. Daniels, J. D., Pettigrew, J. D., and Norman, J. L. (1978): Development of single-neuron responses in kitten's lateral geniculate nucleus. *J. Neurophysiol.*, 41:1373–1393.
19. Revzin, A. M. (1980): Effects of organophosphate pesticides and alcohol on visual mechanisms. In: *Neurotoxicity of the Visual System*, edited by W. H. Merigan and B. Weiss, pp. 255–268. Raven Press, New York.
20. Dyer, R. S., Eccles, C. U., Swartzwelder, H. S., Fechter, L. D., and Annau, Z. (1979): Prenatal carbon monoxide and adult evoked potentials in rats. *J. Environ. Sci. Health*, C13(2):107–120.
21. Verzeano, M. (1970): Evoked responses and network dynamics. In: *The Neural Control of Behavior*, edited by R. E. Whalen, R. F. Thompson, M. Verzeano, and N. M. Weinberger, pp. 27–54. Academic Press, New York.
22. Klorman, R., Thompson, L., and Ellingson, R. (1978): Event related brain potentials across the life span. In: *Event-Related Brain Potentials in Man*, edited by E. Callaway, P. Tueting, and S. Koslow, pp. 511–570. Academic Press, New York.
23. Dyer, R. S., Eccles, C. U., and Annau, Z. (1978): Evoked potential alterations following prenatal methyl mercury exposure. *Pharmacol. Biochem. Behav.*, 8:137–141.

24. Bigler, E. D. (1977): Neurophysiology, neuropharmacology and behavioral relationships of visual system evoked after-discharges: A review. *Biobehav. Rev.*, 1:95–112.

25. Shearer, D. E., and Creel, D. (1978): The photically evoked afterdischarge: Current concepts and potential applications. *Physiol. Psychol.*, 6:369–376.

26. Sillito, A. M. (1975): The contribution of inhibitory mechanisms to the receptive field properties of neurones in the striate cortex of the cat. *J. Physiol. (Lond.)*, 250:305–329.

27. Pettigrew, J. D., and Daniels, J. D. (1973): Gamma-aminobutyric acid antagonism in visual cortex: Different effects on simple, complex, and hypercomplex neurons. *Science*, 182:81–83.

28. Brown, D. L., and Salinger, W. L. (1975): Loss of X-cells in lateral geniculate nucleus with monocular paralysis: Neural plasticity in the adult cat. *Science*, 189:1011–1012.

29. Kasamatsu, T., and Pettigrew, J. D. (1976): Depletion of brain catecholamines: Failure of ocular dominance shift after monocular occlusion in kittens. *Science*, 194:206–209.

30. Kasamatsu, T., Pettigrew, J. D., and Ary, M. (1979): Restoration of visual cortical plasticity by local microperfusion of norepinephrine. *J. Comp. Neurol.*, 185:163–181.

31. Pettigrew, J. D., and Kasamatsu, T. (1978): Local perfusion of noradrenaline maintains visual cortical plasticity. *Nature*, 271:761–763.

32. Muir, D. W., and Mitchell, D. E. (1973): Visual resolution and experience: Acuity deficits in cats following early selective visual deprivation. *Science*, 180:420–422.

33. Mitchell, D. E., Giffin, F., and Timney, B. (1977): A behavioral technique for the rapid assessment of the visual capabilities of kittens. *Perception*, 6:181–193.

34. Blake, R., and Hirsch, H. V. B. (1975): Deficits in binocular depth perception in cats after alternating monocular deprivation. *Science*, 190:1114–1116.

Toxicology of the Eye, Ear, and Other Special Senses, edited by A. W. Hayes. Raven Press, New York © 1985.

Assessment of Chemically Induced Ocular Toxicity: A Survey of Methods

*Ping-Kwong Chan and **A. Wallace Hayes

*Toxicology Department, Rohm and Haas Company, Research Laboratories, Spring House, Pennsylvania 19477; and **R. J. Reynolds Industries, Inc., Bowman Gray Technical Center, Winston-Salem, North Carolina 27102*

The eye is an organ that can capture visible light energy and convert it into neurosignals which then are transmitted to the intricate central neuronetworks. Like other sensory neurosignals, light neurosignals are processed in the central nervous system where appropriate motor responses are generated. The ability to transform light into neuroimages (vision) marks a great step in evolution of the animal kingdom, especially in higher primates that have developed an even more complex ability to perceive their external environment via color vision.

There are three basic components of vision: the optics, the photoreceptors, and the conducting nerves. All three components must function properly to form a clear and sharp neuroimage in the visual cortex. The optics of the eye (cornea, aqueous humor, iris, lens, and vitreous humor) must remain transparent and be able to refract and focus light on the right position on the photoreceptors. The photoreceptors (the cones and rods) of the retina must be able to undergo photolysis and convert light energy into neuropotential impulses. The optic nerves must be able to carry these neuroimpulses to the visual cortex.

Because the eye is constantly exposed to the external environment, its cornea must be protected from drying, dust, and microorganisms. The eyelids, the lacrimal system, and the somatosensory response of the cornea all work together to protect this outermost structure of the eye. Like other organs, the major portion of the eye is nourished by blood vessels. The retinal, circumcorneal, and uveal vessels also nourish and help maintain the eye. These vessels are so arranged and constructed that they normally do not alter the transparency of the ocular optics. Nutrients reach the transport tissues of the eye via tears, the aqueous humor, and vitreous fluids.

Normal ocular functions are in delicate balance and are interdependent. Any traumatic insult—chemical or physical—can upset one or many of these ocular functions, thus creating a disturbance in vision. Depending on the extent of the traumatic injury (ranging from drying of the tear film to corneal ulceration or optic nerve damage), partial or complete loss of vision can result. Besides ocular injury resulting from accidental physical trauma and radiation, chemically induced ocular damage is a concern in modern society.

Chemicals can cause ocular damage locally by accidental exposure to the eye, or systemically by ingestion of chemicals such as contaminants, dietary chemical residues, and drugs. Because many chemicals can produce ocular damage either locally or systemically (51,62,93,115), it is important for industries to take responsibility in testing their products for ocular effects before exposing workers during manufacturing and, ultimately, before subjecting consumers to products on the market.

Conducting ocular tests in humans is generally impractical and is often considered unethical. Consequently, many methods and techniques have been developed over the years for testing ocular effects in animals. This chapter is intended to provide a survey of current methods and techniques for assessing chemically induced ocular toxicity in animals. (This survey is by no means complete and does not provide great detail or in-depth information; readers interested in experimental details should consult the references cited throughout.) It is the authors' intention for readers to benefit from this survey by understanding the basic principles, limitations, and some of the problems surrounding these animal testing methods.

THE DRAIZE TEST

The Draize test is a gross generalized irritation test (33) derived from the work of Friedenwald et al. (42). Its popularity arose from the fact that it is a simple, easy to conduct animal test that can identify most of the moderate to severe human eye irritants.

In the Draize test, a standard 0.1 ml or 0.1 g of a test substance is applied to the conjunctival sac of a rabbit's eye. The eyelid is held together for a few seconds and then released. The degree or extent of opacity of the cornea, the redness of the iris, and the chemosis and discharge on the conjunctiva are scored subjectively according to an arbitrary scale at preselected intervals after exposure. Scoring is based on the degree of the effects caused by the testing substance. More emphasis is placed on the opacity of the cornea, which has a maximum score of 80, whereas emphasis is progressively less with other effects: conjunctival changes (maximum score of 20) and iritis (maximum score of 10) (18,49,86).

The Draize test has become a subject of controversy among animal activist groups (61,117) and even among the scientific community (11,18,49,53,63,86, 112,120,139). This test has been widely criticized for its dose volume, use of animals as models, methods of exposure, irrigation, number of animals, observation and scoring including laboratory procedure variability, and interpretation of results, all of which will now be discussed in more detail.

Dose Volume

The maximal volume that the cul-de-sac of a rabbit's eye can hold is 30 to 50 µl (97), whereas the standard dose volume used in the Draize test is 0.1 ml, which is considered by many investigators as excessive. Hence, a smaller volume such as 0.01 ml or equivalent weight has been recommended (53,141). This recommended volume is not only justified on the basis of the 30 to 50 μl maximal volume the conjunctiva can hold, but it also allows better discrimination of the relative eye irritancy of different closely related materials. In addition, results of irritation from rabbits given the smaller dose volume correlated better with human exposure experience than when the larger dose volume was given: only one of 27 materials tested with the smaller dose volume was inconsistent with the human exposure experience, as compared with 10 of 27 of the same materials that were inconsistent when tested at the 0.1 ml dose volume (53).

Although a smaller dose volume appeared to be more appropriate in predicting human eye irritancy, understanding the dose-response of eye irritancy is just as important (104) for assessing the hazards of the substance. Unfortunately most of the regulatory guidelines still insist on testing eye irritancy under unreasonable maximal test conditions. Williams et al. (141) have pointed out that by reducing the volume of the test liquid, the eye irritation could be moderated, but the rank correlation of severity would not be affected.

Animal Models

For ethical and legal reasons, conducting ocular irritancy tests in humans is impractical; therefore, testing ocular irritancy in animals is currently the only practical model available. As in other toxicologic testing in animals, prime concerns of testing ocular irritancy in animals are similarity and predictability. Recognizing that there are anatomic, physiologic, and biochemical differences between human and animal eyes, researchers are confronted with the difficult task of selecting the appropriate animal model and suitable test conditions to identify potential human eye irritants. For example, the corneal thickness of dogs and rhesus monkeys is similar to that of humans (approximately 0.5 mm) (86,90,98), while rabbit corneal thickness is somewhat thinner (0.37 mm) (86). There is a lack of recognizable Bowman's membrane in rabbits, but they have a well-developed nictitating membrane (an additional target tissue), thick fur around the eye, loose eyelids susceptible to mild irritants, ineffective tear drainage system, and a poorly developed blinking mechanism (104). There are also species differences in biochemistry, e.g., variation in enzyme contents (80), and penetration rates of various substances (85).

Even though there are shortcomings and exceptions in predictability, the rabbit has been selected for most eye irritancy studies. There are some obvious advantages of choosing the rabbit: a wide data base, economy, availability, ease of handling, and large, unpigmented eyes suitable for various ophthalmologic examinations. With some exceptions (52,112), the rabbit eye is generally more sensitive to irritating materials than human or monkey eyes (8,19). Thus, there are built-in safety factors for making extrapolation and assessment of hazards to humans.

In addition to rabbits, dogs and primates are often used for ocular testing. Eye irritancy in primates generally is more closely correlated with the exposure experience in humans, although dogs are also suitable under certain circumstances (12). Because they are much more expensive and less available, dogs and primates are only used occasionally to assess eye irritancy, usually at the later developmental phase of a chemical.

Regardless of which animal is used, the investigator should always have a clear picture of the animal eye being observed. Background ocular findings, if not observed prior to exposure, sometimes can be falsely recorded as a chemically induced damage.

Methods of Exposure

Basically, there are two ways of applying a test substance to the eye: applying the test material into the cul-de-sac of the conjunctiva or applying it directly onto the cornea. The conjunctival exposure method has been adopted historically because of ease in application. It has also been perceived as being accurate in dosing. However, it has been our experience and that of others (12,53) that conjunctival exposure is inappropriate under many circumstances, especially when the test material is a solid powder. The possibility exists of having the test material trapped in the conjunctival sac, thus producing some undesirable mechanical effects and making the interpretation of the results more difficult. In addition, it has been our experience that when a considerable amount of even the standard 0.1 ml or 0.1 g dose is applied (especially as a solid powder), it either falls or is blinked from the eye once the animal's eyelid is released. These findings demonstrate that the claim that conjunctival dosing is more accurate is no longer valid. The corneal exposure method, on the other hand, mimics more closely the actual accidental exposure experienced in humans. When assessing the hazard of most chemical accidents, this method should be considered except when such chemicals are intended for pharmaceutical use (104). Applicators developed for the corneal exposure method have been used in some studies (8,19). A more uniform corneal lesion was observed, resulting in less observation variability (8). For a study as specific as corneal wound healing, a corneal applicator is recommended (102). However, for hazard assessment, it is desirable to apply the test substance directly onto the cornea while the lids of the test eye are gently held open; this action generally mimics the actual exposure more closely (53).

Compared with conjunctival exposure, the corneal method of exposure is just as convenient and reliable. Basically, a specific amount of test substance is measured in a piece of weighing paper or in a disposable syringe. The animal is restrained and the eyelid is held open while the entire amount of the test substance is placed onto the cornea carefully so that the cornea is not accidentally touched. The lid is held open for a few seconds, then released. It is essential that the entire cornea be covered by the test substance, although some may fall or be blinked out.

Irrigation

Washing the eye is a topical emergency measure after accidental exposure to chemical substances. In experimental studies, the treated eye is usually irrigated

20 to 30 sec after exposure to the test substance. Water is rapidly but gently squeezed from a plastic bottle to produce a constant gentle stream of water irrigating the entire treated eye. Irrigation generally lasts for 1 min.

The effect of irrigation on the interpretation of test results has been the subject of many studies (8,10,12,14,28,41,52,54,107,124). While irrigation of the treated eye right after exposure can prevent or minimize eye irritation in rabbits, the effectiveness of irrigation is dependent on the chemical, the concentration, the time lag between exposure and initiation of the irrigation, and the volume of irrigation. Early washing (less than 1 min) is generally recommended to reduce irritation (28,41,54,124), but in some cases increased irritation has been observed after irrigation with water (45,124). In other cases, ocular damage was almost instantaneous if irrigation did not begin after just a few seconds (8).

Number of Animals

It is generally true in experimental studies that the larger the group size the more accurate the test results. However, economic considerations are important factors in determining the number of animals used in a test group. The number of animals tested in a study should be determined by a balance between economic considerations and reliability of test results.

For eye irritation studies, a group size of 9 rabbits was recommended in the original Draize test, and group sizes of at least 6, 3, 3, and 4 rabbits have been recommended by the Federal Hazards Substances Act (FHSA), Interagency Regulatory Liaison Group (IRLG), Organization for Economic Cooperation and Development (OECD), and National Academy of Sciences (NAS) Committees, respectively. The relationships of variability, classification, and group size are addressed throughout the literature (10,54,140). With a larger group size, a smaller variability in results has been noted (140), whereas with decreased group size, lesser differentiation of irritancy has been suggested (10). Recognizing these facts, Guillot et al. (54) suggested a compromised approach, and with 3 rabbits in an initial study, there was a 96% chance that a positive or negative eye irritation result would be obtained.

Nevertheless, 6 rabbits have been routinely used in many laboratories to discriminate the degree of irritancy. Although greater accuracy could be achieved with more than 6 rabbits, this number appears to be sufficient for most practical purposes. If doubt exists about the test results from the 6 animals, the test should be repeated with an additional 6 rabbits.

Observation and Scoring

Reversibility and severity of eye irritancy are the two major remaining criteria used in the Draize test. Reversibility refers to the time needed for all ocular effects to disappear and for the eye to return to its normal state. To determine this reference time, treated eyes are examined periodically at 24-hr intervals, on day 7 after exposure, or at longer intervals if needed to establish reversibility (33). The observation period varies for different guidelines. For example, 24-, 48-, and 72-hr time spans are used in FHSA (40); 1-, 24-, 48-, and 72-hr, and, if needed, extended observations in OECD; and 1, 3, 7, 14, and 21 days in NAS (publication 1138) (104). In our opinion, the observation period should be flexible so that one can confidently assess the persistence of ocular effects and fully characterize the degree of involvement, since the onset and healing of ocular effects often are unpredictable (52).

The assessment of severity of different ocular effects is subjective. This subjective evaluation is the major source of error for intra- and interlaboratory variation (139). Therefore, to minimize at least the intralaboratory variability in scoring, uniformity in scoring techniques must exist among investigators regardless of which scoring system is followed. Pictorial references such as those prepared by the FDA (39) and some descriptive guides can be extremely helpful. Proper controls, both negative and positive, are also essential.

The types of ocular effects evaluated in the Draize test involve those on the cornea, iris, nictitating membrane, and conjunctiva. A grading system was originally proposed by Draize et al. (33), and subsequently a number of modifications were proposed (39,104). Basically, the intensity and area of involvement on the cornea are graded separately on a 0 to 4 scale. The sum of the two scores is multiplied by 5 to obtain a weighted corneal score. The congestion, swelling, circumcorneal injection, hemorrhage, and iridal failure of reactions to light are graded collectively on a scale of 0 to 2, and the score is multiplied by 5 to obtain a weighted iridal score. The redness, chemosis, and discharge of the conjunctivae are graded on a scale of 0 to 3, 0 to 4, and 0 to 3, respectively. The sum of the conjunctival scores is then multiplied by 5 to obtain a weighted conjunctival score. Other lesions are also recorded, such as pannus (corneal neovascularization), phlyctena, and rupture of the eyeball. Various aids are used at times to facilitate or increase the resolution power of the observation. These aids include fluorescein staining and ophthalmoscopic or slit lamp microscopic examinations (described later in this chapter). Other scoring systems have been proposed for lacrimation, blephamitis, chemosis, injection of conjunctival blood vessels, iritis, kerectasis, and corneal neovascularization (6).

Interpretation of Results

There are essentially four levels of data, generated from the Draize test, to be considered when interpreting results of ocular testing: what kind of ocular effects, their severity, their reversibility, and their rate of incidence. Weighting the scores in the original Draize test has, to some extent, taken the first level into consideration, yet it biases toward the cornea—one of the most critical ocular tissues. Severity is measured according to a graded scoring system, while reversibility is expressed as the time needed for the affected ocular tissues to return to their normal state. Incidence is the number of animals showing some kind of ocular effects during the study. Interpretation of such data is a multiple and factorial undertaking. All four levels of data are somewhat interrelated with each other.

Interpretation of eye irritation was not considered as the major contributing factor to interlaboratory variability (139). This is not surprising so long as everyone adheres to the same interpretation criteria; but the question is, what are the appropriate criteria for interpreting eye irritation results that would have an impact on placing eye irritants into different categories.

Many classification systems for eye irritants have been proposed. Some have been published (40,52,54,75,104), and yet there are many others in addition that have been used in individual laboratories. There is practically no disagreement on how test substances should be classified when no irritation is observed or if persistent severe irritation is seen; the classification of irritancy in between these two extremes is very subjective and unavoidably opinionated. Depending on how the data are evaluated, different conclusions can be reached.

Because of the complexity of eye irritancy data and their interdependence, some investigators chose to simplify the interpretation to a positive or negative approach. For example, in the FHSA guideline (40), if 4 or more of 6 test rabbits showing ocular effects within 72 hr after a conjunctival sac exposure (0.1 ml or 100 ml of the test material), the test material is considered a positive eye irritant. The ocular effects in consideration are "ulceration of the cornea (other than a fine stippling), corneal opacity (other than a slight deepening of the normal luster), inflammation of the iris (other than deepening of folds), an obvious swelling with partial eversion of the lids, or a diffuse crimson-red with individual vessels but not easily discernible" (40). If only 1 of the 6 tested animals shows the ocular effects within 72 hr, the test is considered negative. If 2 or 3 of the 6 tested animals show the ocular effects, the test should be repeated. The test substance is considered a positive irritant if 3 or more animals show ocular effects in the repeated test; otherwise, the test is repeated another time. Any positive ocular effect observed in the third test automatically classifies the test substance as an irritant.

A similar approach has been adopted in the IRLG guideline (71), but in it an option is given to declare a test positive when 2 or 3 of 6 rabbits tested show a positive ocular effect and the test is not repeated. This pass or fail interpretation is too simplistic, however, and no consideration is given to separate eye irritants, especially those that fall between the two extreme irritancy categories (from nonirritating to severely irritating).

Green et al. (52) used a different approach. Eye irritancy was classified into four easily recognizable categories based on the most severe responder in a group:

Nonirritation: Exposure of the eye to the material under the specified conditions causes no significant ocular changes. No tissue staining with fluorescein was observed. Any changes that did occur cleared within 24 hr and were no greater than those caused by normal saline under the same conditions.

Irritation: Exposure of the eye to the material under the specified conditions causes minor, superficial, and transient changes of the cornea, iris, or conjunctiva as determined by external or slit lamp examination with fluorescein staining. The appearance at any grading interval of any of the following changes was sufficient to characterize a response as an irritation: opacity of the cornea (other than a slight dulling of the normal luster), hyperemia of the iris, or swelling of the conjunctiva. Any changes that were seen cleared within 7 days.

Harmfulness: Exposure of the eye to the material under specified conditions causes significant injury to the eye, such as loss of the corneal epithelium, corneal opacity, iritis (other than a slight infection), conjunctivitis, pannus, or bullae. The effects healed or cleared within 21 days.

Corrosion: Exposure of the eye to the material under specified conditions results in the types of injury described in the previous category and also results in significant tissue destruction (necrosis) or injuries that adversely affect the visual process. Injuries persisted for 21 days or more.

The classification system has taken into consideration the kinds of ocular effects, the reversibility, and, to a certain extent, the qualitative severity, but not the incidence. The committee that revised NAS publication 1138 (104) put forward a system of classification similar to that of Green et al. (52). The categories are named differently: inconsequential or complete lack of irritation, moderate irritation, substantial irritation, and severe or corrosive irritation. The classification also is based on the most severe responder, and incidence is not considered. A provision for repeating the test is given as an option to increase the confidence level in making a judgment in some borderline cases. This eye irritancy classification system has been widely adopted in many laboratories.

One shortcoming of the NAS system is too wide a spectrum of moderate irritancy, which may sometimes lead to desensitization to the cautionary term "moderate." In order to fill the gap between the inconsequential or nonirritating and the moderate irritation categories, we have modified the classification system, taking into consideration the relative importance of ocular effects for visual function (Table 1). Basically, the conjunctival effect is deemphasized and the nature of ocular effects is also further qualified in our system. A slight irritation category is introduced to bridge the gap between inconsequential and moderate irritations. To be qualified for the "slight" category, the observed ocular effects must be conjunctival and all must disappear within a 72-hr period. Interpretation of neovascularization often proves to be frustrating. Neovascularization is generally considered part of the corneal healing process, but under some circumstances can interfere with the normal visual function by changing the transparency or hydration of the cornea. Recognizing this fact, we set up strict criteria for the interpretation of blood vessels seen on the cornea. Neovascularization is considered a corneal ocular effect, with some exceptions. Such exceptions are made because small vessels less than or equal to 1 mm in length, or a single vessel greater than 1 mm, are not considered to affect vision significantly (L. Rubin, *private communication*). Our system also is based on the most severe responder, but as in the original NAS classification, the test can be repeated to increase confidence. In some borderline cases, judgments have to be made based on the investigator's expertise.

TABLE 1. *Classification of eye irritancy (modified from Revised NAS Publication 1138, ref. 104)*

Eye irritancy classification	Criteria[a]
Inconsequential	No effect at 24 hr
Slight	Conjunctival effect only and reversible within 72 hr but not within 24 hr
Moderate	Corneal or iridal effects at 24 hr but not at 7 days; or conjunctival effects reversible within 7 days but not within 72 hr
Substantial	All effects reversible within 21 days but not within 7 days
Severe	Any effect present at 21 days or beyond
Corrosive	Grossly visible destruction of ocular tissue

[a]Additional Criteria:
A. Neovascularization is considered a corneal effect except for the following:
   1. Slight thickening ($\leqslant 1$ mm) of the limbus.
   2. Persistence of a few, distinct, and short ($\leqslant 1$ mm) blood vessels on the cornea.
   3. Persistence of one or two corneal trunk(s) of a blood vessel without a capillary bed.
B. Areas on the cornea stained by fluorescein should be considered in the classification of eye irritancy. The presence of stippled and stained areas on the cornea may be interpreted to indicate ulcerations of the cornea and is considered for classification. However, a few isolated, minute, nonuniform, and very faintly stained pinpoint spots on the cornea are not used for classification.

Griffith et al. (53) disagreed with using the most severe responder for classification of eye irritancy, claiming that there was no epidemiologic evidence to suggest that the most severe rabbit responder would correlate to the worst possible cases of human exposure experience. Instead, these investigators used the median time for recovery for classification according to the same temporal criteria as in the NAS system. The underlying logic is that the incidence of responders is being indirectly considered.

The classification systems of Green et al. (52), Griffith et al. (53), and NAS (104) apparently have not taken into account the severity of irritancy. Although there is a perception of a direct relationship between severity and reversibility, we have examined the data of Griffith et al. (53) and found that a direct correlation of median time to recovery and the severity of irritancy did occur (Table 2).

Kay and Colandra (75) proposed yet another rating system based on the Draize's scores, taking into account the extent and persistence of irritation and the overall consistency of the data. A similar system was proposed by Guillot et al. (54). Here, the greatest mean irritation score within an observation period is identified. On the basis of this score, the test substance is classified into six categories, ranging from nonirritating to maximum or extremely irritating. To maintain this initial rating, the data must also meet the arbitrary criteria for reversibility and frequency of occurrence, otherwise the rating is upgraded one category. The Kay and Colandra system has not been well verified for correlation to human exposure experience, nor has it been compared with other classification systems. Guillot et al. made an attempt to compare the rating with the OECD protocol. They claimed that one-third of the 56 materials tested could be classified into a lower category by the

TABLE 2. *Correlation of severity and reversibility of eye irritancy[a]*

Test substance	Dose volume (ml)	Mean irritation score ($\pm$ SD)	Median day to clear	Correlation coefficients
Hexane, 100%	0.01(9)[b]	0 $\pm$ 0	1	A. For 0.01 ml dose
	0.03	0 $\pm$ 0	1	volume = 0.9345
	0.10	0 $\pm$ 0	1	
Benzalkonium chloride,	0.01	0 $\pm$ 0	1	B. For 0.03 ml dose
0.1%	0.03	0 $\pm$ 0	1	volume = 0.81
	0.10	0 $\pm$ 0	1	
				C. For 0.10 ml dose
				volume = 0.93
Triethanolamine, 98%	0.01	0 $\pm$ 0	1	
	0.03	1 $\pm$ 1	1	
	0.10	4 $\pm$ 1	3	
Silver nitrate, 1%	0.01	2 $\pm$ 1	1	
	0.03	3 $\pm$ 1	3	
	0.10	12 $\pm$ 3	3	
Acetic acid, 3%	0.01[a]	4 $\pm$ 0	3	
	0.03	23 $\pm$ 4	7	
	0.10	36 $\pm$ 2	14	
Sodium hypochlorite,	0.01	11 $\pm$ 3	7	
5%	0.03	28 $\pm$ 3	18	
	0.10	31 $\pm$ 2	>21	
Sodium lauryl sulfate,	0.01[a]	25 $\pm$ 2	7	
10%	0.03	36 $\pm$ 1	7	
	0.10	40 $\pm$ 2	7	
Sodium lauryl sulfate,	0.01	35 $\pm$ 2	14	
29%	0.03	38 $\pm$ 2	>21	
	0.10	40 $\pm$ 2	>21	
Acetic acid, 10%	0.01	38 $\pm$ 2	>21	
	0.03	43 $\pm$ 2	>21	
	0.10	54 $\pm$ 2	>21	
Calcium hydroxide,	0.01	45 $\pm$ 6	>21	
10%	0.03	72 $\pm$ 8	c	
	0.10	90 (1)	c	
Formaldehyde, 38%	0.01	57 $\pm$ 4	c	
	0.03	56 $\pm$ 4	c	
	0.10	56 $\pm$ 5	c	

[a]Data from Griffith et al. (53).
[b]Mean sum of Draize's irritancy scores in a group of 6 animals (unless otherwise indicated in parentheses) 24 hr after exposure.
[c]Terminated before 21 days, but it was judged that the injury would not have cleared.

OECD protocol. Unfortunately, details have not been given as to how they reached such a conclusion. OECD guidelines do not specify a classification system, leaving the interpretation to the researcher. In our opinion, further studies are needed to verify such a classification system.

SPECIAL AIDS AND OPHTHALMOLOGIC TECHNIQUES

Draize's test, as stated previously, is a generalized gross test concentrating on the effects on the cornea, iris, and conjunctiva. Examination is usually performed by naked eye under a hand light. Accurate gross observations are limited by the experience and training of the investigator. Subtle ocular changes may be missed. If these subtle changes are to be detected and ambiguous gross observations resolved, or if internal tissues (e.g., the lens and the retina) are to be examined, the investigator must rely on special aids and techniques. Many such aids and techniques have been developed over the years, most of which are more objective than the gross examination itself. In the following sections, the basic principles and some practical considerations of some of these special aids and techniques are described.

The Uses of Fluorescein in the Assessment of Ocular Functions

Chemical and Biologic Properties

Fluorescein is a weak organic acid (Fig. 1) and is only slightly soluble in water, but its sodium salt is moderately soluble in water. It is very efficient in absorbing ultraviolet light and emitting fluorescent light. The maximum absorption is 490 μm (excitation) in the violet region and its maximum emission is 520 μm in the green region of the spectrum. Its un-ionized form is less fluorescent than its ionized form. At a pH of 7.4, fluorescein does not seem to bind to tissue and is also nontoxic in animals, making it an ideal marker for an ocular fluid dynamics study. Because fluorescein is a deeply colored and highly fluorescent chemical, it can be detected at very low concentrations in biologic tissues or fluid; however, its detection sensitivity is often limited by the background fluorescence of biologic tissues.

Because sodium fluorescein is a polar molecule, it does not readily traverse lipophilic membranes, but easily diffuses into any aqueous medium. For example, if ulceration occurs on the cornea, the lipophilic membrane barrier is broken down and the fluorescein is freely diffused through and is either dissolved or suspended in the aqueous medium of the stroma. More detailed information on the chemical and biologic properties of fluorescein is provided in two excellent reviews (88,100).

Uses in Assessment of Ocular Effects

Since its first use in studying the origin of aqueous humor secretion a century ago (38), fluorescein has become an important aid. It has been used as a marker in detecting obstructions in the nasolacrimal drainage systems, for studying changes in the flow dynamics of different ocular fluids, for demonstrating leakages of retinal vessels in angiography, for estimating permeability of the cornea and lens, and for identifying ulcerations on the cornea (88). These uses are discussed separately.

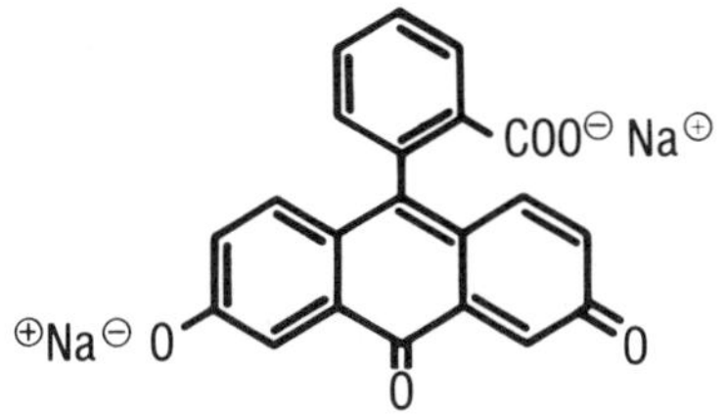

FIG. 1. Chemical structure of fluorescein as sodium salt.

Staining for Corneal Epithelial Damages

Fluorescein staining is one of the most important diagnostic aids for detecting changes that occur on the corneal epithelium (26,68). The corneal epithelium is a lipophilic barrier to sodium fluorescein, but such a barrier is broken when there is an ulceration or change in membrane structure. Some amount of fluorescein applied on the cornea will penetrate into the intercellular spaces of the stroma, which constitute a water-soluble layer of the stroma. When light is cast on the cornea, fluorescence is detected on the damaged area of the epithelium. Once the fluorescein enters the stroma, it will eventually pass through Descemet's membrane and the endothelium into the aqueous humor.

Fluorescein staining is usually accomplished either by solution or impregnated paper strips. Fluorescein solution is commercially available at several concentrations of 2, 1, or 0.25% sodium salt solutions. Preservatives are common in these commercially available solutions to minimize bacterial contamination (24). Usually a drop of the solution is instilled onto the eye and excessive fluorescein is flushed immediately with a sufficient amount of water. The eye can then be examined under a cobalt-filtered light for any epithelial defects.

Fluorescein is also available in impregnated paper strips (79). These strips are free of contamination and are easy to use. Moistened with collyria, a strip is lightly touched to the dorsal bulbar conjunctiva. The small amount of fluorescein should distribute uniformly on the cornea by either diffusion or blinking. Flushing is not usually necessary with the strips if applied properly. Nonetheless, if the strip touches the cornea, it then becomes necessary for the cornea to be flushed with water before examination. Better results are generally obtained with the fluorescein-impregnated strip when examination is by slit lamp microscopy.

Although fluorescein staining can detect very subtle corneal epithelial changes, one can be easily misled by some very noticeable background staining. Because of the delicacy of this examination, proper training and adequate experience are necessary for practitioners to reliably, reproducibly, and consistently benefit from using fluorescein staining. In general, it is not necessary to stain lesions that are obvious and grossly evident. It is when lesions would otherwise go grossly undetected that fluorescein staining is of value.

Nasolacrimal Apparatus Examination

The nasolateral apparatus, including secretory and excretory components, is extremely important for normal optical functions of the eye. The tear film can form an optically uniform layer over the microscopically irregular surface of the epithelial cells, and can continuously flush cellular debris or foreign bodies from the eye. The tear flow also lubricates the corneal surface from mechanical friction caused by blinking, provides nutrition to the cornea, and causes antibacterial activities by proteolytic enzymes and immunoglobulins.

Fluorescein can be used to assess both the secretory and excretory functions of the nasolacrimal system (72,94,143). The rate of tear formation can be estimated by measuring the dilution of an applied amount of fluorescein in the eye (143). The volume of tears formed within a period of time is proportional to the dilution in color of the dye. Appearance of fluorescein in the inferior nasal turbinate indicates normal excretory drainage of the lacrimal system, and can be monitored with a cotton-tipped applicator moistened with 1:1,000 epinephrine and 5% cocaine, applied 1 min after instillation of the dye and at subsequent intervals up to 5 min (72). Delay or absence of the dye appearance does not necessarily indicate a complete blockage. If the upper drainage system is normal, subsequent flushing of the eye with normal saline 5 min after dye instillation will force the dye through the upper drainage channel into the external nares (46).

Fluorescein sometimes is used in measuring tear film breakup time, an indirect method of estimating the secretion of mucin in the tear (94). This is done by instilling a drop of fluorescein solution into the conjunctival sac. The cornea is then scanned by a slit lamp microscope with cobalt blue illumination. The time at which the first sign of fluorescein-free area appears is the tear film breakup time. Normal breakup time is approximately 15 to 30 sec. A breakup time of less than 10 sec may indicate deficiency in secretion of mucin by the goblet cells. A normal amount of mucin, as a wetting agent for the tear, is important in maintaining the stability of a normal layering of tear film; that is, the outermost layer consists of an oily substance and is maintained to limit evaporation of the tear film.

Corneal Permeability

Fluorescein also has been used to study the permeabilty of the cornea (88,98,100). The changes in concentration of fluorescein are monitored with a specially designed fluorophotometer attached to a slit lamp microscope. This apparatus provides the exact location of the tissue where fluorescein concentration is measured with the fluorophotometer. Thus the transport of fluorescein across the cornea can be monitored quantitatively. The success of using such a procedure is greatly dependent on the sensitivity of the fluorophotometer. This method was used by Easty and Mathalone (34) to evaluate the ocular toxicity of 1,8,9-triacetoxyanthracene in rabbits. It is a more objective test for ocular injury.

Epithelial permeability

The integrity of the corneal epithelium sometimes can be evaluated by determining the permeability of various substances. Sodium fluorescein, for example, is an ideal marker because it has low toxicity to the cellular membrane, is moderately soluble in water, does not bind to tissue, and is highly fluorescent, allowing detection at very low concentrations. Epithelial permeability of fluorescein in humans was measured by monitoring fluorescein concentration in the anterior chamber. A permeability coefficient (transfer coefficient) of 1.5×10^{-5} cm/hr was obtained (88).

Endothelial permeability

The endothelium is perhaps the most metabolically active cellular layer of the cornea, and its integrity is vital for the maintenance of proper hydration of the cornea, which in turn affects the turgescence and transparency of the cornea. The proper water content in the cornea is maintained by passive processes and an active pump. The permeability of fluorescein at the endothelium, a layer of cells separating the cornea and aqueous humor, was first measured in rabbits by Mishima and Maurice (100). Ota et al. (108) described a more convenient and noninvasive technique by injecting fluorescein intravenously into the rabbit. The concentration in both cornea and aqueous humor was periodically determined with a slit lamp fluorophotometer. The basic transfer kinetics is described by the following equation (96):

$$\frac{dF_c}{dt} = k_{ac}(F_a - r_{ac} \cdot F_c)$$

where F_c is the concentration in the cornea (g/ml), F_a the concentration in the aqueous humor (g/ml), k_{ac} the transfer coefficient from the aqueous humor to the cornea, r_{ac} the steady state distribution of fluorescein between the aqueous humor and the cornea, i.e., F_a/F_c at a steady state, and

$$\text{permeability of the endothelium} = k_{ac} \frac{(V_c)}{(A)} = k_{ac} \cdot q$$

where V_c is the volume of the cornea, A the area of the cornea, and q the corneal thickness.

After some mathematical manipulations, the following linear function equation is obtained, assuming that r_{ac} and k_{ac} are constants:

$$\frac{\int_{t2}^{t_1} (F_a \, dt)}{\int_{t2}^{t_1} (F_c \, dt)} = r_{ac} + \frac{1}{k_{ac}} \frac{F_c(t_2 - t_1)}{\int_{t2}^{t_1} (F_c \, dt)}$$

where $\int_{t2}^{t_1} (F_a \, dt)$ and $\int_{t2}^{t_1} (F_c \, dt)$ are the areas under the curve (AUC) of the "fluorescein concentration versus time" curve in the aqueous humor and the cornea, respectively. AUC can be obtained by graphic integration. This graphic plotting of the ratio of AUC (aqueous humor)/AUC (cornea) versus the ratio of $(F_c t_2 - F_c t_1)/$ AUC (cornea) yields a straight line (linear):

$$\text{slope} = 1/k_{ac} \qquad \text{intercept} = r_{ac}$$

Thus, permeability of the endothelium is given by

$$\frac{1}{\text{slope}} \cdot q$$

The permeability of the endothelium can then be calculated if the corneal thickness q is known. Corneal thickness can be measured with a slit lamp microscope. Using this approach, Ito et al. (109) obtained a normal corneal transfer coefficient (k_{ac}) of 0.23 hr^{-1} for humans and 0.51 hr^{-1} for rabbits, and an average distribution ratio (r_{ac}) of 0.64 for humans and 0.61 for rabbits. When normal corneal thickness measurement was used, the calculated endothelial permeability coefficient was 3.0×10^{-6} cm/sec for humans and 5.1×10^{-6} cm/sec for rabbits. These values were very close to those determined by more complicated *in vitro* techniques (100,137).

Intraocular Pressure Measurement

Fluorescein is used in applanation tonometry (applanometry), a widely used method for determining intraocular pressure. The principle behind this method is rather simple. When a small flattened surface is applied on the cornea (applanation), there are four forces acting on the surface: (a) the application force (weights applied), (b) the surface tension force resulting from tear displacement on the cornea, (c) the resistance force opposing the applied weight, and (d) the deformation force of the cornea opposing the surface tension force. All four forces are in static balance at a circular applanation diameter of 3 to 4 mm. The applied force (weight) is equal to the resistance pressure times the area of the flattened surface, and the surface tension and deformation forces cancel each other. The resistance pressure is actually the intraocular pressure acting on the corneal surface. Therefore, if this balance point can be found by varying the applied force on a specific flattened surface area (e.g., 3.04 mm diameter on the plunger of an applanometer), the intraocular pressure can be calculated (applied weight divided by surface area) or obtained from a calibrated curve. For this principle to work, the surface must be flat and not indented. Fluorescein is used to ensure that when a specific area (e.g., 3 mm in diameter) of a flat object (the plunger) is applied with a specific weight (applied force), the resulting contact surface on the cornea is flat and not indented, and the flattened area on the cornea is exactly equal to the specific area.

The tear film on the cornea is stained with fluorescein. When the flat plunger is applied on the corneal surface, the stained tear film within the area is displaced. If the area is indeed flat, it will appear blue and be rimmed by the greenish fluorescein-stained tear film when the field is viewed under a blue light. For more discussion on various types of applanometers and their advantages or limitations, the reader is referred to Moses (101).

Angiography

Perhaps the most important clinical use of fluorescein is in angiography, a study of retinal circulation. Several excellent review articles on the use of fluorescein in angiography in animals have been published (13,48,56,60,109,116). This technique has been an essential diagnostic tool for diabetic retinopathy, inflammations, retinal detachments, hypertension, vascular anomalies, and neoplasm. In animals, fluorescein is injected rapidly in either the jugular, tail, or cephalic vein. The fundus then can be viewed by an ophthalmoscope or monitored by fundus photography with appropriate filters. Five to 15 seconds after injection, fluorescein appears on the fundus (64,105). Fluorescein will not enter the neurosensory retina under normal conditions because of the tight intercellular junctions between the retinal pigment epithelial cells, nor will it leak from retinal arteries, capillaries, or venules. However, fluorescein will leak into the retina if damage occurs.

According to the sequence of appearance of fluorescein in the fundus after injection, the angiogram is divided into the following phases: choroidal (usually masked by tapetal autofluorescence in some species), the retinal anteriolar, capillary, venular, and recirculation. The bright and faint images of the vessels closely follow the antomic arrangement. These phases are usually followed by series photography with an auto advance camera. The intensity of the fluorescent images will reflect the status of ocular vasculature. Hyperfluorescence may be related to specific leakages in the retinal vasculature, retinal pigment epithelial defects, or blood vessel abnormalities, such as retinal tortuosity, dilatation, neovascularization, aneurysms, telangiectasis, shunts, subretinal neovascularization, and tumors. Hypofluorescence may be related to blockage, hemorrhage, exudates, transudates, edema, retinal degeneration, or vascular occlusion (109).

Direct Ophthalmoscopy

The ophthalmoscope was developed over a century ago mainly for examaining the fundus. The principle is simple. A real, inverted, and smaller image of an external object is usually formed on the fundus by the optics of the eye. On the other hand, if the fundus is illuminated, the optics of the eye can help to form an image of the fundus. With intervening lenses of the ophthalmoscope, the images of the fundus can be focused and reviewed by an observer. A direct ophthalmoscope thus consists of a light source, a mirror or prism to reflect the light to illuminate the fundus, and a viewing hole with a series of different strengths (diopter) of convex and concave lenses to focus the reflected and magnified images of the fundus. With some other attachments such as red-free (green) filter, grid, and slit, specific conditions of the fundus such as hemorrhage, size of lesion, and elevated depression of a lesion can be detected. For example, with a slit option, a depressed lesion can be detected if it is focused with a 5-diopter lens and the retina is in focus at 0 diopters. More detailed descriptions of the use of the direct ophthalmoscope are available (7,20,50).

Indirect Ophthalmoscopy

Indirect and direct ophthalmoscopy are fairly similar techniques. One difference with indirect ophthalmoscopy is that it uses high diopter corrective lenses (usually as a hand condensing lens) between the observing biomicroscope (binocular) and the observed eye. The fundus images formed by the condensing lens are inverted, real, and can be seen on an opaque film held at the focal plane of the lens. While the image is smaller than that seen in direct ophthalmoscopy, the field view is larger, making it easier to detect some important gross lesions such as tumors. In addition, the light source is brighter, making it possible to traverse even some relatively translucent media. The eyepiece on this ophthalmoscope is binoculars with prisms that can split the reflected light so that it is easier and more convenient to manipulate the examination. The distance between the examiner and the eyes to be examined is longer, making it safer to examine some animals. More detailed descriptions of indirect ophthalmoscopy are available (118,135).

Slit Lamp Biomicroscopy

The slit lamp biomicroscope is a very important instrument for studying many ocular tissues, especially the cornea. As its name suggests, a slit lamp biomicroscope consists of a microscope that views optical sections of different layers of the cornea made by an intense light beam acting as a surgical knife or microtome. Thus, many grossly undetected lesions can be observed with the slit lamp biomicroscope. Newer models of slit lamp microscopes not only can observe the different layers of the cornea, but they can also examine other transparent parts of the eye such as the aqueous humor, lens, and vitreous body.

The illuminating components and the microscope itself are both movable and adjustable so that the eye can be illuminated and observed at different angles with different width and height adjustments of the slit light beam. The incidence of light beam and the microscope can be aligned and focused at the same point on the cornea, thus simultaneously illuminating and magnifying the area being examined. The light beam also can be directed at the area in different fashions, providing different views of the same area.

Basically, there are two types of slit images used for illumination: parallelepiped and optical section (92). For parallelepiped slit image, a rectangular light beam (approximately 1–2 mm wide and 5–10 mm high) is projected on the cornea. The shape of the illuminated area is similar to a parallelepiped prism where outer and inner surfaces are curved because of the curvature of the cornea. For optical section slit image, the width (20 μm) of the light beam is narrowed to its minimum and is projected onto the cornea, providing a sagittal view similar to a thin histologic section.

There are seven basic types of illumination techiques (Fig. 2): diffuse illumination, sclerotic scatter, direct and focal illumination, direct and indirect retroillumination, and specular reflection (92,128).

Diffuse Illumination

In diffuse illumination, a slightly out-of-focus wide beam is used to scan and localize any gross lesions of a large area of the eye. It is usually the first step in examining the eye under a microscope for gross lesions and their extent of change. This technique is similar to observing the eye with a hand light, except that the observation is made under the microscope (Fig. 2a).

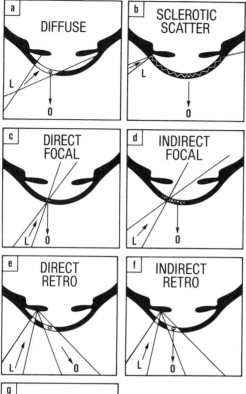

FIG. 2. Seven basic methods of illumination in slit lamp microscopy: **(a)** diffuse illumination; **(b)** sclerotic scatter; **(c)** direct focal
illumination; **(d)** indirect focal illumination; **(e)** direct retroillumination; **(f)** indirect retroillumination; and **(g)** specular reflection. O,
observer; L, illuminator light. (Modified from ref. 128, with permission.)

Sclerotic Scatter Illumination

In sclerotic scatter illumination (Fig. 2b), a narrow light beam is directed at the
temporal limbus, and the microscope is focused centrally at the cornea on the area
to be examined. The light reflected from the sclera will transmit within the cornea
by total reflection. Under normal conditions nothing will be seen, but if only minor
changes are present the reflected light will be obstructed and the damaged area
(e.g., mild corneal edema) will be illuminated. This techique is useful in detecting
minimal changes in the cornea.

Direct Focal Illumination

In direct focal illumination, the light beam and the microscope are sharply
focused at the same point of interest in the same plane (Fig. 2c). If a rectangular

slit image is used for illumination and focused on the cornea, three general areas are seen when the parallelepiped is formed on the cornea: the epithelium (the anterior bright line), the stroma (the central clear marble-like area), and the endothelium (the posterior thin bright line). If an optical section slit image is used for illumination, the corneal layers seen from anterior to posterior are a thin bright layer, a thin dark layer, a granular layer, and another thin bright layer. These correspond to the tear film, the epithelium, the stroma, and the endothelium, respectively. Altering the angle of incidence of the light beam decreases or increases the reflections. This allows for the detection of the lesion depth. Opacities on the different layers can be easily detected as obstruction of the incident light beam.

Indirect Focal Illumination

Indirect focal illumination (Fig. 2d) is done by a narrow beam of light directed at an opaque area of the cornea. Changes in, for example, blood vessels at the cornea adjacent to the opaque area are illuminated and can be detected by focusing the microscope at these areas.

Retroillumination

In direct (Fig 2e) and indirect (Fig. 2f) retroillumination, the light beam is directed at some tissues behind the cornea, e.g., the iris or the fundus. The reflection light illuminates the area of interest of the corneal tissue and can be focused under the microscope. The microscope can be directly located on the path of the reflection light (direct retroillumination), thus permitting subtle changes to be observed against a contrasting background. Any optical obstruction by lesions such as scars, pigment, or vessels located along the reflection light path will appear as darker areas on a brighter background. Lesions such as corneal edema and precipitates that can scatter the reflection light will show up as a brighter area against a darker background. When the microscope is located off the reflection light path (indirect retroillumination), the corneal structure is observed against a dark background such as the pupil or iris. Indirect retroillumination is better for observing opaque structures, whereas direct illumination is often used to detect corneal edema and precipitates.

Specular Reflection Illumination

Specular reflection (Fig. 2g) is the most difficult of the illumination techniques, but it is the most useful in studying the endothelium and precorneal tear film. This technique makes use of the difference in refractive properties between the corneal surface and the adjacent medium of the posterior and anterior surfaces of the cornea. The microscope is focused on the cornea adjacent to the incident slit light beam path. By alternating the angle of incidence, a point can be reached such that a total reflection is obtained on the junction between the aqueous medium and the most posterior corneal surface, thus illuminating endothelial cell patterns and Descemet's membrane. Similar techniques can be performed on the anterior corneal surface to visualize precorneal tear film.

By using the slit lamp, microscopic techniques can reveal many subtle changes that could not otherwise be observed in the Draize test. A different scoring system must be developed to reflect such subtle changes. Baldwin et al. (3) proposed a scoring system for the cornea, anterior chamber, iris, and lens. Subsequently the NAS committee (104) developed a scoring system for slit-lamp examinations similar to the Draize system, placing emphasis on the cornea, iris, and conjunctiva. Basically, in the NAS system the intensity and the area involved are the two main criteria for scoring. Using such a scoring system, the investigator must have a clear mental picture of a normal eye. Like the Draize score, the NAS system is also based on corneal effects; total maximal corneal score is 20 as compared with 11 and 15 for the iridal and conjunctival scores. A detailed scoring scale and criteria are listed in Table 3.

Local Anesthetics

Primarily for humane reasons, some guidelines such as those of IRLG and OECD provide options for using local anesthetics in eye irritation studies. Tetracaine, lidocaine, butacaine, proparacaine, and cocaine have all been tested for their interaction with eye irritation. Results seem to be mixed and inconclusive (Table 4). While most of these anesthetics can alleviate pain, they can also inhibit or reduce the somatosensory area of the eye and the blinking reflex. Tear flow is also reduced causing the test substance to be trapped and remain undiluted on the cornea instead of being blinked from the eye or diluted and flushed away by the tear flow. The blinking and tearing reflexes are important defense mechanisms, especially among higher primates, upon accidental exposure to any test substance (63). Some local anesthetics also can cause delay in corneal epithelial regeneration and loss of surface cells from the cornea (55). However, at least one study has shown that a 0.5% tetracaine solution apparently had no effect on corneal healing (110). Further research is needed to reveal the interaction of local anesthetics and chemically induced ocular effects. Local anesthesia is sometimes useful to induce akinesia of the eyelid during eye examination.

PHYSIOCHEMICAL APPROACHES IN THE ASSESSMENT OF OCULAR TOXICITY

Many physiologic and biochemical parameters are often indicative of the functional status of the cornea. Because these physiobiochemical parameters can be quantitatively measured, such an approach to the assessment of ocular toxicity is more objective and thus more reproducible. Changes in these parameters take place much earlier than does the appearance of gross lesions. Therefore, mild eye irritants that may go undetected by gross observation or even microscopic examination can be identified.

Examination of the Tear Film

Proper tear formation and drainage as well as the stability of the precorneal tear film are important for a normal precorneal optical surface, lubrication, nutrition

TABLE 3. *Scoring criteria for ocular effects observed in slit lamp microscopy*

Location of observations	Grades
Corneal observations	
Intensity	
Only epithelial edema (with only slight stromal edema or without stromal edema)	1
Corneal thickness 1.5 × normal	2
Corneal thickness 2 × normal	3
Cornea entirely opaque so that corneal thickness cannot be determined	4
Area involved	
≤25% of total corneal surface	1
>25% but ≤50%	2
>50% but ≤75%	3
>75%	4
Fluorescein staining	1
≤25% of total corneal surface	1
>25% but ≤50%	2
>50% but ≤75%	3
>75%	4
Neovascularization and pigment migration	
≤25% of total corneal surface	1
>25% but ≤50%	2
>50% but ≤75%	3
>75%	4
Perforation	4
Maximal corneal score	20
Iridal observations	
Iritis is quantitated by the cells and flare in the anterior chamber, iris, hyperemia, and capillary light reflex	
Cells in aqueous chamber	
A few	1
A moderate number	2
Many	3
Aqueous flare (Tyndall effect)	
Slight	1
Moderate	2
Marked	3
Iris hyperemia	
Slight	1
Moderate	2
Marked	3
Pupillary reflex	
Sluggish	1
Absent	2
Total maximal iridal score	11
Conjunctival observations	
Hyperemia	
Slight	1
Moderate	2
Marked	3
Chemosis	
Slight	1
Moderate	2
Marked	3
Fluorescein staining	
Slight	1
Moderate	2
Marked	3
Ulceration	
Slight	1
Moderate	2
Marked	3

TABLE 4. *Effect of local anesthetics on eye irritancy studies*

Local anesthetics	Animal	Effects	Reference
Butacaine sulfate	Rabbits	Higher corneal opacity score in anesthetized eyes exposed to 10% acetic acid or ammonia, relative to unanesthetized eye	134
		Higher corneal water content in anesthetized eyes exposed to 5% acetic acid or 1% ammonia	134
Proparacaine (0.5%)	Rabbits	Intensity of ocular effects increased but no prolonged effect	63
	Monkeys	Increased the severity of ocular effects and prolonged their duration	63
Butacaine sulfate Larocaine hydrochloride Cocaine hydrochloride Tetracaine hydrochloride Phenacaine hydrochloride (repeated doses)	Guinea pigs	Healing inhibition on mechanical abrasion of the cornea was dependent on the type, concentration, and toxicity of the local anesthetics; 0.5% tetracaine and 1.0% phenacaine hydrochloride solution had the least effect on corneal epithelial regeneration	55
Proparacaine (0.5%) Tetracaine (0.5%) (single dose)	Rabbits	No effects on the cornea were observed by scanning electron microscopy	110
Cocaine (4.0%)	Rabbits	Loss of epithelial cells and plasma membrane injury were observed by scanning electron microscopy	110

for the cornea, removal of bacteria and debris from the cornea, and antibacterial activity on the cornea. Reduction of tear formation or increase in the stability of the tear film layers can often lead to a dry eye, mechanical friction, irritation, or infection. The use of fluorescein to evaluate the nasolacrimal system and the tear film breakup time has been described in previous sections.

Reduction or total lack of tear formation is often measured by the Schirmer's tear test (122). The rate of tear formation is measured by the amount of wetting on a filter paper inserted in the lower conjunctival fornix at the outer half of the palpebral fissure. A standard Schirmer's test kit was developed for clinical use in 1961, consisting of strips of 0.5×35-mm Whatman No. 41 filter paper with a 55-mm folder over at one end (57). The wetting of the exposed portion of the paper strip over a period of time (1 to 4 min) is a measure of the rate of tear secretion. Basic secretion can be estimated by using a local anesthetic to eliminate secretion due to reflex stimuli. The Schirmer II test can be used to examine the integrity of reflex secretion. This test measures tear formation under stimulation of the nasal mucosa with an irritant such as ammonia, a wisp of cotton, and other mechanical means. The Schirmer II test has been used in many animal studies

(47,59,113,114,119). In dogs, normal wetting ranges from 10 to 25 mm/min, and a value of 5 mm/min is considered abnormal.

Assessment of Corneal Function

The cornea is a powerful refractive biologic optic. Its refractive power is dependent on its being transparent and in proper hydration. Maintenance of proper transparency and hydration is dependent on many mechanisms, for example, proper tear flow, absence of deposits and blood vessels, proper arrangement of collagen fibrils, unimpaired nutritional supply for metabolic active pump [(Na$^+$-K$^+$) pump], and proper intraocular pressure. Decreased transparency or hydration can be a result of corneal scars (decreased corneal thickness) or corneal edema (increased corneal thickness). Corneal edema can be caused by epithelial damage, endothelial damage, increased intraocular pressure, lack of oxygen, or inhibition of the electrolyte balance pump [(Na$^+$-K$^+$)-activated ATPase], which is located mainly in the endothelial membrane but is also found in the epithelium. All these physiologic parameters are potentially useful for the evaluation of corneal damages.

Corneal Curvature

Changes in the curvature of the corneal surface will affect refraction and image formation by the optics of the eye, since curvature is related to the hydration of the cornea. The normal curvature radius of the anterior surface centrally is about 7.8 mm. A shorter radius may indicate myopia and keratosis.

The value of curvature is needed for estimating corneal thickness (95,98). Corneal curvature is usually measured by keratometer or ophthalmometer (128). The surface of the cornea is similar to a convex mirror. An object in front of a convex mirror will form a visual (unreal) image. When the distance and the size of the object are known, the size of the virtual image is proportional to the radius of the corneal curvature. The image is seen by the keratometer and its size can be measured by the instrument; thus, when calibrated, the radius of corneal curvature can be read directly from the instrument. By knowing the radius of corneal curvature, the refractive power of the cornea can be calculated by the following equation:

$$D = \frac{n - 1}{r}$$

where D is the refractive power of the cornea, r the radius of curvature, and n the index of refraction.

Corneal Thickness

The corneal thickness is very sensitive to many factors that affect the hydration and transparency of the cornea. It is thus a very sensitive endpoint to assess the integrity of the cornea. Changes in corneal thickness have been used by many researchers to assess chemically induced corneal damages (22,23,27,34,138). Burton (22) noted that corneal swelling, expressed as the corneal thickness determined before and after treatment, correlated well with corneal opacity and the total corneal Draize's scores; persistence of corneal damage also correlated with corneal swelling for 4 days. Conquet et al. (27) found good correlation between corneal thickness and the Draize's corneal scores at 2 and 24 hr, but poor correlation at 3, 7, and 11 days. Maximal response in corneal thickness was seen earlier than maximal Draize's scores (138).

Optical methods for measuring corneal thickness have been reviewed comprehensively by Mishima (95). All modern methods use image-doubling devices of various types attached to a slit lamp microscope. Of all the optical methods used for measuring corneal thickness, two have been recommended (95): the Maurice-Giardini method (90) and the newer Haag-Streit pachometer method (98).

Maurice–Giardini method

The principle of this method (Fig. 3) is similar to that of the first optical method of Von Bahr (136). The single plexiglas plate with a central aperture covered by a blue filter is placed in front of a bright slit lamp light beam. The slit lamp light

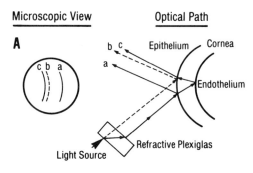

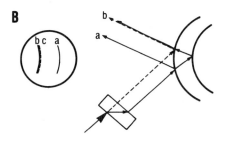

FIG. 3. Optical principle of Maurice and Giardini. Methods for measuring corneal thickness (98). **A:** Displaced (——) and nondisplaced (----) light beams reflected from the endothelium and epithelium surface, respectively. **B:** Displaced (——) and nondisplaced (----) light beams reflected from the epithelium and endothelium surface are in alignment.

beam and the observing microscope are set at a 60° angle. Part of the slit lamp beam passes through the aperture without displacement and is focused on the epithelial surface and reflects to the observing microscope. The other part of the slit lamp light beam passes through the plexiglas, becomes displaced, and is then refracted to focus on the endothelial surface. A portion of this displaced light beam is also reflected by the epithelial surface. With the proper amount of displacement by rotating the plexiglas, the displaced beam reflected from the endothelium is brought in alignment with the undisplaced beam reflected from the epithelial surface. The rotation angle is dependent on the curvature, the thickness, and the refractive index of the cornea. Thus, by knowing the angle of rotation of the plexiglas, the corneal thickness can be directly obtained from a calibrated curve which is obtained by using glass rods of known thickness and with the same curvature and refractive index as those of the cornea. The corneal thickness can then be obtained from a standard calibrated curve.

Haag-Streit pachometer

The Haag-Streit pachometer has been the most popular optical method for measuring corneal thickness. The principle is illustrated in Fig. 4. A narrow slit lamp light beam is cast on the cornea, creating a vertical optical section. The optical section is observed with only one microscope (the right objective lens) at a 40° angle. The apparent corneal thickness can be measured by the split image optical principle. This method differs from the Maurice–Giardini method in that a refractive glass is used to displace both the endothelial and the epithelial reflected light beams. Two glass plates are placed in front of the objective lens of the microscope. One plate is fixed and covers the lower half of the objective lens, and

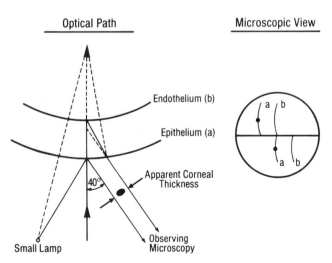

FIG. 4. Optical principle of Haag-Streit pachometer. (Modified from Mishima and Hedbys, ref. 98, with permission.)

the other plate is rotatable and covers the upper half of the objective lens. A split image eyepiece with a prism divides the visual field into upper and lower halves. Therefore, images of the optical section of the corneal layers are formed on both the lower and upper visual fields. When the upper glass is rotated, the light beam is displaced through the upper glass plate. With proper rotation of the upper glass plate, the image of endothelial surface on the upper visual field is displaced to align with the image of the lower fixed visual field. The displacement (rotation) is related to the apparent (under the microscope) corneal thickness. The actual corneal thickness can be calculated from the angle of rotation, the refractive index of the glass plate and the cornea, and the curvature of the cornea, or it can be read directly from the scale on the instrument. The actual corneal thickness is not linearly related to the rotation of the glass plate; thus, a correction has to be made to obtain the actual corneal thickness. Correction tables are available for most of the pachometers.

In this method, the slit lamp beam must be perpendicular to the cornea. To ensure the exact vertical positioning of the slit lamp beam on the corneal surface, two small lights are placed at the same distance from the slit lamp as from the microscope to the slit lamp. If the slit lamp beam is perpendicular to the surface, the images of the two small lights should be seen on the epithelium on both the upper and lower fields.

Intraocular Pressure

Increased intraocular pressure can cause stromal edema and an increase in corneal thickness. Increased pressure in the aqueous and vitreous humor is usually a result of (a) obstruction or stenosis of aqueous outflow channel of the ocular chambers, (b) increased production of the aqueous from ciliary capillary, or (c) possibly increased protein and other solute in the aqueous humor. Prolonged increases in ocular pressure can cause damage to the corneal endothelium as well as to the retina and other ocular tissues.

The relationship of ocular pressure and chemically induced eye irritation has not been fully investigated. Nonetheless, some correlation was reported between an increase in ocular pressure and gross eye irritation produced by 10% sodium lauryl sulfate in rabbit eyes anesthetized with 0.5% proparacaine (63). The intraocular pressure was measured with a calibrated hand-held tonometer via the applanation method with a drop of milk for visualization of the applanation ring. Ballantyne et al. (4) showed a transient increase in ocular pressure when an irritant was applied to rabbit eyes. Maul and Sears (87) also showed a dose-response relationship of increased ocular pressure by nitrogen mustard.

There are three methods for measuring intraocular pressure (tonometry): the digital palpation, the indentation, and the applanation methods. Digital palpation is the simplest but also the most subjective. It is heavily dependent on the investigator's experience and skill in using fingers to feel the ocular pressure. In the indentation method, a Schiotz tonometer is used. This method is primarily used in animals. The weight plunger of the Schiotz tonometer slides through the center of a concave footplate and depresses an indented area on the cornea. The depth of the indentation is related to the ocular pressure, which can be easily read from a calibrated scale. The principle of the applanation tonometer is described in the section, Uses of Fluorescein in the Assessment of Ocular Functions.

Blood/Aqueous Humor Barrier

Inflammation in the ocular tissues can change the permeability of the blood vessels supplying them. One of the changes in these blood vessels is increased permeability leakage, which disrupts the barrier between the blood and intercellular fluid and the fluid in the ocular chambers (i.e., the blood/aqueous humor barrier). Proteins and other blood constituents that leak into the aqueous humor when inflammation occurs will increase the osmotic force. As a result, water infiltration is increased, as is ocular pressure. Theoretically, this blood/aqueous barrier can be evaluated, which can reveal the potential of the ocular toxicity of materials that can cause inflammation in the eye before gross changes occur.

To study the blood/aqueous humor barrier, Davson and Quilliam (29) used low-toxicity dyes with a high affinity for protein. The dyes were injected intraveneously. The protein-bound dye detected in the aqueous humor indicated protein leakage. Lallier et al. (82) adopted such an approach to examine increased disruption of the blood/aqueous humor barrier. A 50-mg/kg dose of Evan blue (a highly protein-bound dye) was injected intravenously in rabbits 24 hr after the exposure of eye irritants. The aqueous humor concentration of Evan blue was assayed by a micro-spectrophotometer at a wavelength of 620 nm. While this approach can be potentially useful in identifying mild eye irritants, it is an invasive test and can only be performed in animals.

Dry Weights of Ocular Tissue as an Indicator for Edema in Ocular Tissues

Some researchers have compared the ratio of dry weight to wet weight of an ocular tissue to quantitate edema in ocular tissue (82,134,142). The tissue (e.g., the isolated cornea) was dried either by submersion in acetone followed by 24-hr storage over silica gel in a vacuum desiccator (82), or by lyophilization. Such a method, although objective in nature, is also an invasive test and can only be applied to animals. Furthermore, there are many potential experimental errors during trimming, drying, and weighing.

Active Transport Enzyme (Na^+-K^+) ATPase

Corneal endothelium is rich in the active transport enzyme (ATPase). The maintenance of proper hydration of the cornea has been attributed to the activity of the enzyme, which catalyzes an active pump (15,76,84). Ouabain is a potent inhibitor of (Na^+-K^+)-activated ATPase, and when injected into the aqueous humor it increases corneal hydration (17). Using isolated corneas, Trenberth and Mishima

(132) found that ouabain, when applied directly to the endothelium, causes corneal swelling. Because such an approach involves the basic biochemical activity in the membrane at a molecular level, it is a potentially useful method for identifying eye irritants.

Measuring the activity of (Na^+-K^+)-activated ATPase in tissues is not difficult. It can be easily assayed colorimetrically. An excellent review is available (111).

Corneal Endothelial Damage

It is considerably more difficult to assess damage on the endothelium than on the epithelium. Most studies of the endothelium have been done on *in vitro* isolated corneas with saline perfusion on the endothelial side. Corneas are then examined by slit lamp specular microscopy (89,91,121). Corneal thickness has also been measured and examined by scanning electron microscopy (30,35–37,91). The end points for endothelial damage were increased corneal thickness and microscopic changes seen by electron microscopy.

Other Methods

Other physiobiochemical methods used to assess corneal toxicity include measuring the increase in temperature associated with ocular inflammation by an infrared thermometer (2) and by enzyme histochemistry to evaluate the cytotoxicity of the cornea and endothelium (44).

Assessment of Corneal Healing

The cornea is an active tissue. If injury occurs and is not extensive, ordinarily the cornea will regenerate the wounded tissue. This healing process is particularly active in the epithelium. The reversibility of eye irritation is dependent on the efficiency of the healing process. Furthermore, many ophthalmic pharmaceuticals are used in diseased eyes, and knowing the effect of these drugs on ocular healing is important. Detailed reviews on this subject are available (58,77,81,83,127,133).

The healing process in the epithelium starts as soon as 1 hr after exposure (78). Epithelial cells (primarily the wing cells) adjacent to the wound slide continuously by ameboid movements across the wounded area until that area is completely covered (81). Eventually, mitosis of the migrated epithelial cells will fill the wounded area. Finally, the epithelium adheres firmly to the stroma, thereby reestablishing the epithelial barrier (81). The normal rate of this epithelial regeneration process ranges from 0.80 to 1.42 mm^2/hr (102,133). A relatively intact basement is needed for this healing process so that the newly regenerated epithelial cells can adhere to it (65,66,77). When the damaged epithelium is covered by regenerated cells, stromal repairs start by the migration of adjacent keratocytes to the wounded area where the cells are transformed into the connective tissues, thus reestablishing the matrix of stroma. The polysaccharide content in the stroma also changes as the wound heals (83). Endothelial healing starts only hours after the injury, also by migration or enlargement of the adjacent endothelial cells over the wounded area; a new Descemet's membrane is synthesized within 1 to 2 weeks.

The mechanism that triggers corneal healing is not understood, but there is evidence that the process involves cyclic AMP and other growth factors (67,73,74).

The healing process of the epithelium is by far the most studied. A good review is available (133). Basically, an epithelial wound (approximately 7 mm in diameter) is made on the corneal epithelium by acid (sulfuric acid), alkali (sodium hydroxide), chemical solvent (*n*-heptanol), iodine, keratectomy, or scraping (25,66,67,102,131). The rate of healing then is determined by either periodic measurements of the fluorescein-stained area or by measurements of other quantitative end points such as corneal thickness (133).

Because the wound must be uniform in size and have a significant amount of injury for healing studies, some specific wounding procedures have been developed:

Mechanical wounds: This procedure has been recommended for studying different factors that affect the normal healing process of the cornea and for studying the mechanism of wound healing when chemical interaction is to be avoided (133). For such wounding, a mark approximately 0.05 mm deep and 7 mm in diameter is made with a surgical trephine. The epithelium is then stained with fluorescein to highlight the cut mark. The epithelium within the cut mark is carefully removed by scraping with a No. 64 Beaver blade or a No. 10 Bord Parker blade (133). It is recommended that this procedure be performed under a microscope.

Chemical wounds: Iodine plus cocaine, iodine vapor, *n*-heptanol, sulfuric acid, and sodium hydroxide have been used in chemical wound procedures. For iodine wounds (65,66), a 7-mm trephine is held firmly against the epithelium forming a well, followed by instillation of 0.1 mm of 2% iodine tincture solution into the well. After 60 sec, the treated area is vigorously irrigated with a balanced salt solution with the trephine still sitting on the cornea. After removing the trephine, 0.25 ml of a 4% cocaine hydrochloride solution is applied to bind the iodine complex, and the resulting opaque sheet of corneal epithelium can be gently removed with a saline-moistened, cotton-tipped applicator.

A more convenient method of obtaining iodine wounds has been described by Moses et al. (102). In this method, an iodine applicator is used consisting of a glass tube in which iodine crystals are placed. The end of the tube is plugged with glass wool. To produce a uniform wound, the end of the tube is held against an anesthetized eye for a short period of time followed by rinsing then removal of the wounded epithelium as described above. For a heptanol wound, a 6-mm diameter (approximately) filter disc (Whatman No. 50 filter paper), distorted into the shape of a contact lens and saturated with *n*-heptanol, is carefully placed onto the corneal surface of the rabbit's eye. The disc is removed after 60 sec and the cornea is rinsed thoroughly with normal saline solution. Any remaining debris is wiped off with a saline-moistened, cotton-tipped swab (25).

Similar techniques with sodium hydroxide (4 N) can be employed to obtain a chemical burn on the cornea (66). Sodium hydroxide can produce deeper wounds than *n*-heptanol but, more often than not, the stroma is involved. For an acid burn wound, 0.1 ml of sulfuric acid (18 N) is instilled into a trephine-created well on the cornea as previously described. After 10 sec, the area is irrigated with a balanced salt solution (66).

The healing rate is usually monitored by measuring the size of the wound periodically. The wounds can be stained with a drop of 2% fluorescein solution followed by water flushing. The stained wounds are photographed with a single lens reflex camera fitted with a cobalt light source. The negatives are then projected onto a white paper at a specific distance, and the boundary of the stained wounds is traced on the paper. The areas within the boundary of the wound are determined by either a planimeter or a computer planimetry program and graphics tables (133).

A damaged corneal epithelial barrier allows tears to enter the stroma and cause swelling. Gradual return to a normal state takes place once the epithelial barrier is reestablished by the healing process. Thus it is logical to quantify the degree of healing by measuring corneal thickness periodically. As previously discussed, corneal thickness can be measured with a pachometer attached to a slit lamp microscope.

Other techniques have been used to follow the healing process. For example, phase contrast, light microscopy, and slit lamp techiques are used to observe and grade the wounded area. Serial corneal biopsy specimens fixed in glutaraldehyde-formaldehyde solution and epoxy-embedded semithin sections stained with para-phenylenediamine and examined by transmission electron microscopy are also used (65,66).

Assessment of Somatosensory Sensations

Innervation of the cornea is rich and abundant. Most of the corneal nerve fibers originate from ciliary branches of the ophthalmic nerve. In addition, the sclera, iris, ciliary body, and conjunctiva are all richly innervated with somatosensory nerves. All somatosensory nerve connections are extremely important for protecting the cornea. These nerve endings function as pain, touch, pressure, sting, pH, or temperature receptors. Registration of these noxious changes will elicit such reflexes as blinking and tear secretion to minimize or neutralize damage to the eye. These discomfort sensations usually occur much earlier than gross lesions and at lower concentrations. Identifying such eye discomfort caused by low concentration chemicals in consumer products is extremely important.

Experimental somatosensory responses can be followed by electrophysiologic techniques, but simpler behavioral techniques are more convenient and probably are just as reliable in identifying chemicals that can cause ocular discomfort. Many animal models for testing have been proposed, but the mouse writhing test is the one most used in the assessment of ocular pain or stinging sensation. Using this approach, Shanahan and Ward (125) have noted a reasonably good correlation with the results of stinging studies in humans. In their test, diluted shampoo was injected intraperitoneally at 0.2 ml/mouse. The animals were then observed for "writhing syndrome" occurrences that indicate pain, stinging, and discomfort sensations. A combination of signs is indicative of the writhing syndrome: contraction of abdominal muscles (tension and flexion), ataxia, high stepping gait, reduced motor exploratory activities, and excessive preening and licking of the injection site.

In another study, an increased blinking rate was found to be the most important irritating response for low-concentration exposure to formaldehyde in humans (123). Ballantyne and Swanston (5) compared the sensitivity of blepharospasm (uncontrollable winking) in animals and humans. They concluded that humans were much more sensitive than rabbits or guinea pigs. Consequently, the blepharospasm test run in animals was not suitable for identifying materials that can cause ocular discomfort in humans.

The upper respiratory tract test (1) is another useful test in identifying chemicals that can cause eye discomfort in humans. A qualitative correlation in this test was noted between the respiratory rate (or increased duration of expiration) and the sensory potential of eye irritants.

Assessment of Lenticular Damage

Other than the cornea, the lens is the most important refractive optics of the eye. The focus of images on the retina depends on the transparency of the crystalline lens and its ability to accommodate for far and near distance vision. The lens is avascular and its nutrition comes from its surrounding fluids—the aqueous humor and vitreous body. The outermost layer of the lens is a capsule rich in glycoprotein. The lens also consists of the epithelium (under the anterior capsule), a monolayer of cuboidal cells having the highest metabolic rate of the lens; the central bulk of nuclear fibers composed of water-soluble glycoproteins, glycolipids, phospholipids, a small amount of acidic mucopolysaccharides, and sulfhydryl proteins; and the thin zonular filaments from which the lens is suspended. The capsular layer restricts penetration of molecules by size and lipid solubility, and it functions as the basement membrane for the underlying epithelium.

The epithelium is the transport site for electrolytes, carbohydrates, and amino acids by the (Na^+-K^+)ATPase pump and other facilitated or active transport systems. The epithelium also is an important transport site for proteins and glutathione and provides the most important source of soluble sulfhydryls. The fibers make up the bulk of the lens. Only a small amount of fibers in the membrane is insoluble; most fibers and proteins are water soluble. Fibers also provide the elasticity of the lens for accommodating for far and near vision.

Unlike the cornea, the transparency of the lens does not depend on the geometric arrangement of the fibers but rather on the maintenance of proper density, osmolarity, pH, the solubility of its fibers and proteins, and its negligible extracellular spaces. Any toxic insults that can create an imbalance of the normal physiologic or biochemical processes needed for maintaining the proper solubility, hydration, density, and composition of the lens will produce opacity or cataracts of the lens. For example, cataracts can result from inhibition of enzymes (quinone), accumulation of metabolites or particles, dietary insufficiency, physical trauma, vacuole formation, etc. (51).

Most of the gross defects such as opacification of the lens (cataracts) are detected by observation with a slit lamp microscope. The density of the lens has also been measured as an indicator of damage in the lens (32). Graded increase in density of the lens was observed with different degrees of lenticular opacity. Thus the opacity of the lens can be quantified by the densitometric recordings. Most of our understanding of the function of the lens comes from *in vitro* biochemical and physiologic studies that go beyond the scope of this chapter.

Assessment of Retinal Damage

The retina is the site for conversion of light to neurosignals. In the retina the light receptors are rod and cone cells with synpases to the central nervous system. Anatomic and physiologic aspects of the retina are described in many physiology textbooks. Anatomic examination of the fundus by direct and indirect ophthalmoscopy and by fundus fluorescein angiography has been described previously in this chapter.

The functional integrity of the retina is usually examined by electroretinography (ERG), electrooculography (EOG), or visually evoked response (VER). Procedures and interpretations of these tests are detailed elsewhere (43,70), but brief descriptions of the examination techniques are provided in the following sections.

Electroretinography (ERG)

The ERG technique records the changes in electropotential across the retina upon a flash stimulus. Ideally, the potential is measured across the two sides of the retina itself, but this is possible only in animals. A noninvasive approach is to place a recording electrode (in the shape of a contact lens) on the cornea and a reference electrode on the forehead. When a flash of light is cast on the retina, its resting potential is changed rapidly. Such an action potential only lasts a short time. The recorded ERG is an algebraic sum of four basic components, the "a," "b," "c," and "d" waves, that correspond to the responses of different layers of cells in the retina (Fig. 5). A "a" wave is from the rods and cones (photoreceptors), the "b" wave is from the bipolar cell layer (inner nuclear layer), the "c" wave is from the junction between the photoreceptors and the pigmented epithelial layer, and the "d" wave is from the cones when the flash is turned off. Usually under intense light stimulation, only the "a" and "b" waves are evident on the ERG, especially when the eye is well adapted to the dark. Because the rods and cones are sensitive to different wavelengths of light, the recorded "a" and "b" waves are actually the sum of two components of each wave (i.e., "a_1" and "b_1"; "a_2" and "b_2") that correspond to phototopic components (cones, sensitive to longer wavelengths) and scotopic components (rods, sensitive to shorter wavelengths). To differentiate between the phototopic and scotopic components, the ERG can be recorded under two conditions: light-adapted eyes exposed to an intense flash to stimulate the cones and dark-adapted eyes exposed to a weaker flash to stimulate the rods. The cones also have higher temporal discrimination when fusing the waves of higher flickering

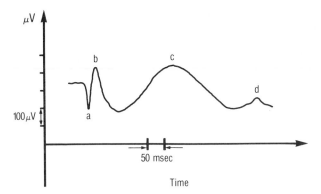

FIG. 5. A normal electroretinogram: *(a)* rods and cones (photoreceptors); *(b)* bipolar cell layer (inner nuclear layer); *(c)* junction between photoreceptors and pigmented epithelial layer; and *(d)* cones when flash is turned off. (Adapted from Galloway, ref. 43, with permission.)

frequency (successive flash stimuli). The flickering approach is used more often in clinical evaluation of the cones.

Electroretinography is useful in evaluating the integrity of the cones, rods, bipolar layer, and pigmented epithelium. Lesions beyond that (from ganglion to the visual cortex) cannot be detected by ERG.

Visually Evoked Response (VER)

Theoretically, to evaluate the conductivity of various visual neuropathways, two electrodes can be placed at the points of interest to record the neurosignals passing through. Again, this is possible only in animals. A noninvasive technique is often used based on the assumption that the occipital lobe of the cortex receives large portions of its neurosignals from the retina. Thus, measuring the electrical activities on the scalp at the occipital area will represent the general activity of the visual cortex. The VER technique is actually a visually evoked electroencephalogram (EEG). Abnormalities in the VER indicate abnormalities in the retina, the visual neural pathways, or the visual cortex. The analysis of VER is a complicated task, but it is a valuable tool complementary to other tests in identifying lesions at various levels of visual dysfunction.

Electrooculography (EOG)

The EOG technique is based on the resting potential between the cornea and the fundus. This large resting potential, approximately 6 mV in the normal eye, is positive at the cornea and negative at the fundus. This is different from the flash action potential in the ERG technique. Such a resting potential is generated at the retinal receptors and the pigmented epithelium. Factors that can alter this resting potential include hypoxia, retinotopic drugs, retinal illumination, and ocular movement. EOG also is an important tool in detecting diseased retinal layers involved in photolysis. The electrodes are placed on the skin on either side of the eye at the medial and lateral canthi, and an indifferent electrode is placed on the forehead. Any two-channel electroencephalographic recorder with preamplifiers having a bandwidth of 1 to 50 Hz can be employed for recording the change of the resting potential.

A normal EOG depends on the anatomic and physiologic integrity of the photoreceptors and pigmented epithelium and an adequate blood supply to the retina. Reduced or even abolished light-induced (retinal illumination) potential results if these components of the retina are damaged. In some cases of severe retinal degeneration, even the potential is decreased, and in some mild cases, the peak of light-induced potential is delayed.

HISTOLOGIC APPROACHES

Histologic examination of the eyes has been routinely included in subchronic and chronic toxicity studies, but because it is time consuming and costly, this test is performed only occasionally in eye irritation studies. Also, results may not be as informative as those from observations and measurements used in other techniques. However, histologic examination of ocular tissue under proper conditions can reveal the type of damage, tissues involved, and subtle changes in ocular tissue.

Both electron and light microscopic examinations have been used to evaluate local ocular injuries (21,52,73,74,115,129,130,137). A review of this subject is available (63). Although such methods can sometimes reveal morphologic changes of different parts of the cornea, conjunctiva, lens, retina, and visual nerve degeneration, shortcomings are not uncommon. Among the many problems are sectioning the precise lesion, problems in slide preparation, and subjective interpretation of observations. A particularly important problem is that histologic examination must be made on dehydrated tissue (21), which makes some conditions, such as corneal edema, difficult to detect. However, histologic examination of ocular tissues in local eye irritation studies has been considered an objective method because of its high sensitivity in detecting very mild ocular effects (63).

IN VITRO ALTERNATIVE METHODS FOR THE ASSESSMENT OF LOCAL EYE IRRITATION

Recent humane concerns about using animals in chemical-induced eye irritation tests have prompted many investigators to turn to alternative methods. Although the development of such alternatives is still in its infancy, organizations such as the Johns Hopkins Center for Alternatives to Animal Testing, the Rockefeller Laboratory Animal Research Center, and the Fund for Replacement of Animals in Medical Research (FRAME) of England have been very active in promoting alternatives. These attempts are successful in at least drawing the attention of many scientists. Consequently, the first generation of alternative methods for eye irritation testing has been surfacing.

Recent research has focused on validation of methods, most of which are *in vitro*. Basically, the current approaches for *in vitro* methods can be grouped into two categories: perfused organs (or tissues) and cell cultures. Many physiologic and biochemical markers of cellular function have been proposed. They include cytomorphology, enzyme leakage, corneal thickness and swelling, uptake of radioactive exogenous and endogenous chemicals, synthesis of tissue-specific proteins, and inflammatory parameters such as macrophage migration. All of these are in one way or another indicators of the integrity of the cellular membrane and cytotoxicity.

As early as 1956, Shapiro (126) used isolated corneas from rabbits to study the effect of sodium hydroxide solution on corneal swelling. Later, Mishima and Kudo (99), Hull (69), and Edelhauser et al. (35–37) used a perfused cornea to study the toxicity of selected chemicals on the corneal endothelium. In these studies, corneal thickness was the major end point measured. Besides specular microscopy, cytomorphologic examinations were also performed. In 1981 Burton et al. (23) used similar endpoints to validate the *in vivo* and *in vitro* irritancy of a number of chemicals, and a broad correlation was noted.

The first successful corneal cell culture was achieved by Baum et al. in 1979 (9). The *in vitro* corneal culture technique was used later by Norton-Root et al. (106) to validate the irritancy of a series of surfactants. The endpoint measured was cytotoxicity. About 400 rabbit corneal cells were suspended in an incubating growth medium for 18 hr at 38°C. A solution of the surfactant or control medium was then added. The treated culture cells were incubated again for 7 to 8 days to allow surviving cells to form colonies. The colonies were fixed with 10% formalin and stained with 0.1% crystal violet, and the number of colonies was counted. A fairly good rank correlation was observed between their *in vitro* results (cytotoxicity) and the reported *in vivo* irritancy of surfactants by the Draize test.

Borenfreund et al. (16) and Shopsis and Sathe (126a) used Hep G_2 cells (human epithelial hepatoma cell line) and Balb/C.353 cells (murine fibroblast cell line) to validate the irritancy of different alcohols. Two endpoints were measured: cytotoxicity and membrane transport. Cytotoxicity was observed by phase microscopy for morphologic alterations such as changes in cell shape, vascularization and granularity, detachment and loss of viability as indicated by cell lysis, and trypan blue dye exclusion. Membrane transport was measured by ^{3}H-uridine uptake, which has been related to the status of membrane integrity and the metabolic phosphorylation process of cultured cells. A good rank correlation was noted between the *in vivo* irritancy by the Draize test and *in vitro* UI_{50} values (concentration at which a 50% inhibition of uridine uptake was observed).

Muir et al (103) recently demonstrated that cytotoxicity, in terms of hemolytic potency *in vitro* of eight surfactants, did not correlate with *in vivo* eye irritation in rabbits. However, the ability of these surfactants to block spontaneous contractions of isolated mouse or rabbit ilea correlated better with the *in vivo* eye irritancy of these surfactants.

At a recent symposium organized by the Society of Comparative Ophthalmology, Douglas (31) presented data indicating that radioactive ^{51}Cr can be a useful tool for *in vitro* studies. With this method, cultured corneal endothelial cells from calves were first saturated with ^{51}Cr by incubating them in radioactive sodium chromate medium. After treating the cultured cells with a test substance, the cells were washed and reincubated; the amount of ^{51}Cr released from the cell was measured. A fairly good rank correlation was noted between the *in vitro* ^{51}Cr release and the *in vivo* irritancy by Draize's test.

This survey of current *in vitro* eye irritation method development is by no means complete. Many unpublished reports of ongoing studies include macrophage migration, histamine release from mast cells, chorioallantoic membrane of the chick embryo, plasminogen activator secretion, etc. Much of this work is expected to reach the literature by the time this book is published.

Although the idea of replacing *in vivo* testing in animals is admirable and the current thrust in method development and validation is encouraging, there are many inherent problems and shortcomings in these alternative *in vitro* methods. For example, most *in vitro* techniques have problems with the solubility of certain chemicals. Correlation between *in vitro* and *in vivo* data appears to be good only within certain classes of chemicals. Validation of different types and classes of chemicals is needed. Most current *in vitro* techniques are not suitable to establish reversibility of eye irritation, which is extremely important in the classification of eye irritants. It is fair to state in summary that, at the present time, none of the *in vitro* techniques appear to be able to replace *in vivo* testing in animals.

In this chapter we have surveyed the techniques used in the assessment of various ocular effects. The widely used Draize test is described and critiqued. Some of the principles behind the various aids and techniques that have been used in ocular toxicity testing are described. Physiologic and biochemical approaches for evaluation of conjunctival, corneal, lenticular, and retinal functions are useful methods for assessing ocular toxicity of chemicals. Histologic approaches are useful in detecting morphologic changes, and sometimes in detecting subtle changes in the ocular tissues. *In vitro* alternatives are still in the infancy stage. Method development and validation studies are needed before such tests are adopted for routine ocular toxicity evaluations.

REFERENCES

1. Alarie, Y. (1966): Irritating properties of airborne materials to the upper respiratory tract. *Arch. Environ. Health*, 13:433–449.
2. Ashford, J. J., and Lambel, J. W. (1974): A detailed assessment procedure of antiinflammatory effects of drugs on experimental immunogenic uveitis in rabbits. *Invest. Ophthalmol.*, 13:414–421.
3. Baldwin, H. A., McDonald, T. D., and Beasley, C. H. (1973): Slit-lamp examination of experimental animal eyes. II. Grading scales and photographic evaluation of induced pathological conditions. *J. Soc. Cosmet. Chem.*, 24:181–195.
4. Ballantyne, B., Gazzard, M. F., and Swanston, D. W. (1972): Effects of solvents and irritants on intraocular tension in the rabbit. *J. Physiol.*, 226:12P–14P.
5. Ballantyne, B., and Swanston, D. W. (1973): The irritant potential of dilute solutions of ortho-chlorobenzylidene malononitrile (CS) on the eye and tongue. *Acta Pharmacol. Toxicol.*, 32:266–277.
6. Ballantyne, B., and Swanston, D. W. (1974): The irritant effects of dilute solutions of dibenzoxyazepine (CR) on the eye and tongue. *Acta Pharmacol. Toxicol.*, 35:412–423.

7. Barnett, K. C. (1967): Principles of ophthalmoscopy. *Vet. Scope*, 62:56.
8. Battista, S. P., and McSweeney, E. S. (1965): Approaches to a quantitative method for testing eye irritation. *J. Soc. Cosmet. Chem.*, 16:199–301.
9. Baum, J. L., Niedra, R., Davis, C., and Yue, D. (1979): Mass culture of human corneal endothelial cells. *Arch. Ophthalmol.*, 97:1136–1140.
10. Bayard, S., and Hehir, R. M. (1976): Evaluation of proposed changes in the modified Draize rabbit irritation test. *Toxicol. Appl. Pharmacol.*, 37:186.
11. Beckeley, J. H. (1965): Critique of the Draize eye test, now and then—Eighteen, nine or six rabbits. *Am. Perf. Cosmet.*, 80:51–54.
12. Beckley, J. H. (1965): Comparative eye testing: Man vs. animal. *Toxicol. Appl. Pharmacol.*, 7:93–101.
13. Bellhorn, R. W. (1973): Fluorescein fundus photography in veterinary ophthalmology. *J. Am. Anim. Hosp. Assoc.*, 9:277.
14. Bonfield, C. T., and Scala, R. A. (1965): The paradox in testing for eye irritation. A report on thirteen shampoos. *Proc. Sci. Sect. Toilet Goods Assoc.*, 43:34–43.
15. Bonting, S. L., Simon, K. A., and Hawkins, N. M. (1961): Studies on sodium-potassium-activated adenosine triphosphatase. I. Quantitiative distribution in several tissues of the rat. *Arch. Biochem.*, 95:416–423.
16. Borenfreund, E., Shopsis, C., Barrero, O., and Sathe, S. (1983): *In vitro* alternative irritancy assays: Comparison of cytotoxic and membrane transport effects of alcohols. *Ann. NY Acad. Sci.*, 407:416–419.
17. Brown, S. I., and Hedbys, B. O. (1965): The effect of ouabain on the hydration of the cornea. *Invest. Ophthalmol.*, 4:216–221.
18. Buehler, E. V. (1974): Testing to predict potential ocular hazards of household chemicals. In: *Toxicology Annual*, edited by C. L. Winek, pp. 53–69. Marcel Dekker, Inc., New York.
19. Buehler, E. V., and Newman, E. A. (1964): A comparison of eye irritation in monkeys and rabbits. *Toxicol. Appl. Pharmacol.*, 6:701–710.
20. Bunce, D. F. (1955): The use of the ophthalmoscope in veterinary practice. *Vet. Med.*, 50:599.
21. Burnstein, N. L. (1980): Corneal cytotoxicity of topically applied drugs, vehicles, and preservatives. *Surv. Ophthalmol.*, 25:15–30.
22. Burton, A. B. G. (1972): A method for the objective assessment of eye irritation. *Fd. Cosmet. Toxicol.*, 10:209–217.
23. Burton, A. B. G., York, M., and Lawrence, R. S. (1981): The *in vitro* assessment of severe eye irritant. *Fd. Cosmet. Toxicol.*, 19:471–480.
24. Cello, R. M., and Lasmanis, J. (1958): Pseudomonas infection of the eye of the dog resulting from the use of contaminated fluorescein solution. *J. Am. Vet. Med. Assoc.*, 132:297.
25. Cintron, C., Hassinger, L., Kablin, C. L., and Friend, J. (1979): A simple method for the removal of rabbit corneal epithelium utilizing *n*-heptanol. *Ophthalmic Res.*, 11:90–96.
26. Cohen, I. J. (1983): Use of fluorescein in eye injuries. *J. Occup. Med.*, 5:540.
27. Conquet, G. D., Laillier, J., and Plazonnet, B. (1977): Evaluation of ocular irritation in the rabbit: Objective versus subjective assessment. *Toxicol. Appl. Pharmacol.*, 39:129–139.
28. Davies, R. G., Kynoch, S. R., and Liggett, M. P. (1976): Eye irritation tests—An assessment of the maximum delay time for remedial irrigation. *J. Soc. Cosmet. Chem.*, 27:301–306.
29. Davson, H., and Quilliam, J. P. (1947): The effects of nitrogen mustard on the permeability of the blood-aqueous humour barrier to Evan blue. *Br. J. Ophthalmol.*, 31:717–721.
30. Dickstein, S., and Maurice, D. M. (1972): The metabolic basis to the fluid pump in the cornea. *J. Physiol.*, 221:29.
31. Douglas, W. (1983): The use of corneal cell culture for identification of ocular irritants. *Annual Meeting of the Society of Comparative Ophthalmology*, April 22, 1983, Newark, NJ.
32. Dragomirescu, V., Hockwin, O., Koch, H. R., and Sassaki, K. (1978): Development of a new equipment for rotating slit image photography according to Scheimpflug's principle. *Interdis. Top. Gerontol.*, 13:118–130.
33. Draize, J. H., Woodward, G., and Calvery, H. O. (1944): Methods for the study of irritation and toxicity of substances applied topically to the skin and mucous membranes. *J. Pharmacol. Exp. Ther.*, 82:377–390.
34. Easty, D. L., and Mathalone, M. B. R. (1969): Toxicity of 1,8,9-triacetoxyanthracene to the cornea in rabbits. *Br. J. Ophthalmol.*, 53:819–823.

35. Edelhauser, H. F., Gonnerings, R., and Van Horn, D. L. (1978): Intraocular irrigation solutions: A comparative study of BSS plus and lactated Ringer's solution. *Arch. Ophthalmol.*, 96:516.
36. Edelhauser, H. F., Van Horn, D. L., Hyndink, R. A., and Schultz, R. O. (1975): Intraocular irrigating solutions: Their effect on the corneal endothelium. *Arch. Ophthalmol.*, 93:648.
37. Edelhauser, H. F., Van Horn, D. L., Schultz, R. O., and Hyndink, R. A. (1976): Comparative toxicity of intraocular irrigating solution on the corneal endothelium. *Am. J. Ophthalmol.*, 81:473–481.
38. Ehrlich, P. (1882): Über provocirte fluorescenzer - Scheinungen am Auge. *Dtsch. Med. Wochenschr.*, 2:21.
39. FDA (1976): Illustrated guide for grading eye irritation by hazardous substances.
40. FHSA (1979): Regulations under the Federal Hazardous Substance Act. Chapter II. Title 16. *Code of Federal Regulations.*
41. Floyd, E. P., and Stockinger, H. G. (1958): Toxicity studies of certain organic peroxides and hydroperoxides. *Am. Indust. Hyg. Assoc. J.*, 19:205–212.
42. Friedenwald, J. S., Hughes, W. F., and Hermann, H. (1944): Acid-base tolerance of the cornea. *Arch. Ophthalmol.*, 31:279–283.
43. Galloway, N. R. (1975): *Ophthalmic Electrodiagnosis.* W. B. Saunders Company, Ltd., London.
44. Gasset, A. R., Ishii, Y., Kaufman, H. E., and Miller, T. (1974): Cytotoxicity of ophthalmic preservatives. *Am. J. Ophthalmol.*, 78:98–105.
45. Gaunt, I. F., and Harper, K. H. (1964): The potential irritancy to rabbit eye mucosa of certain commercially available shampoos. *J. Soc. Cosmet. Chem.*, 15:209–230.
46. Gelatt, K. N. (1974): *Diagnostic Procedures in Comparative Ophthalmology*, 2nd ed. American Animal Association, South Bend, IN.
47. Gelatt, K. N. (1975): Evaluation of tear formation in dog using a modification of the Schirmer tear test. *J. Am. Vet. Med. Assoc.*, 166:368.
48. Gelatt, K. N., Henderson, J. D., Jr., and Steffen, G. R. (1976): Fluorescein angiography of the normal and diseased ocular fundi of the laboratory dog. *J. Am. Vet. Med. Assoc.*, 169:980.
49. Giovacchini, R. P. (1972): Old and new issues in the safety evaluation of cosmetics and toiletries. *CRC Crit. Rev. Toxicol.*, 1:361–378.
50. Gordon, D. M. (1973): Fundamentals of ophthalmoscopy. *Vet. Scope*, 11:1.
51. Grant, W. M. (1974): *Toxicology of the Eye*, 2nd ed., Charles C Thomas Publisher, Springfield, IL.
52. Green, W. R., Sullivan, J. B., Hehir, R. M., Scharpf, L. F., and Dickinson, A. W. (1978): *A Chemically-Induced Eye Injury in the Albino Rabbit and Rhesus Monkey.* The Soap and Detergent Association, New York.
53. Griffith, J. F., Nixon, G. A., Bruce, R. D., Reer, P. J., and Bannan, E. A. (1980): Dose-response studies with chemical irritants in the albino rabbit eye as a basis for selecting optimum testing conditions for predicting hazard to human eye. *Toxicol. Appl. Pharmacol.*, 55:501–513.
54. Guillot, J., Gonnet, J. F., and Clement, C. (1982): Evaluation of the ocular irritation potential of 56 compounds. *Fd. Chem. Toxicicol.*, 20:573–582.
55. Gundersen, T., and Liebman, S. D. (1944): Effect of local anesthetics on regeneration of corneal epithelium. *Arch. Ophthalmol.*, 31:29–33.
56. Haining, D. W. (1966): Diagnostic value of intravenous fluorescein studies. *Br. J. Ophthalmol.*, 50:587.
57. Halberg, G. P., and Berens, C. (1961): Standardized Schirmer tear test kit. *Am. J. Ophthalmol.*, 51:840.
58. Hanna, C. (1966): Proliferation and migration of epithelial cells during corneal wound repair in the rabbit and the rat. *Am. J. Ophthalmol.*, 61:55–63.
59. Harker, D. B. (1970): A modified Schirmer tear test technique. *Vet. Rec.*, 86:196.
60. Harris, L. S., Toyofuku, H., and Shimmyo, M. (1972): Fluorescein iris angiography in albino rabbit. *Arch. Ophthalmol.*, 88:193.
61. Harriton, L. (1981): Conversation with Henry Spira: Draize test activist. *Lab. Anim.*, 10:16–22.
62. Henkes, H., and Canta, L. R. (1973): Drug-induced disorders of the eye. In: *Excerpta Medica 14: Proceedings of the European Society for the Study of Drug Toxicity*, edited by W. A. M. Duncan, pp. 146–153. Elsevier North Holland, Inc., New York.
63. Heywood, R., and James, R. W. (1978): Towards objectivity in the assessment of eye irritation. *J. Soc. Cosmet. Chem.*, 29:25–29.

64. Hill, D. W., and Young, S. (1973): Arterial fluorescence angiography of fundus oculi of the cat: Appearances and measurements. *Exp. Eye Res.*, 16:457.

65. Hirst, L. W., Fogle, J. A., Kenyon, K. R., and Stark, W. J. (1982): Corneal epithelial regeneration and adhesion following acid burns in the rhesus monkey. *Invest. Ophthalmol. Vis. Sci.*, 23:764–773.

66. Hirst, L. W., Kenyon, K. R., Fogle, J. A., Hanninen, L., and Stark, W. J. (1981): Comparative studies of corneal surface injury in the monkey and rabbit. *Arch. Ophthalmol.*, 99:1066–1073.

67. Ho, P. C., Davis, W. H., Elliot, J. H., and Cohen, S. (1974): Kinetics of corneal epithelial regeneration and epidermal growth factors. *Invest. Ophthalmol.*, 13:804–809.

68. Holland, M. C. (1964): Fluorescein staining of the cornea. *JAMA*, 188:81.

69. Hull, D. S. (1979): Effects of epinephrine, benzalkonium chloride, and intraocular miotics on corneal endothelium. *South. Med. J.*, 2:1380–1381.

70. Ikeda, H., and Friedmann, A. I. (1972): Electrooculography, electroretinography, and the visually evoked occipital response. In: *Modern Ophthalmology, Vol. 1*, 2nd ed., edited by A. Sorsky, pp. 543–556. J. B. Lippincott Company, Philadelphia.

71. IRLG (Interagency Regulatory Liaison Group) (1981): Recommended guideline for acute eye irritation test.

72. Jones, L. T., and Marquis, M. M. (1972): Lacrimal function. *Am. J. Ophthalmol.*, 73:658.

73. Jumblatt, M. M., Fogle, J. A., and Neufeld, A. H. (1980): Cholera toxin stimulates adenosine 3′5′-monophosphate synthesis and epithelial wound closure in the rabbit cornea. *Invest. Ophthalmol. Vis. Sci.*, 19:1321–1329.

74. Jumblatt, M. M., and Neufeld, A. H. (1981): Characterization of cyclic AMP-mediated wound closure of the rabbit corneal epithelium. *Curr. Eye Res.*, 1:189–195.

75. Kay, J. H., and Calandra, J. C. (1962): Interpretation of eye irritation tests. *J. Soc. Cosmet. Chem.*, 13:281–289.

76. Kaye, G. I., and Tice, L. W. (1966): Studies on the cornea. V. Electron microscopic localization of adenosine triphosphatase activity in the rabbit cornea in relation to transport. *Invest. Ophthalmol.*, 5:22–32.

77. Khodadounst, A. A., and Green, K. (1976): Physiological function of regenerating endothelium. *Invest. Ophthalmol.*, 15:96.

78. Khodadounst, A. A., Silverman, A. M., Kenyon, K. R., and Dowling, J. E. (1968): Adhesion of regenerating epithelium. *Am. J. Ophthalmol.*, 65:339.

79. Kimura, S. J. (1951): Fluorescein paper: Simple means of insuring use of sterile fluorescein. *Am. J. Ophthalmol.*, 34:446.

80. Kuhlman, R. E. (1959): Species variation in the enzyme content of corneal epithelium. *J. Cell. Comp. Physiol.*, 53:313–326.

81. Kuwabara, T., Perkins, D. G., and Cogan, D. G. (1976): Sliding of the epithelium in experimental corneal wounds. *Invest. Ophthalmol.*, 15:4.

82. Lallier, J., Plazonne, B., and LeDouarec, J. C. (1975): Evaluation of ocular irritation in the rabbit: Development of an objective method of studying eye irritation. *Proceedings of European Society of Toxicology*, 17:336–350.

83. Lemp, M. A. (1976): Cornea and sclera: Animal review. *Arch. Ophthalmol.*, 94:473.

84. Maeda, K., and Sakagudin, K. (1965): Studies on sodium-potassium-activated adenosine triphosphatase in the cornea. Electron-microscopic observations on the rat cornea. *Jpn. J. Ophthalmol.*, 9:195–199.

85. Marzulli, F. N. (1965): New data on eye and skin tests. *Toxicol. Appl. Pharmacol.*, 7:79–85.

86. Marzulli, F. N., and Simmon, M. E. (1971): Eye irritation from topically applied drugs and cosmetics: Preclinical studies. *Am. J. Optom.*, 48:61–79.

87. Maul, E., and Sears, M. L. (1976): Objective evaluation of experimental ocular irritation. *Invest. Ophthalmol.*, 15:308–312.

88. Maurice, D. M. (1967): The use of fluorescein in ophthalmological research. *Invest. Ophthalmol.*, 6:465–477.

89. Maurice, D. M. (1968): Cellular membrane activity in the corneal endothelium of the intact eye. *Experimentia*, 24:1094–1095.

90. Maurice, D. M., and Giardini, A. A. (1951): A simple optical apparatus for measuring the corneal thickness, and the average thickness of the human cornea. *Br. J. Ophthalmol.*, 35:169–177.

91. McCarey, B. E., Edelhauser, H. F., and Van Horn, D. L. (1973): Functional and structural changes in the corneal endothelium during *in vitro* perfusion. *Invest. Ophthalmol.*, 12:40.

92. McDonald, T. O., Baldwin, H. A., and Beasley, C. H. (1973): Slit-lamp examination of experimental animal eyes. I. Techniques of illumination and the normal eye. *J. Soc. Cosmet. Chem.*, 24:163–180.
93. Meier-Ruge, W. (1973): Eye toxicity. In: *Excerpta Medica 14: Proceedings of the European Society for the Study of Drug Toxicity*, edited by W. A. M. Duncan, pp. 133–145. Elsevier North Holland Inc., New York.
94. Milder, B. (1981): The lacrimal apparatus. In: *Adler's Physiology of the Eye: Clinical Application*, edited by R. A. Moses, p. 24. C. V. Mosby Company, St. Louis.
95. Mishima, S. (1968): Corneal thickness. *Surv. Ophthalmol.*, 13:57–96.
96. Mishima, S. (1975): *In vivo* determination of fluorescein permeability of the corneal endothelium. *Arch. Ophthalmol. (Paris)*, 35:191–196.
97. Mishima, S. (1981): Clinical pharmacokinetics of the eye. *Invest. Ophthalmol. Vis. Sci.*, 21:504.
98. Mishima, S., and Hedbys, B. O. (1968): Measurement of corneal thickness with the Haag-Streit pachometer. *Arch. Ophthalmol.*, 80:710–713.
99. Mishima, S., and Kudo, T. (1967): *In vitro* incubation of rabbit cornea. *Invest. Ophthalmol. Vis. Sci.* 6:329–339.
100. Mishima, S., and Maurice, D. M. (1971): *In vivo* determination of the endothelial permeability to fluorescein. *Acta Soc. Ophthalmol. (Japan)*, 75:236–243.
101. Moses, R. A. (1981): Intraocular pressure. In: *Adler's Physiology of the Eye: Clinical Application*, edited by R. A. Moses, pp. 227–254. C. V. Mosby Company, St. Louis.
102. Moses, R. A., Parkinson, G., and Schuchardt, R. (1979): A standard large wound of the corneal epithelium in rabbits. *Invest. Ophthalmol. Vis. Sci.* 18:103–106.
103. Muir, C. K., Flower, C., and Van Abbe, N. J. (1983): A novel approach to the search for *in vitro* alternatives to *in vivo* eye irritancy testing. *Toxicol. Lett.*, 18:1–5.
104. NAS Committee for Revision of NAS Publication 1138 (1977): Dermal and eye toxicity tests. In: *Principles and Procedures for Evaluating the Toxicity of Household Substances*, pp. 41–54. National Academy of Sciences, Washington, DC.
105. Newsom, W. A., Levereh, S. D., Jr., and Kirkland, V. G. (1968): Retinal fluorescein angiography of the rhesus monkey. *Arch. Ophthalmol.*, 79:768.
106. Norton-Root, H., Yackovich, F., Demetrulias, J., Gacula, M., Jr., and Heinze, J. G. (1982): Evaluation of an *in vitro* cell toxicity test using rabbit corneal cells to predict the eye irritation potential of surfactants. *Toxicol. Lett.*, 14:207–212.
107. Olson, K. J., Dupree, R. W., Plomer, E. T., and Rerve, V. (1962): Toxicological properties of several commercially available surfactants. *J. Soc. Cosmet. Chem.*, 13:469–476.
108. Ota, Y., Mishima, S., and Maurice, D. M. (1974): Endothelial permeability of the living cornea to fluorescein. *Invest. Ophthalmol.*, 13:945–949.
109. Patz, A., and Fine, S. L. (1977): Interpretation of the fundus fluorescein angiogram. *Int. Ophthalmol. Clin.*, 17:1.
110. Pfister, R. R., and Burstein, N. (1976): The effects of ophthalmic drugs, vehicles, and preservatives on corneal epithelium: A scanning electron microscope study. *Invest. Ophthalmol.*, 15:246–258.
111. Phillips, T. D., Fedorowski, A., and Hayes, A. W. (1982): Techniques in membrane toxicology. In: *Principles and Methods of Toxicology*, edited by A. W. Hayes, pp. 587–608. Raven Press, New York.
112. Rieger, M. M., and Battista, G. W. (1964): Some experiences in the safety testing of cosmetics. *J. Soc. Cosmet. Chem.*, 15:161–172.
113. Roberts, S. R. (1962): Abnormal tear secretion in the dog. *Mod. Vet. Pract.*, 43:37.
114. Roberts, S. R., and Erickson, O. F. (1962): Dog tear secretion and tear proteins. *J. Small Anim. Pract., 3:1.*
115. Roeig, D. L., Hasegawa, A. T., Harris, G. J., Lynch, K. L., and Wang, R. I. H. (1980): Occurrence of corneal opacities in rats after acute administration of *l*-α-acetylmethadol. *Toxicol. Appl. Pharmacol.*, 56:155–163.
116. Rosen, E. S. (1969): *Fluorescence Photography of the Eye.* Butterworths, London.
117. Rowan, A. (1981): The Draize test: Political and scientific issues. *Cosmet. Tech.*, 3(7):32–48.
118. Rubin, L. F. (1960): Indirect ophthalmoscopy. *J. Am. Vet. Med. Assoc.*, 137:648.
119. Rubin, L. F., Lynch, R. K., and Stockman, W. W. (1965): Clinical estimation of lacrimal function in dogs. *J. Am. Vet. Med. Assoc.* 147:946.
120. Russell, K. L., and Hock, S. G. (1962): Product development and rabbit eye irritation. *Proc. Sci. Sect. Toilet Goods Assoc.*, 37:27–32.

121. Schimmelpfenning, B. H. (1979): Long-term perfusion of human corneas. *Invest. Ophthalmol. Vis. Sci.*, 18:107.
122. Schirmer, O. (1903): Studien zur Physiologie und Pathologie der Tranenabsonderung und Tranenabfur. *Grafes Arch. Ophthalmol.*, 56:197.
123. Schuck, E. A., Stephens, E. R., and Middleton, J. T. (1966): Eye irritation response at low concentrations of irritants. *Arch. Environ. Health*, 13:570–575.
124. Seabrough, V. M., Osterberg, R. E., Hoheisel, C. A., Murphy, J. C., and Bierbower, G. W. (1976): A comparative study of rabbit ocular reactions to various exposure times to chemicals. *Society of Toxicology, 15th Annual Meeting,* Atlanta, Georgia.
125. Shanahan, R. W., and Ward, C. O. (1975): An animal model for estimating the relative sting potential of shampoos. *J. Soc. Cosmet. Chem.*, 26:581–592.
126. Shapiro, H. (1956): Swelling and dissolution of the rabbit cornea in alkali. *Am. J. Ophthalmol.*, 42:292–298.
126a.Shopsis, C., and Sathe, S. (1984): Uridine uptake inhibition as a cytotoxicity test: correlation with the Draize test. *Toxicology*, 29:195–206.
127. Sigelman, S., Dohlman, C. H., and Friedenwald, J. S. (1954): Miotic and wound healing activities in rat corneal epithelium. *Arch. Ophthalmol.*, 52:751–757.
128. Sugar, J. (1980): Corneal examination. In: *Principles and Practice of Ophthalmology, Vol. 1,* edited by G. A. Peyman, D. R. Sanders, and M. F. Goldberg, pp. 393–395. W. B. Saunders Company, Philadelphia.
129. Tanaka, N., Ohkawa, T., Hiyama, T., and Nakajima, A. (1982): Evaluation of ocular toxicity of two beta blocking drugs, cereteolol and practolol, in beagle dogs. *J. Pharmacol. Exp. Ther.*, 224:424–430.
130. Tonjum, A. M. (1975): Effects of benzalkonium chloride upon the corneal epithelium: Studies with scanning electron microscopy. *Acta Ophthalmol.*, 53:358–366.
131. Thoft, R. A., and Friend, J. (1977): Biochemical transformation of the regenerating ocular surface epithelium. *Invest. Ophthalmol.*, 16:14.
132. Trenberth, S. M., and Mishima, S. (1968): The effect of ouabain on the rabbit corneal endothelium. *Invest. Ophthalmol.*, 7:44–52.
133. Ubels, J. L., Edelhauser, H. F., and Shaw, D. (1982): Measurement of corneal epithelial healing rates and corneal thickness for evaluation of ocular toxicity of chemical toxicity of chemical substances. *J. Toxicol. Cut. Ocular Toxicol.*, 1:133–145.
134. Ulsamer, A. G., Wright, P. L., and Osterberg, R. E. (1977): A comparison of the effects of model irritants on anesthetized and non-anesthetized rabbit eyes (Abstr.). *16th Annual Meeting of Society of Toxicology*, 143.
135. Vierheller, R. C. (1966): Clinical experience with indirect ophthalmoscopy. *Mod. Vet. Pract.*, 47:41.
136. Von Bahr, G. (1948): Measurement of the thickness of the cornea. *Acta Ophthalmol.*, 26:247–266.
137. Waltman, S. R., and Kaufman, H. E. (1970): *In vivo* studies of human corneal and endothelial permeability. *Am. J. Ophthalmol.*, 70:45–47.
138. Walton, R. M., and Heywood, R. (1978): Applanation tonometry in the assessment of eye irritation. *J. Soc. Cosmet. Chem.*, 29:365–368.
139. Weil, C. S., and Scala, R. A. (1971): Study of intra- and inter-laboratory variability in the results of rabbit eye and skin irritation tests. *Toxicol. Appl. Pharmacol.*, 19:276–360.
140. Weltman, A. S., Sharber, S. B., and Jurtshuk, T. (1968): Comparative evaluation and influence of various factors on eye irritation scores. *Toxicol. Appl. Pharmacol.*, 7:308–319.
141. Williams, S. J., Grapel, G. J., and Kennedy, G. L. (1982): Evaluation of ocular irritancy: Potential intra-laboratory variability and effect of dosage volume. *Toxicol. Lett.*, 12:235–241.
142. Wright, P. L., Ulsamer, A. G., and Osterberg, R. E. (1976): Effect of model eye irritants on corneal proteins and water content (Abstr.). *15th Annual Meeting of Society of Toxicology*, 226.
143. Zappia, R. J., and Milder, B. (1972): Lacrimal drainage function. II. The fluorescein dye disappearance test. *Am. J. Ophthalmol.*, 74:160.

Toxicology of the Eye, Ear, and Other Special
Senses, edited by A.W. Hayes. Raven Press,
New York © 1985.

Developmental Periods of Susceptibility to Auditory Trauma in Laboratory Animals

*James C. Saunders and **Chia-Shong Chen

*Department of Otorhinolaryngology and Human Communication, University of
Pennsylvania, Philadelphia, Pennsylvania 19104; and **Department of Psychology,
Monash University, Clayton, Victoria, Australia

The question of whether the developing ear is more vulnerable to auditory trauma than the adult ear is an issue with a relatively short history. During the past decade, however, animal models of early auditory trauma have provided some interesting observations. Early damage to the ear can come from many sources, but it is the purpose of this chapter to consider only that which arises from acoustic or ototoxic trauma. Other reviews of this problem offering additional detail may be found elsewhere. The interested reader is referred to papers by Saunders (33), Saunders and Bock (34), Chen and Willott (10), and, particularly, the recent review by Henry (20).

IS THE DEVELOPING EAR MORE SUSCEPTIBLE TO ACOUSTIC TRAUMA?

Data from five mammalian species support the hypothesis that exposure to intense sound in the developing ear is more traumatic than in the adult ear. These data will be examined with respect to exposures that produce either a permanent or a temporary hearing loss. We will also consider whether the receptor organ, during early development, passes through a precisely defined sensitive period of enhanced susceptibility to acoustic trauma. The central consequences of this trauma will also be noted.

PERMANENT DAMAGE

The cochlear microphonic (CM) response was measured in 8-week-old kittens and adult cats 30 days after exposure to intense pure tones [50 min of a 5.0-kHz tone at a sound pressure level (SPL) that varied somewhat between test groups, but that was typically 105 dB]. The results, for certain stimulus levels, showed a loss in CM sensitivity in the kittens that was greater than in the adults (29). The CM response reflects the integrity of the cochlear receptor cells (particularly the outer hair cells) and it is likely that the kitten hair cells were more traumatized by the exposure than those in the adult. Noise exposure in neonatal guinea pigs (30 hr of white noise at 120 dB SPL) beginning at either 2 or 8 days postpartum has also been shown to produce significantly greater cochlear pathology than the same exposure in 8-month-old adults (16). After a month of recovery, an evaluation of the inner ear by the surface preparation technique (17) revealed that there was a 24% loss of outer hair cells for the pups exposed at 2 days, a 37% loss after exposure at 8 days, and only a 7% loss for the adults. The reduction in inner hair cells and supporting pillar cells was 3%, 1.5%, and less than 1% in the respective groups. Nonexposed, age-matched, control animals showed negligible losses in all of these cell types.

The above observations have been extended to much less traumatic noise exposures in the guinea pig (80 dB SPL of white noise). Cochlear examination showed that the outer hair cell loss in 1-week-old pups was greater than in adults (14). In addition, apical turn outer hair cell loss in animals exposed between 3 and 8 weeks of age proved to be greater than in noise-exposed adults aged between 8 and 16 weeks (13). In another study two 48-hr-old guinea pig pups were exposed to narrow-band noise for 1 hr at 115 dB SPL (12). This noise was centered at 4.0 kHz. At 120 days of age another 2 animals were exposed to the same stimulus for 1 hr. All 4 animals, plus 2 additional nonexposed controls, were trained with a conditioned suppression technique when 6 months old. The suppression behavior was used to obtain an estimate of the quiet threshold at 8.0 kHz. The threshold in the exposed pups averaged 25 dB SPL, while those of the exposed adults and controls were 7.5 and 2.5 dB, respectively. Since the pups had nearly 6 months to recover, the 20 dB threshold shift, relative to the other 2 groups, must be considered a permanent hearing loss. Although the sample size and test conditions were limited in this study, the results remain unique. Finally, it has recently been shown that the auditory system of the fetal guinea pig is also susceptible, *in utero*, to noise exposure (11).

In all of these studies, regardless of whether cochlear physiology, cochlear anatomy, or behavioral discriminations were measured, it appeared that the neonatal ear was more susceptible to permanent trauma than the adult ear. Moreover, the guinea pig experiments suggest that the locus of this early trauma lies in the inner ear, particularly at the level of the outer hair cells. Unfortunately, it is not clear why these cells should be so sensitive early in life. Indeed, there is only one feature of the developing inner ear that appears dynamically related to acoustic trauma: the locus of frequency coding along the basilar papilla of the neonatal chick shifts early in life (30,32). Thus hair cells, which are sensitive to one frequency shortly after hatching, are sensitive to another frequency several weeks later. It is not known whether a similar phenomenon occurs in the developing mammalian cochlea, or whether this observation bears on the early susceptibility of the cochlea to acoustic trauma.

It is important to recognize that the studies cited above tell us that the neonatal ear is more at risk than the adult ear. Since the age at exposure was not specifically varied, the temporal course of that risk remains unknown. In the following sections, however, studies will be described in which the exposure age was specifically manipulated.

TEMPORARY FATIGUE

The permanent losses in cochlear function cited in the preceding section may be only one aspect of a more general process. Younger ears may also be susceptible to overstimulation at sound levels that do not cause permanent hearing loss. The possibility that young ears more readily exhibit temporary threshold shift from exposure to intense sound was addressed in the following experiment (5). Auditory fatigue was examined in 5 groups of neonatal hamsters at selected ages between 15 and 85 days. A recording electrode was placed in the inferior colliculus of anesthetized animals, and the ear was exposed to intense pure tones (10 min of a 3.0 kHz tone at 110 dB SPL). The "visual detection level" of inferior colliculus evoked responses was used to estimate auditory thresholds at a variety of test frequencies. The amount of threshold shift at 4.0 kHz 1 min postexposure was lowest in the 15- and 85-day-old groups and showed complete recovery to preexposure thresholds within 100 min. The threshold shift was significantly greater, and recovery took much longer than 100 min, when 40-day-old pups were exposed to the tone. These data are important, because they indicate that the young cochlea is sensitive to overstimulation at both high and moderate levels of sound exposure. Moreover, the results demonstrate a period of enhanced susceptibility to temporary auditory fatigue that showed a peak around 40 days of age.

SENSITIVE PERIODS

The observation of a heightened period of susceptibility to acoustic trauma as demonstrated in the hamster (5) has also been shown in experiments with other species. These studies, conducted with mice, hamsters, and rats, systematically varied the neonatal age at which the animals were exposed. The recovery interval (between 5 and 14 days), as well as all other test conditions, was held constant for each age group. It has long been known that certain strains of mice can be rendered susceptible to audiogenic seizures by exposure to sound during a specifically defined time after birth (10,21,34). The noise exposure that renders these mice susceptible to seizures is remarkably mild, given the profound effect it has on the animal (90–120 sec of wide- or narrow-band noise between 90 and 110 dB SPL). The frequency range of the noise is also important. In the mouse, for example, exposure to an 8.0- to 16.0-kHz noise band was much more effective than a 2.5- to 5.0-kHz noise band (both were equated for SPL) in producing both seizure behavior and hearing loss (3). It would appear that the most damaging sounds lie in the region of best sensitivity in the animal's audibility curve.

Recent work investigating the physiologic basis of the sensitive period showed that the mouse cochlea was severely damaged by noise exposure during the critical period (27). Furthermore, CM-isopotential thresholds or cochlear nucleus evoked-response thresholds showed a loss between 25 and 40 dB following noise exposure during the sensitive period (35–37). Exposure to the same noise in older animals (40–50 days) had relatively little effect on thresholds (37). The peak of the sensitive period to noise trauma in the C57BL/6J mouse appears to lie between 17 and 19 days, while in the BALB/c mouse it occurs between 21 and 23 days (10). Similar studies have revealed a sensitive period for acoustic trauma in the hamster that is greatest between 30 and 40 days (4,40), and in the rat between 20 and 25 days (23). No traumatic effect was observed in sound-exposed hamsters older than 65 days or rats older than 40 days. The characteristic time course of the sensitive period for acoustic trauma in these three species is illustrated in Fig. 1. In this figure, the percent of maximum threshold loss at the most affected frequency was plotted as a function of age. This frequency varies among species and the reader is referred to the original articles for specific details.

In the mouse, rat, and hamster, the peak of the sensitive period corresponds well with the final stages of functional and structural maturation of the cochlea. The cochlear histopathology observed in both rat and mouse after noise exposure during the sensitive period is generally the same. There is massive outer hair cell damage widely distributed throughout the cochlea (24,27,41). Preliminary evidence also indicates that the same is probably true for the hamster. Remarkably, the inner hair cells appear undamaged. These observations were similar to those reported in the kitten and guinea pig; however, the degree of outer hair cell loss was much greater for the mouse and rat. In the kitten and guinea pig, the age at exposure was not manipulated specifically. As a consequence, the results reported in those investigations may be from neonates, whose age at testing was outside of the most effective time in the sensitive period.

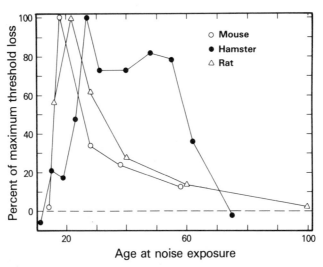

FIG. 1. Time course of the sensitive period for mouse, rat, and hamster. Each curve represents the percent of maximum threshold loss observed, at the most affected frequency, as a function of age. (Redrawn from Saunders and Tilney, ref. 39, with permission.)

Why should hair cells be so susceptible during the sensitive period? There is no answer to this question yet, but several possible explanations exist. Outer hair cells are probably subject to greater mechanical stress than inner hair cells, during stimulation, because of their location on the basilar membrane. Indeed, the outer hair cells are almost always the first to show damage in adult studies of acoustic trauma. Furthermore, the occurrence of outer hair cell damage in neonates could be due to basilar membrane immaturity. If the neonatal basilar membrane were unusually compliant, then its mechanical displacement might be greater than when it is fully developed. It is also hypothesized that outer hair cell damage from acoustic trauma (in adults) may arise from metabolic imbalance in the cell due to overstimulation. Perhaps the metabolic machinery of the neonatal outer hair cell is less well developed than in the adult, and thus it is more sensitive to trauma from acoustic insult. These and other possibilities need to be explored in future work concerned with the underlying mechanisms of the sensitive period.

CENTRAL CONSEQUENCES

In two of the species studied (hamster and mouse), an interesting phenomenon in the central auditory pathway accompanies the loss in peripheral auditory function. There is evidence that outer hair cell pathology in the neonate is correlated with an abnormal growth of auditory evoked-response intensity in central auditory nuclei, and with an abnormal behavioral judgment of loudness (18). These observations are associated with the clinical condition of loudness recruitment (34). Abnormal growth in evoked-response amplitude, with increasing stimulus intensity, has been observed in the inferior colliculus and cochlear nucleus of the mouse and hamster (34,36,46). The interesting feature of this abnormal growth is that at high stimulus levels (i.e., above 100 dB SPL) the response far exceeds that seen in control animals. For example, in the BALB/c mouse exposed to noise at 21 days of age (and tested at 27 days of age), the cochlear nucleus evoked response to a click stimulus at 95 dB SPL averaged 220 μV. Nonexposed control animals at the same age showed a similar evoked-response amplitude to a 95-dB click. At 110 dB SPL, however, the noise-treated subjects exhibited a 510-μV response, whereas the control animals showed only a 305-μV response. This abnormally large response to intense sound in the noise-exposed neonate was called overrecruitment (36). An example of changing evoked response amplitude with stimulus intensity, in control and noise-exposed mice, is presented in Fig. 2. Evoked-response indications of overrecruitment have been observed by others in noise-exposed neonatal animals (19,22,46).

A single-cell analogue of this phenomenon has, unfortunately, not yet emerged. However, in a recent study, sustained afterdischarges in the poststimulus time histograms of inferior colliculus cells were demonstrated in noise-exposed neonatal mice (42). Similar afterdischarges were not seen in inferior colliculus cells of nonexposed control animals. Whether or not this is the cellular counterpart of overrecruitment has yet to be determined. Furthermore, whether or not the occur-

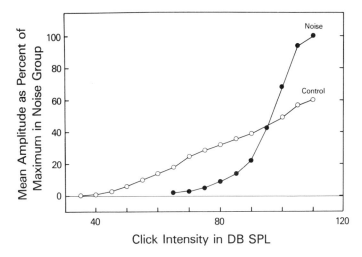

FIG. 2. Growth in evoked-response amplitude as a function of stimulus level. Data were recorded from the cochlear nucleus for a group of noise-exposed and control BALB/c mice. Noise exposure occurred at the height of the sensitive period for this species. Amplitude is plotted as a percent of the maximum response in the noise group. (Redrawn from Saunders and Bock, ref. 34, with permission.)

rence of overrecruitment has a strictly peripheral (cochlear) or central origin is also unresolved. Other aspects of single-cell responses observed after neonatal noise exposure have been considered elsewhere (45).

IS THE DEVELOPING EAR MORE SUSCEPTIBLE TO OTOTOXIC TRAUMA?

Recent evidence suggests that there is a sensitive period for ototoxic insult to the cochlea. Mice of the BALB/c strain were treated with the ototoxic aminoglycoside kanamycin for 16 days (one injection of 400 mg/g per day). Treatment between 5 and 21 days of age resulted in a 40 to 60% loss of outer hair cells in the apical turn, and a 70 to 90% loss in the basal cochlear turn. A 10-day treatment from 17 to 27 days produced a 40% loss of outer hair cells throughout the cochlea (27). In both instances the inner hair cells appeared normal. Unfortunately, age and number of injections were confounded in this study, thus making it difficult to conclude whether the pathology was due to age or to number of injections. Similar massive outer hair cell damage was reported in another study after kanamycin treatment in the neonatal mouse (41).

It has been shown that ototoxic poisoning (typically with kanamycin) can be used to "prime" neonatal mice for audiogenic seizure behavior (6,8,27,41). In addition, measures of the severity of audiogenic seizure behavior following age-dependent injections of kanamycin revealed that BALB/c neonates were at the peak of ototoxic sensitivity between 10 and 14 days of age (7). Kanamycin injections

(400 mg/kg), in a more recent study, were administered over a 4-day interval to mice in three age groups (6–9 days, 10–13 days, and 15–18 days). Fifteen days after the last injection the animals were killed. Scanning electron microscopy was used to evaluate the presence or absence of hair cells along the organ of Corti. Extensive damage to the outer hair cell system was reported in the 10- to 13-day-old group. Some damage to outer hair cells was observed in the 6- to 9-day-old group, and almost no hair-cell pathology was seen in the oldest group (8). In all groups, the inner hair cells appeared normal.

Thus, in BALB/c and C57BL/6J mice it has been shown that audiogenic seizure behavior is in part dependent on the time of ototoxic treatment. Moreover, as with noise exposure, the locus of trauma seen in the receptor organ is centered on the outer hair cells. In both these strains the sensitive period is between 10 and 13 to 14 days postpartum. Electrophysiologic measures from the cochlear nucleus of the C57BL/6J mice (treated from 10 to 13 days and tested at 25 days) revealed an evoked-response threshold shift for test frequencies between 8.0 and 20.0 kHz that averaged about 45 dB. However, unlike early noise exposure, kanamycin treatment did not produce abnormal augmentation of cochlear nucleus evoked-response amplitude at high stimulus levels. There was no indication of overrecruitment (9). This result is not entirely surprising, since it has been shown for some other conditions of early trauma in mice that seizure behavior is always accompanied by threshold loss, but not necessarily by overrecruitment (20). Finally, it is interesting to note that a 16-day treatment (400 mg/kg) of kanamycin in C3H mice caused only minimal outer hair cell loss in the extreme base of the cochlea. These animals were aged between 3 and 4 months at the onset of treatment (15).

Data from the rat have also shown profound hair cell pathology and loss in auditory function following kanamycin treatment between days 11 and 20 postpartum. Identical treatment between days 1 and 10 or between days 15 and 23 had relatively little effect on auditory function or on cochlear structures (28). This sensitive period, defined between 11 and 20 days, has been related to the onset of auditory function in the rat (25).

The profound loss of outer hair cells in these ototoxic poisoning experiments was similar to that observed after noise exposure during the sensitive period. The sensitive period to ototoxic trauma, however, is more difficult to determine precisely, but the initial evidence suggests that it precedes the sensitive period to acoustic trauma in both the mouse and the rat. The observation of a difference in sensitive period timing is important and needs further elaboration, since it suggests different underlying developmental mechanisms for these two traumatic agents. Similarly, the absence of overrecruitment responses in the auditory central nervous system following neonatal kanamycin treatment also needs to be described further. As a final point, there may be a sensitive period for ototoxic exposure in the fetal guinea pig. Drug administration to the mother is very effective in altering the fetal auditory system during the last 3 weeks of pregnancy (43). Unlike the mouse and rat, cochlear development in the guinea pig occurs prior to birth (31).

CONCLUSIONS

The data in rat, mouse, and hamster indicate that the sensitive period of greatest susceptibility to auditory trauma occurs around the time that the cochlea enters its final stages of maturation. If this observation can be generalized to all mammalian ears, then the cochlea of humans may be susceptible to trauma as it reaches its final stages of development between the eleventh and eighth weeks before birth. It must be strongly emphasized, however, that the authors are unaware of direct evidence supporting a period of enhanced susceptibility to acoustic trauma in the human fetus or premature infant. Furthermore, the situation in placental mammals whose inner ear develops during fetal life is complicated by the complexity of the acoustic pathways to the fetal ear. The attenuating properties of the abdominal wall and placental fluids, and the fact that the middle ear is fluid-filled, make it difficult to precisely specify the effective stimulus reaching the fetal ear (1,2,44). These arguments, of course, do not apply to the premature infant. Similarly, antibiotic drug treatment administered to the mother during the last trimester of pregnancy may have a profound influence on the developing cochlea. It has also been suggested that the human neonate and child may be at heightened risk to acoustic trauma (20, 26), and if this is true, it may be due to immaturity in the outer and middle ear rather than enhanced susceptibility of the cochlear receptor cells to trauma (38).

ACKNOWLEDGMENT

This work was supported in part by research awards from the Deafness Research Foundation, the Pennsylvania Lions Hearing Research Foundation, the NINCDS (NS-14843-05), and the Australian Research Grants Committee. Dr. Chen was on leave from the Department of Psychology, Monash University, Clayton, Victoria, Australia. The authors greatly appreciate the assistance of Monica Goodwin and Joseph Locala.

REFERENCES

1. Armitage, S. E., Baldwin, B. A., and Vince, M. A. (1980): The fetal sound environment of sheep. *Science*, 208:1173–1174.
2. Bench, J. (1968): Sound transmission to the human foetus through the maternal abdominal wall. *J. Genet. Psychol.*, 113:85–87.
3. Bock, G. R., and Saunders, J. C. (1976): Effects of low and high frequency noise bands in producing a physiologic correlate of loudness recruitment in mice. *Trans. Am. Acad. Ophthal. Otolaryngol.*, 82:356–362.
4. Bock, G. R., and Saunders, J. C. (1977): A critical period for acoustic trauma in the hamster and its relation to cochlear development. *Science*, 197:396–398.
5. Bock, G. R., and Seifter, E. J. (1978): Developmental changes of susceptibility to auditory fatigue in young hamsters. *Audiology*, 17:193–203.
6. Chen, C.-S., and Aberdeen, G. C. (1980): Potentiation of noise-induced audiogenic seizure risk by salicylate in mice as a function of salicylate-noise exposure interval. *Acta Otolaryngol.*, 90:61–68.
7. Chen, C.-S., and Aberdeen, D. C. (1981): The sensitive period for induction of susceptibility to audiogenic seizures by kanamycin in mice. *Arch. Otorhinolaryngol.*, 232:215–220.
8. Chen, C.-S., and Saunders, J. C. (1983): The sensitive period for ototoxicity of kanamycin in mice: Morphological evidence. *Arch. Otorhinolaryngol.*, 238:217–223.

9. Chen, C.-S., and Saunders, J. C. (1984): Effects of kanamycin on cochlear nuclear evoked responses and behavioral responses in C57BL/6J mice. *Exp. Neurol.*, 83:461–467.
10. Chen, C.-S., and Willott, J. F. (1983): Developmental plasticity: Acoustic priming for audiogenic seizures. In: *The Auditory Psychobiology of the Mouse*, edited by J. F. Willott, pp. 426–469. Charles C. Thomas, Springfield, IL.
11. Cook, R. O., Konishi, T., Salt, A. N., and Hamm, C. W., Lebetkin, E. H., and Koo, J. (1982): Brainstem evoked responses of guinea pigs exposed to high noise levels *in utero*. *Devel. Psychobiol.*, 15:95–104.
12. Danto, J., and Carazzo, A. J. (1977): Auditory effects of noise on infant and adult guinea pigs. *J. Am. Audiol. Soc.*, 3:99–101.
13. Dodson, H. C., Bannister, L. H., and Douek, E. E. (1978): Further studies of the effects of continuous white noise of moderate intensity (70–80 dB SPL) on the cochlea in young guinea pigs. *Acta Otolaryngol.*, 86:195–200.
14. Douek, E., Bannister, L. H., Dodson, H. C., Ashcroft, P., and Humphries, K. N. (1976): The effects of incubator noise on the cochlea of the newborn. *Lancet*, 2:1110–1113.
15. Ehret, G. (1979): Correlations between cochlear hair cell loss and shifts of masked and absolute behavioral thresholds in the house mouse. *Acta Otolaryngol.*, 87:28–36.
16. Falk, S. A., Cook, R. V., Haseman, J. D., and Sanders, G. M. (1974): Noise-induced inner ear damage in newborn and adult guinea pigs. *Laryngoscope*, 84:444–453.
17. Hawkins, J. E, Jr., and Johnson, L.-G. (1976): Microdissection and surface preparation of the inner ear. In: *Handbook of Auditory and Vestibular Research Methods*, edited by C. A. Smith and J. A. Vernon, pp. 5–22. Charles C. Thomas, Springfield, IL.
18. Henry, K. R. (1972): Pinna reflex thresholds and audiogenic seizures: Developmental changes after acoustic priming. *J. Comp. Physiol. Psychol.*, 79:77–81.
19. Henry, K. R. (1972): Unilateral increase of auditory sensitivity following early auditory exposure. *Science*, 176:689–690.
20. Henry, K. R. (1983): Abnormal auditory development resulting from exposure to ototoxic chemicals, noise, and auditory restriction. In: *Development of Auditory and Vestibular Systems*, edited by R. Romand, pp. 273–308. Academic Press, New York.
21. Henry, K. R., and Bowman, R. E. (1970): Acoustic priming of audiogenic seizures in mice. In: *Physiological Effects of Noise*, edited by B. L. Welch and A. S. Welch, pp. 185–203. Plenum Press, New York.
22. Henry, K. R., and Saleh, M. (1973): Recruitment deafness: Functional effect of priming-induced audiogenic seizures in mice. *J. Comp. Physiol. Psychol.*, 84:430–435.
23. Lenoir, M., Bock, G. R., and Pujol, R. (1979): Supra-normal susceptibility to acoustic trauma of the rat pup cochlea. *J. Physiol. (Paris)*, 75:521–524.
24. Lenoir, M., and Pujol, R. (1980): Sensitive period to acoustic trauma in the rat pup cochlea. *Acta Otolaryngol.*, 89:357–362.
25. Marot, M., Uziel, A., and Romand, R. (1980): Ototoxicity of kanamycin in developing rats: Relationship with the onset of auditory function. *Hearing Res.*, 2:111–113.
26. Mills, J. H. (1975): Noise and children: A review of literature. *J. Acoust. Soc. Am.*, 58:767–779.
27. Norris, C. H., Cawthon, T. H., and Carroll, R. C. (1977): Kanamycin priming for audiogenic seizures in mice. *Neuropharmacology*, 16:375–380.
28. Osako, S., Tokimoto, T., and Matsuura, S. (1979): Effects of kanamycin on the auditory evoked responses during postnatal development of the hearing of the rat. *Acta Otolaryngol.*, 88:359–366.
29. Price, G. R. (1976): Age as a factor in susceptibility to hearing loss: Young versus adult ears. *J. Acoust. Soc. Am.*, 60:886–892.
30. Rebillard, G., Ryals, B. M., and Rubel, E. W. (1982): Relationship between hair cell loss on the chick basilar papilla and threshold shift after acoustic overstimulation. *Hearing Res.*, 8:77–81.
31. Romand, R. (1971): Maturation des potentiels cochléaires dans la période périnatale chez le chat et chez le coboye. *J. Physiol. (Paris)*, 63:763–782.
32. Rubel, E. W., and Ryals, B. M. (1983): Development of the place principle: Acoustic trauma. *Science*, 219:512–513.
33. Saunders, J. C. (1974): The physiological effect of priming for audiogenic seizure in mice. *Laryngoscope*, 84:750–756.
34. Saunders, J. C., and Bock, G. R. (1978): Influences of early auditory trauma on auditory development. In: *Studies on the Development of Behavior and the Nervous System, Vol. 4: Early Influences*, edited by G. Gottlieb, pp. 249–287. Academic Press, New York.

35. Saunders, J. C., Bock, G. R., Chen, C. S., and Gates, G. R. (1972): The effects of priming for audiogenic seizures on cochlear and behavioral responses in BALB/c mice. *Exp. Neurol.*, 36:426–436.
36. Saunders, J. C., Bock, G. R., James, R., and Chen, C. S. (1972): The effects of priming for audiogenic seizures on auditory evoked responses in the cochlear nucleus and inferior colliculus of BALB/mice. *Exp. Neurol.*, 37:388–394.
37. Saunders, J. C., and Hirsch, K. A. (1976): Changes in cochlear microphonic sensitivity after priming C57BL/6J mice at various ages for audiogenic seizures. *J. Comp. Physiol. Psychol.*, 90:212–220.
38. Saunders, J. C., Kaltenbach, J. A., and Relkin, E. M. (1983): The structural and functional development of the outer and middle ear. In: *Development of the Auditory and Vestibular Systems*, edited by R. Romand, pp. 3–25. Academic Press, New York.
39. Saunders, J. C., and Tilney, L. G. (1982): Species differences in susceptibility to noise exposure. In: *New Perspectives on Noise-Induced Hearing Loss*, edited by R. P. Hamernik, D. Henderson, and R. Salvi, pp. 229–248. Raven Press, New York.
40. Stanek, R., Bock, G. R., Goran, M. L., and Saunders, J. C. (1977): Age dependent susceptibility to auditory trauma in the hamster: Behavioral and electrophysiologic consequences. *Trans. Am. Acad. Ophthalmol. Otolaryngol.*, 84:465–472.
41. Tepper, J. M., and Schlesinger, K. (1980): Acoustic priming and kanamycin-induced cochlear damage. *Brain Res.*, 187:81–95.
42. Urban, G. P., and Willott, J. F. (1979): Response properties of neurons in the inferior colliculi of mice made susceptible to audiogenic seizures by acoustic priming. *Exp. Neurol.*, 63:229–243.
43. Uziel, A., Romand, R., and Marot, M. (1979): Electrophysiological study of the ototoxicity of kanamycin during development in guinea pigs. *Hearing Res.*, 1:203–207.
44. Walker, D., Grimwade, J., and Wood, C. (1971): Intrauterine noise: A component of the fetal environment. *Am. J. Obstet. Gynecol.*, 109:91–95.
45. Willott, J. F. (1983): Central nervous system physiology. In: *The Auditory Psychobiology of the Mouse*, edited by J. F. Willott, pp. 305–340. Charles C. Thomas, Springfield, IL.
46. Willott, J. F., and Henry, K. R. (1974): Auditory evoked potentials: Developmental changes of threshold and amplitude following early acoustic trauma. *J. Comp. Physiol. Psychol.*, 86:1–7.

Toxicology of the Eye, Ear, and Other Special Senses, edited by A. W. Hayes. Raven Press, New York © 1985.

Clinical Assessment of Auditory Dysfunction

William G. Thomas

Division of Otolaryngology, School of Medicine, University of North Carolina, Chapel Hill, North Carolina 27514

Clinical assessment of auditory dysfunction is a broad topic, potentially covering many different methods of assessment and many types of auditory dysfunction. It is well known that auditory dysfunction can be caused by literally hundreds of different problems or pathologies. Auditory dysfunction can occur as a result of peripheral or central pathologies, or it can occur as a local manifestation of some systemic disease. Auditory dysfunction can be caused by extrinsic factors (infections, drugs, trauma, tumors, neurologic diseases, metabolic diseases, etc.) or intrinsic factors (genetic, etc.). Auditory dysfunction may be congenital or acquired. If congenital, it may be genetic, with hearing loss occurring alone, as in the case of Mondini's aplasia; in the form of a syndrome with other abnormalities, such as Usher's syndrome; or as a chromosomal abnormality. It may also be congenital but nongenetic, with hearing loss occurring alone, in the case of many ototoxic agents; or occurring with a host of other abnormalities, as in the case of maternal rubella, anoxia, bacterial infections, and metabolic disorders. As indicated, auditory dysfunction may also be acquired: either genetic or nongenetic. If genetic, hearing loss may occur alone, as in the case of familial progressive sensorineural deafness; or it may occur in conjunction with other abnormalities, as in the case of Alport's syndrome. If nongenetic, hearing loss may occur as a result of numerous pathologies, including inflammatory diseases, ototoxicity, neoplastic disorders, traumatic injury, metabolic disorders, vascular insufficiency, or central nervous system diseases (e.g., multiple sclerosis).

It is obvious that the exact cause of a specific auditory dysfunction is frequently impossible to determine. It is also of interest to note that toxic agents may cause congenital or acquired auditory dysfunction. The topic of concern here is ototoxicity. Therefore, the remainder of this chapter will deal specifically with this topic. It should be remembered, however, that the same clinical assessment is appropriate to a wide range of auditory dysfunctions and not specific to those caused by ototoxicity.

OTOTOXICITY

It is probably safe to say that the action of any substance on an organ or cell can be either detrimental or beneficial, depending on many factors. Some controversy continues, however, as to whether any chemical, drug, substance, or agent has a beneficial effect on the inner ear. Recent literature would indicate that nearly 200 substances have some documentation in the medical literature of ototoxicity (11,40,41). Although these cannot be fully described in this chapter, they can be separated into general categories. These include chemicals (carbon monoxide, alcohol, nicotine, arsenic, potassium bromate, etc.), heavy metals (lead, tin, gold, mercury, etc.), antibiotics, diuretics, analgesics and antipyretics (salicylates, quinine, etc.), antineoplastics (bleomycin, nitrogen mustard, *cis*-platinum), and miscellaneous drugs (pentobarbital, hexadine, etc.). The literature on chemical or drug ototoxicity for antibiotics and diuretics is extensive. The aminoglycosides have received the majority of attention; however, other antibiotics, such as vancomycin, erythromycin, chloramphenicol, polymyxin B, and ampicillin, have also been indicated as potentially ototoxic. Diuretics have also received substantial research as potentially ototoxic. Specifically, furosemide and ethacrynic acid have been shown to have ototoxic properties, or at least to potentiate ototoxicity. However, other diuretics, such as mannitol and the mercurials, may be ototoxic. Perhaps the greatest body of literature with regard to ototoxic effects concerns exposure to noise. Auditory dysfunction following noise exposure has been documented for more than 100 years.

It is an understatement, but also an accurate statement, to describe the action of any chemical, drug, or other agent as extremely complex, with many variables contributing to potential ototoxic effects. The mechanisms of action of ototoxic substances or agents may involve the entire organ, specific cells within the organ, components of specific cells, or individual biochemical pathways. The action has been related to overall dose, duration of exposure, blood serum levels in the case of chemicals, drugs, or heavy metals, general health of the subject and underlying disease, age of subject, prior exposure, renal impairment, individual susceptibility, and, of course, possible potentiation and synergistic effects of combinations of chemicals, drugs, and other agents. All of these factors create a rather confusing picture with regard to true ototoxic effects and may explain, to some extent, apparent disagreements within the literature.

Auditory dysfunctions resulting from ototoxic agents usually present as tinnitus, hearing loss, and/or vertigo. Cochlear damage usually results from an orderly progression of hair cell loss in the organ of Corti beginning in the basal turn and progressing toward the apex. Injury to other cochlear structures has been demonstrated, including changes in the stria vascularis, suprastrial portion of the spiral ligament, pericapillary tissues of the spiral prominence, outer sulcus cells, and Reissner's membrane. In addition, vestibular damage may occur, specifically in the type I hair cells of the cristae ampullaris and in the utricle (15,16). Auditory dysfunction resulting from ototoxic agents almost always results in sensorineural pathology. In most cases this loss is bilateral and symmetric, although there are exceptions reported in the literature. Hearing loss caused by chemical or heavy metal toxicity may involve brainstem or central pathology and is usually associated with a variety of other neurologic manifestations.

CLINICAL TEST BATTERY

Clinical assessment of auditory dysfunction follows an orderly progression of tests to identify the site of disorder. While the shape of the auditory function may give information regarding possible pathology or etiology, auditory tests are designed to give primary information as to site-of-lesion. For example, auditory tests may indicate the primary source of pathology in the cochlea. These results, however, give no indication as to type of pathology (i.e., hair cell damage, damage to stria vascularis, rupture of Reissner's membrane, etc.), nor do they give information regarding possible etiology, since many factors, including ototoxicity, can cause damage to the cochlea. As a point of major differentiation, auditory tests are designed to separate peripheral and central auditory disorders. The major point of demarcation between peripheral and central disorders is the synapse at the cochlear nucleus between the first and second order neurons. With this definition, pathologies in the external ear, middle ear, inner ear, and auditory nerve would be considered peripheral disorders, and pathologies in the brain stem and cortex would be considered central disorders. Other auditory tests are designed to help differentiate site-of-lesion within the peripheral or central auditory system. As defined, auditory dysfunction in the peripheral system might be expected to show the following characteristics: ipsilateral symptoms, usual loss of sensitivity, distortion present in cochlear and auditory nerve disorders, and abnormal adaptation or fatigue in cochlear and auditory nerve disorders. Central auditory dysfunction might be characterized by contralateral symptoms, frequently normal sensitivity, and dysfunction in ability to transmit complex stimuli. Differences in characteristics of peripheral and central auditory dysfunctions have led to development of different auditory test batteries. In peripheral testing, pure tone stimuli can conveniently be used. Central testing, however, usually requires more subtle changes in stimuli and the use of complex stimuli (20).

The classic peripheral auditory test battery contains tests to differentiate between conductive, cochlear, and retrocochlear hearing loss. In addition, tests are available to aid in differentiating sites-of-lesion within these three major areas.[1] A typical test battery might include the following tests:

Pure Tone Thresholds

Pure tone air conduction testing is used to measure the sensitivity of the ear to different frequencies, when compared to normal hearing. Air conduction testing uses the entire auditory system (i.e., external ear, middle ear, inner ear, VIIIth nerve, and central systems). Pure tone bone conduction testing is used to measure the sensitivity of the ear to different frequencies when the external ear and middle ear have been bypassed and sound is transmitted directly to the inner ear, although

---

[1]For a complete description of auditory tests, the reader is referred to several standard audiology textbooks (20,30,33).

this is an oversimplification. The difference between air and bone conduction scores is the first evidence of conductive or sensorineural hearing loss.

Speech Reception Threshold (SRT)

The sensitivity of the ear to speech material is measured. The speech materials generally used are spondee words (i.e., two-syllable words with equal emphasis on each syllable, like baseball, airplane, etc.). The speech reception threshold should agree with the average pure tone air conduction results at 500, 1,000, and 2,000 Hz.

Speech Discrimination (SD)

The ability of a subject to transmit and understand complex stimuli (speech) is measured. Speech discrimination lists are presented at a level above threshold so that they can be heard without difficulty, usually 40 dB sensation level (SL), and the patient's articulation ability is measured. The speech materials generally used are short, single-syllable, phonetically balanced words.

Alternate Binaural Loudness Balance (ABLB)

The presence or absence of loudness recruitment is measured by having the subject balance the loudness of a standard tone in one ear with an alternating tone in the pathologic ear. The presence of loudness recruitment is measured by the growth of loudness in the pathologic ear. One contraindication of this test is that it is difficult to use and the results are questionable in bilaterally symmetrical hearing losses.

Short Increment Sensitivity Index (SISI)

The SISI test measures the ability of a subject to detect a 1 dB change in intensity at a level 20 dB above threshold. This test can be used at any frequency in either ear, regardless of the asymmetry of the hearing loss. A positive SISI score (i.e., above 60%) is an indication of cochlear pathology. Several modifications have been made to the classic SISI procedure (36).

Tone Decay (TD)

Tone decay measures the fatigue or adaptation of the auditory system to a constant stimulus. Tone decay is measured as the decay in decibels from threshold over a 1-min period. A positive tone decay (i.e., greater than 25 dB) is an indication of VIIIth nerve disorder. Modifications to this original technique have been reported in the literature (23,42,49).

Bekesy Tracings

The Bekesy tracings indicate threshold sensitivity measured on an automatic audiometer when the tones are pulsed and when they are continuous. Theoretically, the pathologic auditory system should show more adaptation to a continuous tone than to a pulsed tone. Particular patterns of tracings have been identified with conductive, cochlear, and retrocochlear pathology. The automatic Bekesy audiometer is essentially under the control of the subject. The subject is instructed to press a button when he hears a tone and release the button when the tone disappears. In this way the patient automatically traces his threshold for pulsed and continuous tones. Thus, the audiometer can be used in several different ways:

Sweep Frequency

The audiometer automatically sweeps through frequencies from 100 to 10,000 Hz, with the subject controlling the intensity. Pulse tones are used first, then continuous tones are plotted on the same audiogram, showing the amount of adaptation between pulsed and continuous tones (19).

Fixed Frequency

The audiometer can be set for one particular frequency, and thresholds for pulsed and continuous tones are plotted as a function of time. The purpose is to look at the amount of adaptation occurring at one particular frequency (19).

Backward Sweep

The audiometer can also be swept from 10,000 to 100 Hz, showing whether the adaptation is a function of time or frequency (24).

Most Comfortable Loudness

The subject is instructed to keep the tone at his most comfortable loudness, which makes this a suprathreshold test. This modification is based on the concept that abnormal adaptation first appears only at high intensities and eventually appears at lower levels, until it finally appears at threshold. Abnormal decay of a continuous tone at suprathreshold levels is an indication of VIIIth nerve pathology (23).

Impedance

The study of impedance in the auditory system involves an analysis of the acceptance or rejection by this system of the flow of energy per unit of time. In other words, how much is the flow of energy impeded by this particular system? A system with high impedance rejects or reflects the majority of energy, whereas a system with low impedance accepts or absorbs most of the energy and reflects less. Normally, there are three components that combine to determine the impedance of a particular system—resistance, stiffness, and inertia or mass. In order to accomplish this clinically, a probe is placed in the external canal and sealed. The probe emits a low-frequency tone (usually 220 Hz) and a microphone in the probe measures the reflected sound from the tympanic membrane. The amount of sound reflected gives an indication of the integrity of the middle ear. Normally, four measures may be made—static compliance, tympanometry, acoustic reflex threshold, and acoustic reflex decay.

Static Compliance

Static compliance of the middle ear is a measure of mobility. Mass (inertia), resistance (friction), and stiffness (or its reciprocal, compliance) work together in a complex manner to facilitate or impede motion of the middle ear system, as measured at the tympanic membrane (MT). Historically, static compliance has been termed acoustic impedance or absolute impedance, although the term compliance is a more descriptive term of what is actually measured. Static compliance is used to denote a single number representing the mobility of the middle ear system. Tympanometry is also a measure of compliance; however, this measure is made over numerous values as the MT moves in response to changes in air pressure and thus is a measure of dynamic compliance.

Static compliance of the middle ear system is measured by quantifying the sound energy reflected from the MT. When the middle ear system is stiff, more energy is reflected rather than absorbed or transmitted through the middle ear. Therefore, a stiff middle ear system is said to have low compliance or high resistance. A flaccid middle ear mechanism absorbs more energy and reflects less. Therefore, this system has high compliance or low resistance.

Static compliance can be measured in terms of equivalent volume of air in cubic centimeters or in acoustic ohms. This test requires two measurements: one measurement is made with the MT in a position of low compliance by exerting an air pressure of + 200 mm of water in the external ear relative to the middle ear; the second measurement is made with the MT in a position of maximum compliance (normally at 0 mm of water). Neither of these two measures has any significance when taken alone. However, by subtracting one measure from the other, the external ear canal volume is effectively cancelled, thus allowing a measurement value of the middle ear mechanism. The compliance of the normal middle ear system is influenced by many variables, including age, sex, etc. In general, however, normal static compliance values range between 0.26 and 1.5 cc. A stiff middle ear system should have a compliance less than 0.26 cc, while a flaccid middle ear system should have a compliance greater than 1.5 cc. The normal range of absolute impedance in acoustic ohms is approximately 600 to 3,000 ohms. Absolute values below 600 ohms indicate a very compliant ear, whereas values above 3,000 ohms indicate a resistive middle ear system.

Tympanometry

Tympanometry is the measurement of eardrum compliance as the air pressure is altered in the external ear relative to the middle ear. These measurements are normally recorded on a graph that represents compliance versus air pressure function, called a *tympanogram*. A point of significance is that the MT is at maximum compliance when the air pressure in the middle ear is equal to that in the external ear. Tympanometry can provide an indirect measure of existing middle ear pressure by identifying the air pressure in the external canal at which the eardrum shows its maximum compliance. Subjects who have intact MTs, with no middle ear pathology and adequate eustachian tube function, will show maximum compliance at atmospheric pressure or within ± 50 mm of atmospheric pressure. Subjects with intact MTs and poor eustachian tube function will show maximum compliance at negative air pressure values. Subjects with fluid in the middle ear will usually not reach a point of maximum compliance, to the maximum of the instrumentation, while those with a resistive type middle ear pathology will show very low compliance (high stiffness or resistance) at normal atmospheric pressure.

Acoustic Reflex Threshold

The stapedial muscle contracts reflexively when the ear is stimulated with a sufficiently loud sound. In normal ears, the acoustic reflex can be elicited with stimulation at sensation levels of 70 to 95 dB. Contraction of the middle ear muscles decreases the compliance of the MT. This contraction occurs bilaterally. In the demonstration of the acoustic reflex, the sudden change in the relative compliance of the middle ear created by the muscle contractions is utilized. If the acoustic signal is sufficiently loud to elicit the bilateral acoustic reflex, the resulting contraction of the stapedius muscle in the probe ear will suddenly decrease the compliance at the MT synchronously with the presentation of the stimulus, and this change in relative compliance can be observed as a sudden deflection in the balance meter. The acoustic reflex can be elicited by either contralateral stimulus presentation or ipsilateral stimulus presentation at approximately the same stimulus levels. Also, the reflex may be elicited with pure tone stimuli or with noise.

Reflex Decay

Reflex decay is a truly remarkable phenomenon. In normal ears, contraction of the middle ear muscles to an auditory stimulus of 1,000 Hz or lower can be maintained for up to 45 sec without obvious decay, fatigue, or adaptation. In subjects with retrocochlear lesions and some cochlear lesions, the reflex appears normal when first turned on. When the acoustic stimulus is sustained, however, reflex amplitude declines and may eventually disappear. Klockoff (32) and Anderson et al. (1) advocate the use of reflex decay as an indicator of VIIIth nerve lesions. These authors have reported a decay in the acoustic reflex for patients with VIIIth nerve pathology when a stimulus is presented at a reflex sensation level of 10 dB for 10 sec. When a stimulus is presented in this manner, the amplitude of the reflex decays to a level of 50% or less of the original amplitude in less than 10 sec in pathologic ears. The same results have been found in normal ears at 4,000 Hz, and to a lesser degree at 2,000 Hz. No significant decay is observed in normal ears at 500 and 1,000 Hz, however.

PI-PB Function

The PI-PB function test is a special use of speech discrimination. This abbreviation refers to Performance versus Intensity for Phonetically Balanced words and simply refers to the discrimination test given at several different intensities. In the case of cochlear pathology, the function should reach a plateau with increased intensity and remain there, while in VIIIth nerve pathology, the discrimination score becomes worse at high intensities (22).

Tests for central auditory dysfunction will not be discussed in this chapter. The reader is referred to several excellent texts describing these tests (31,48). The majority of tests used to identify central auditory dysfunction use complex stimuli like speech because changes in the central nervous system are usually subtle. In general, the speech material is changed in some way to reduce its redundancy and increase its ability to detect subtle changes. Tests have been designed that alter speech stimuli in many ways. These include submerging the speech material in a background of noise, combining the speech material with a competing message of different speech material in either the contralateral or ipsilateral ear, filtering the speech material to reduce its intelligibility, interrupting the speech material, accelerating the speech material, presenting different frequency bands of speech to different ears, and presenting two different speech messages simultaneously to the two ears (dichotic speech). Some toxic substances are known to affect the central nervous system more than the peripheral system. These include carbon monoxide and heavy metals. In these cases complete clinical assessment would include central auditory tests.

Several more recent auditory tests appear to show promise in enhancing the clinical assessment of auditory dysfunction. The most prominent appears to be the auditory brainstem evoked response (BSER, BAER, BER, or ABR). This is one of several evoked responses that have been identified in the auditory system. At present, the following responses have been identified: (a) auditory nerve response (latency 1–4 msec), (b) brainstem or fast responses (latency 2–12 msec), (c) middle responses (latency 12–50 msec), (d) sonomotor or muscle responses (latency 10–50 msec), (e) slow auditory responses (latency 50–300 msec), and (f) contingent negative variation (CNV) (latency 300–600 msec) (5,37).

One of the more stable evoked potential measures is the brainstem response. This is a series of vertex-positive waves following a click or tone burst with latencies from 1 to 10 msec (5,6,25–28,37,38). To date, seven different waves have been identified and associated with various nuclei in the auditory brainstem system (37,38). The most prominent and visible wave of this series occurs with a latency of approximately 5.5 msec and has been identified as wave V (17,43,44). It is assumed to originate in the vicinity of the inferior colliculus and is a good candidate for assessing the higher auditory frequency responses occurring in the basal turn of the cochlea. Other waves have been ascribed to the auditory nerve (wave I), cochlear nucleus (wave II), trapezoid body (wave III), lateral lemniscus (wave IV), and medial geniculate (wave VI). The utility of the brainstem response as a clinical tool seems to be enhanced since the response is extremely stable, is not unusually affected by state of sleep, can be recorded from unconscious patients, shows a maturational development, can be recorded in a relatively short period of time, and includes waves that are associated with various nuclei in the auditory system of the brainstem (45,47).

The latencies of the various waves of the brainstem evoked response are extremely stable from test to test in the same subject and between subjects. In fact, the standard deviations around these mean latencies range from 0.1 to 0.3 msec (13,46). In addition, the latency changes in a predictable manner as the intensity of the stimulus is increased or decreased. This latency versus intensity relationship makes the ABR a valuable tool in assessing hearing function of difficult-to-test subjects. For example, the mean latency of the V wave in normal hearing subjects at 70 dB above threshold is approximately 5.5 msec. As intensity is decreased to 10 dB above threshold, the latency increases to approximately 8.0 msec (39). Therefore, a measure of the latency of the V wave in a difficult-to-test subject would give some estimate of the subject's threshold for that particular stimulus. In addition, the latency of the various waves of the ABR, particularly the V wave, has been shown to exhibit recruitment (39). The presence of this phenomenon can give a good indication as to whether the pathology is of cochlear origin.

Another important aspect of the ABR is the neural transmission time. This is a measure of the latency between the I wave (i.e., primary auditory nerve) and the other waves, thus giving a measure of the travel time in the auditory brainstem system. This measure has proved valuable in assessing the site of pathologies in the brainstem, such as acoustic tumors, multiple sclerosis, and brainstem vascular and neoplastic lesions. In very young children, this transmission time is also delayed, probably because of incomplete maturation or myelination of the central auditory pathways. This latency reaches normal adult values, however, around 1 year of age. Increased neural transmission time in older children or adults with normal latencies for the I wave may be an indication of lack of maturation, demyelinating pathologies, or the presence of space-occupying lesions.

Another potentially important addition to the auditory test battery for clinical assessment is the use of high-frequency audiometry. This measurement of auditory function in the frequencies from 8,000 to 20,000 Hz has potential significance for both clinical and research testing. Changes in high-frequency auditory thresholds have been described as an early indication of ototoxic effects of certain drugs and noise exposure (4,12,18). This procedure has been used by several investigators; however, it is not yet completely accepted as a clinical measure because of difficulties in instrumentation (8,10,14,34). This procedure, with adequate and stable instrumentation, could serve as a valuable tool in the early detection of auditory dysfunction resulting from some form of ototoxicity (7,9,35).

CLINICAL ASSESSMENT

As previously stated, clinical assessment of auditory dysfunction usually includes a progressive battery of tests designed to indicate site-of-lesion. The first order of priority is to determine the amount of auditory dysfunction, if any, and the extent of this dysfunction. This is normally accomplished with pure tone thresholds for various frequencies, speech reception thresholds, and speech discrimination scores. By assuming an auditory dysfunction is present, the second order of priority is to determine if this dysfunction is conductive, sensorineural, mixed, or central. A mixed-type hearing loss has components of both conductive and sensorineural origin, since these types of hearing losses are not mutually exclusive. This is normally accomplished with pure tone bone conduction thresholds and the impedance test battery. For a conductive hearing impairment, pure tone bone conduction thresholds should be normal or near normal in the presence of abnormal pure tone air conduction thresholds. Speech reception thresholds should agree within ± 10 dB of average air conduction thresholds at 500, 1,000, and 2,000 Hz, and speech discrimination should be normal (90–100%). The impedance test battery should show abnormal static compliance (either resistive or compliant, depending on the nature of the hearing loss); tympanometry should be abnormal (showing a very compliant system, a very resistive system, negative pressure, or the presence of middle ear effusions, depending on the site and type of dysfunction); acoustic reflex should be absent (depending on extent of conductive hearing loss); and acoustic reflex decay will obviously not be measured if the reflex is absent. Literature has indicated that a very mild conductive hearing loss will cause the absence of the acoustic reflex in the affected ear (21). At this point a specific treatment protocol is indicated, since the majority of conductive hearing losses can be medically or surgically treated. Also, there is no concrete evidence of conductive hearing losses resulting from ototoxicity.

Should auditory tests indicate a sensorineural hearing loss, the third order of priority is to distinguish between cochlear and retrocochlear involvement. In the case of sensorineural hearing loss, pure tone air conduction thresholds should be abnormal, although they may vary from normal to total deafness in retrocochlear lesions. Pure tone bone conduction thresholds should agree reasonably well with air conduction, indicating no involvement of the external or middle ear. Speech reception thresholds should agree with average pure tone thresholds, and speech discrimination will usually be abnormal. In the case of cochlear involvement, speech discrimination will usually vary between 50 and 90%, while it is not unusual for retrocochlear involvement to show speech discrimination scores much lower than 50%. The impedance test battery will usually show specific types of patterns for cochlear and retrocochlear involvements. In both cases, static compliance and tympanometry should be normal, since there is presumably no middle ear involvement. Cochlear involvement, usually accompanied by loudness recruitment, will normally show the presence of an acoustic reflex, assuming the hearing loss does not exceed 75 to 85 dB. One indication of cochlear involvement is the presence of acoustic reflexes at abnormally low levels (21). If the reflex is present in cochlear hearing loss, it will normally show no significant decay. Retrocochlear lesions, on the other hand, will frequently present with an absence of reflex, even in the presence of sufficient hearing to elicit this reflex. If the reflex is present in retrocochlear lesions, it usually decays abnormally.

The use of the classic diagnostic test battery is also helpful in distinguishing between cochlear and retrocochlear lesions. Usually the tests that indicate an abnormal sensitivity to changes in loudness (ABLB, SISI, and, to some extent, the Bekesy) will show abnormal results in cochlear lesions. The ABLB will normally show the presence of loudness recruitment in the affected ear, and the SISI will show a high percentage of small intensity increments detected (greater than 60%). In classic retrocochlear lesions these tests are usually normal, since abnormal sensitivity to loudness changes is associated with cochlear pathology. Tests that show abnormal adaptation, such as the tone decay and, to some extent, the Bekesy, will usually show no abnormal tone decay (less than 25 dB) and a type II Bekesy tracing in cochlear lesions. Retrocochlear lesions will normally indicate abnormal fatigue or adaptation on the tone decay (greater than 25 dB) and show type III or type IV Bekesy tracings. The PI-PB also shows unique results for cochlear and retrocochlear lesions. For cochlear lesions, this function will normally reach a maximum discrimination and plateau or show a very slight decline. For retrocochlear lesions, however, this function will usually reach a maximum, although at a low discrimination level, and show a severe decline or rollover as intensity is increased.

The brainstem evoked response has become one of the most reliable tests in differentiating cochlear and retrocochlear lesions. In conductive hearing losses, the results are often quite variable, since it may be difficult to present stimuli at sufficient levels to elicit adequate responses. In cochlear lesions, especially those exhibiting loudness recruitment, ABR results are usually normal and may even show a decreased latency when compared to the level of stimulation. In retrocochlear lesions, the ABR usually indicates abnormal latency measures, especially for waves III, IV, and V. This test is obviously useful in indicating other types of lesions in the brain stem that might alter amplitude of response or latency of response. These may include space-occupying lesions and demyelinating lesions.

As previously indicated, the majority of ototoxic substances or agents have their direct effect on various parts of the cochlea, with the noted exceptions. Although clinical assessment cannot differentiate between various pathologies or etiologies affecting the cochlea, results should indicate cochlear pathology in the presence of ototoxic substances or agents. The shape of the audiometric function frequently can give an indication of toxic damage to the inner ear. Noise exposure, for example, usually shows a characteristic audiogram with the greatest loss at 3,000, 4,000, or 6,000 Hz, whereas ototoxicity from drugs or chemicals shows a progressive hearing loss as a function of frequency, frequently severe in nature. This hearing loss is usually accompanied by tinnitus and occasionally by vertigo.

In clinical assessment of auditory dysfunction, including that caused by ototoxicity, several points should be made. In this section, descriptions such as frequently, usually, and normally are used repeatedly. This has not resulted from lack of vocabulary, but because of the variability in auditory tests. Review of pertinent literature indicates that any single auditory test, taken alone, shows the classic result in 60 to 90% of cases (2,3,20,29). This means that a relatively high percentage of subjects (10–40%) may show retrocochlear signs on some tests when they have cochlear lesions, or cochlear signs when they have retrocochlear lesions. In addition, the nature of the lesion itself may cause damage in more than one anatomic area. An acoustic tumor, for example, which should indicate a retrocochlear lesion, may also compromise the blood supply to the cochlea, causing cochlear damage. In this case, the test results would be quite variable and show indications on various tests of both cochlear and retrocochlear lesions. The first point, therefore, is that the entire test battery should be considered in the assessment, with less weight to the results of a single test. The percentage of false positive and false negative results drops significantly when expected results are found on two, three, or four of the tests in the battery. The second point is that test results should be interpreted in conjunction with a detailed case history. While an auditory test battery may give an indication as to site-of-lesion, the case history and other pertinent data may shed light on the possible etiology.

The third major point in clinical assessment of auditory dysfunction, particularly in the case of ototoxicity, is the development of adequate testing protocols. Toxic effects on the human auditory system are quite variable and the presence and extent of damage depend on many parameters. Toxic effects may occur immediately, as in the case of many diuretics, within days, as in the case of various drugs and chemicals, or over years, as in the case of heavy metal toxicity and noise exposure. In addition, decrease in auditory function may continue for months after the toxic substance has been removed. Therefore, hearing assessment to detect changes in auditory sensitivity should be on a regular basis, depending on the substance or agent involved. In the case of aminoglycosides, diuretics, and certain antibiotics and antineoplastics, testing should probably occur on a weekly basis while the subject is on the drug, and monthly up to six months after cessation of the drug. In the case of analgesics and antipyretics, monthly to quarterly testing is probably adequate. Exposure to noise or heavy metal toxicity may require annual testing, although testing for heavy metal toxicity may depend on the blood levels. It is also obvious that preexposure assessment would be ideal, to separate changes in auditory function attributed to the ototoxic agent from preexisting auditory dysfunction and to serve as a baseline for comparison of changes in auditory function. However, in many cases of life-threatening illness or infection, documented decreases in auditory function resulting from the therapy may be purely academic.

SUMMARY

Many drugs, chemicals, substances, and agents are potentially toxic to the human auditory system. The extent of toxicity depends on numerous factors. With few exceptions, toxicity in the auditory system affects various organs or cells within the cochlea or vestibular system, with brainstem and other central nervous system involvement reported with some chemicals, substances, and agents. This ototoxicity usually presents as a decrease in auditory sensitivity, tinnitus, and/or vertigo or loss of balance. Classic and newer audiologic techniques used in clinical assessment are beneficial in specifying the site-of-lesion in the cochlea, although auditory test results, themselves, give little information regarding possible pathology or etiology within the cochlea. Typically, ototoxicity results in high-frequency hearing loss, progressive as a function of frequency, usually accompanied by tinnitus and occasionally by vertigo or loss of balance. Auditory testing protocols are necessary to document this loss in auditory function.

REFERENCES

1. Anderson, H., Barr, B., and Wedenberg, E. (1969): Intra-aural reflexes in retrocochlear lesions. Acoustic intra-aural reflexes in clinical diagnosis. In: *Disorders of the Skull Base Region*, edited by C. Hamburg and J. Wershall. Almquist & Wiksell, Stockholm, Sweden.
2. Buxton, F. (1970): Audiological tests in cochlear and retrocochlear diagnosis: A review of the literature. Unpublished Thesis, University of Houston, Houston, Texas.
3. Clemis, J., and Mastricola, P. (1976): Special audiometric test battery in 121 proved acoustic tumors. *Arch. Otolaryngol.*, 102:654–656.
4. Corliss, L. M., Doster, M. E., Simonton, J., and Downs, M. P. (1970): High-frequency and regular audiometry among selected groups of high school students. *J. Sch. Health*, 40:400–404.
5. Davis, H. (1976): Principles of electric response audiometry. *Ann. Otol. Rhinol. Laryngol. (Suppl. 28)*, 85:1–96.
6. Davis, H. (1976): Brain stem and other responses in electric response audiometry. *Ann. Otol.*, 85:3–14.
7. Fausti, S. A., Erickson, D. A., Frey, R. H., Rappaport, B. Z., and Schechter, M. A. (1981): The effects of noise upon human sensitivity from 8000 to 20,000 Hz. *J. Acoust. Soc. Am.*, 69:1343–1349.
8. Fausti, S., Frey, R., Erickson, D., Rappaport, B., Cleary, E., and Brummett, R. (1979): A system for evaluating auditory function from 8000–20,000 Hz. *J. Acoust. Soc. Am.*, 66:1713–1718.
9. Fausti, S. A., Frey, R. H., Rappaport, B. Z., and Erickson, D. A. (1979): An investigation of the effect of bumetanide on high frequency (8–20kHz) hearing in humans. *J. Aud. Res.*, 19:243–250.
10. Fausti, S. A., Rappaport, B. Z., Schechter, M. A., and Frey, R. H. (1982): An investigation of the validity of high-frequency audition. *J. Acoust. Soc. Am.*, 71:646–649.
11. Fee, W. E. (1980): Aminoglycoside ototoxicity in the human. *Laryngoscope (Suppl.)*, 24:1–19.
12. Flottorp, G. (1973): Effects of noise upon the upper frequency limit of hearing. *Acta Otolaryngol.*, 75:329–331.
13. Gilroy, J., Lynn, G., and Ristow, G. (1977): Auditory evoked brain stem potentials in a case of "locked-in" syndrome. *Arch. Neurol.*, 34:492–495.
14. Harris, J. D., and Meyers, C. K. (1971): Tentative audiometric threshold level standards from 8 to 18 kHz. *J. Acoust. Soc. Am.*, 49:600–608.
15. Hawkins, J. E. (1976): Drug ototoxicity. In: *Handbook of Sensory Physiology, Vol. V/3*, edited by W. D. Keidel and W. D. Neff, pp. 707–748. Springer, Heidelberg.
16. Hawkins, J. E., and Preston, R. E. (1975): Vestibular ototoxicity. In: *The Vestibular System*, edited by R. F. Naunton, pp. 321–349. Academic Press, New York.
17. Hecox, K., and Galambos, R. (1974): Brain stem auditory evoked responses in human infants and adults. *Arch. Otolaryngol.*, 99:30–33.
18. Jacobsen, E. J., Downs, M. P., and Fletcher, J. L. (1969): Clinical findings in high frequency thresholds during known ototoxic drug usage. *J. Aud. Res.*, 9:379–385.
19. Jerger, J. (1960): Audiological manifestations of lesions in the auditory nervous system. *Laryngoscope*, 70:417–425.
20. Jerger, J. (1973): Diagnostic audiometry. In: *Modern Developments in Audiology*, Second Edition, edited by J. Jerger, pp. 75–115. Academic Press, New York.
21. Jerger, J. (1975): Diagnostic use of impedance measures. In: *Handbook of Clinical Impedance Audiometry*, edited by J. Jerger, pp. 149–172. American Electromedics Corp., Dobbs Ferry, NY.
22. Jerger, J., and Jerger, S. (1971): Diagnostic significance of PB word function. *Arch. Otolaryngol.*, 93:573–580.

23. Jerger, J., and Jerger, S. (1975): A simplified tone decay test. *Arch. Otolaryngol.*, 101:403–407.
24. Jerger, J., Jerger, S., and Mauldin, L. (1972): The forward-backward discrepancy in Bekesy audiometry. *Arch. Otolaryngol.*, 72:400–406.
25. Jewett, D. (1970): Volume conducted potentials in response to auditory stimuli as detected by averaging in the cat. *Electroencephalogr. Clin. Neurophysiol.*, 28:609–618.
26. Jewett, D., and Romano, M. N. (1972): Neonatal development of auditory system potentials averaged from the scalp of rat and cat. *Brain Res.*, 36:101–115.
27. Jewett, D., Romano, M. N., and Williston, J. S. (1970): Human auditory evoked responses: Possible brain stem components detected on the scalp. *Science*, 167:1517–1518.
28. Jewett, D., and Williston, J. S. (1971): Auditory evoked far fields averaged from the scalp of humans. *Brain*, 94:681–696.
29. Johnson, E. (1968): Auditory findings in 200 cases of acoustic neuromas. *Arch. Otolaryngol.*, 88:598–603.
30. Katz, J., editor (1972): *Handbook of Clinical Audiology.* Williams and Wilkins Co., Baltimore.
31. Keith, R. W., editor (1977): *Central Auditory Dysfunction.* Grune and Stratton, New York.
32. Klockhoff, I. (1961): Middle ear muscle reflex in man. *Acta Orolaryngol. (Suppl.)*, 164:1–94.
33. Martin, F. N. (1981): *Introduction to Audiology.* Prentice-Hall, Englewood Cliffs, NJ.
34. Northern, J. L., Downs, M. P., Rudmose, W., Glorig, A., and Fletcher, J. L. (1972): Recommended high-frequency audiometric threshold levels (8000–18,000 Hz). *J. Acoust. Soc. Am.*, 52:585–595.
35. Osterhammel, D. (1979): High frequency audiometry and noise-induced hearing loss. *J. Soc. Occup. Med.*, 29:152–154.
36. Owens, E. (1965): The SISI test with VIIIth nerve versus cochlear involvement. *J. Speech Hear. Disord.*, 30:252–262.
37. Picton, T. W., and Hillyard, S. A. (1974): Human auditory evoked potentials. II. Effects of attention. *Electroencephalogr. Clin. Neurophysiol.*, 36:191–199.
38. Picton, T. W., Hillyard, S. A., Krausz, H. L., and Galambos, R. (1974): Human auditory evoked potentials. I. Evaluation of components. *Electroencephalogr. Clin. Neurophysiol.*, 36:179–190.
39. Picton, T. W., Woods, D. L., Baribeau-Braun, J., and Healey, T. M. G. (1977): Evoked potential audiometry. *J. Otolaryngol.*, 6:90–119.
40. Prazma, J. (1981): Ototoxicity of aminoglycoside antibiotics. In: *Pharmacology of Hearing*, edited by R. D. Brown, pp. 153–195. John Wiley Interscience, New York.
41. Quick, C. A. (1980): Chemical and drug effects on the inner ear. In: *Otolaryngology*, edited by M. M. Paparella and D. A. Shumrick, pp. 1804–1827. W.B. Saunders Co., Philadelphia.
42. Rosenberg, P. (1958): Rapid clinical measurement of tone decay. Paper presented before American Speech and Hearing Association, New York.
43. Salamy, A., and McKean, C. M. (1976): Postnatal development of human brain stem potentials during the first year of life. *Electroencephalogr. Clin. Neurophysiol.*, 40:418–426.
44. Salamy, A., McKean, C. M., and Buder, F. B. (1975): Maturational changes in auditory transmissions as reflected in human brain stem potentials. *Brain Res.*, 96:361–366.
45. Schulman-Galambos, C., and Galambos, R. (1975): Brain stem auditory evoked responses in premature infants. *J. Speech Hearing Res.*, 18:456–465.
46. Starr, A. (1976): Auditory brain stem responses in brain death. *Brain*, 99:543–554.
47. Starr, A., and Achor, J. (1975): Auditory brain stem responses in neurological disease. *Arch. Neurol.*, 32:761–768.
48. Sullivan, M. D., editor (1974): Proceedings of a symposium on central auditory processing disorders. University of Nebraska Medical Center, Omaha, Nebraska.
49. Yantis, P. (1959): Clinical applications of the temporary threshold shift. *Arch. Otolaryngol.*, 70:779–787.

Toxicology of the Eye, Ear, and Other Special Senses, edited by A.W. Hayes. Raven Press, New York © 1985.

Electrophysiologic Methods for Assessing Hearing Loss

Aage R. Møller

Department of Neurological Surgery, University of Pittsburgh School of Medicine, Pittsburgh, Pennsylvania 15213

Responses from various parts of the auditory nervous system of animals have been recorded electrophysiologically for a long time by researchers interested in how hearing is altered by experimental manipulation of the ear. Before the technique of signal averaging was perfected, it was necessary to place electrodes directly on the cochlea, or on or very close to neural tissue, in order to record the responses of these structures to sound stimuli. Such invasive techniques could not be used for routine study of human auditory responses. However, recent development of such techniques as signal averaging and digital filtering has made it possible to record very small potentials from the human auditory system, despite a background of other electrical activity of much higher amplitude. This chapter describes how these methods have made it possible to record auditory evoked potentials from scalp electrodes and how such recordings can be used to assess hearing in humans. Recently, we developed a technique for recording directly from neural structures of the auditory system in patients undergoing neurosurgical operations; since the auditory nervous system may be injured during such procedures, such monitoring is invaluable in decreasing the potential for such injury.

RESULTS OF ANIMAL EXPERIMENTS

The earliest response that can be recorded from the auditory nervous system in response to a click sound or a brief tone is the compound action potential of the auditory nerve. Recorded from the round window of the cochlea in small animals such as guinea pigs, cats, or rats, it is characterized by two negative peaks known as N_1 and N_2. A typical neural response recorded from the round window of a rat in response to a click sound is shown in Fig. 1. More specifically, the N_1 potential is the compound action potential of the auditory nerve, and the positive trough between the two negative peaks, together with the N_2 potential, is generated in the cochlear nucleus (8). These potentials are evoked by exciting the auditory receptor cells (hair cells), which are located in rows along the basilar membrane of the cochlea.

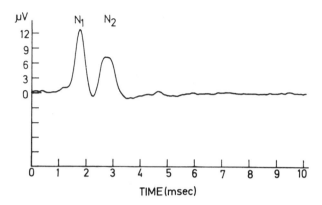

FIG. 1. Typical compound action potentials recorded from the round window of the cochlea in a rat. The stimulus was a brief click delivered to the ear via an earphone. The time scale gives the time in milliseconds after the occurrence of the click.

Excitation of these receptor cells on the basilar membrane takes the form of a traveling wave that moves along the basilar membrane from the base of the cochlea to its apex. When the wave motion has traveled a certain distance its amplitude increases and thereafter rapidly decreases. The distance the wave travels to reach its maximum is a direct function of the frequency of the stimulus sound: high frequencies travel a short distance and low frequencies travel a longer distance. Receptor cells located along the basilar membrane thereby become excited according to the frequency of the sound. In this way the basilar membrane plays an important role in the ear's ability to discriminate sounds of different frequencies.

The receptor cells are transformed epithelial cells, and the bending of the hairs located on the top of these cells is the natural response of these auditory receptors to stimulation. The hair cells connect to auditory nerve fibers via synapses, which delay the response by about 0.7 msec. The wave of motion set up along the basilar membrane in response to sound stimulation is relatively slow, and the time it takes for the sound energy to reach the receptor contributes significantly to the delay between the time the stimulus is presented and the time that the response (N_1N_2) is seen. This delay is called the latency of the neural potentials (N_1N_2). Since different sound frequencies travel different distances on the basilar membrane before they reach their maximal vibration amplitude, this delay differs for different frequencies.

This delay is illustrated in Fig. 2, which presents the family of curves representing the latencies of the two peaks (N_1 and N_2) of the compound action potentials recorded from the round window of a rat. Bandpass-filtered click sounds were used as stimuli. In this figure it can be seen how the latencies decrease as the stimulus intensity increases. When the center frequency of the bandpass filter was set at different frequencies, the latencies of the N_1N_2 peaks changed systematically: the responses to low-frequency sounds have longer latencies than do the responses to high-frequency sounds (bandpass-filtered clicks are similar to short tones with

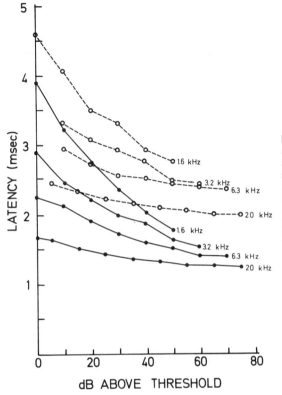

FIG. 2. Latency of the N_1 *(solid lines)* and N_2 *(dashed lines)* peaks of the response to bandpass-filtered click sounds. The results were obtained from a rat and the filter was a $\frac{1}{3}$-octave bandpass filter. The center frequency of the filter is indicated by legend numbers. The duration of the clicks before filtering was 5 μsec (9).

a frequency equal to the center frequency of the bandpass filter). This is because sounds of different frequency take different lengths of time to travel along the basilar membrane. Furthermore, there is a component of latency that is dependent on the stimulus intensity: the rate at which the generator potential in the hair cells rises when a sound is suddenly presented is proportional to the intensity of the stimulus. Thus, the stronger the excitation, the faster the generator potential rises, and the shorter the delay before the threshold of neural firing is reached (6). (It is assumed that the N_1 peak represents synchronized neural discharges in many fibers of the auditory nerve.) The amplitude of the N_1N_2 potential decreases when the stimulus intensity is decreased. Near threshold, the amplitude becomes smaller than the background noise (which consists of noise generated in the amplifiers as well as by the biologic activity of the animal). It therefore becomes necessary to present the same stimulus many times and to average a number of responses to detect the response.

For each frequency there is a stimulus level below which there is no discernible response, even when the responses to a large number of stimuli are averaged. This stimulus level is known as the threshold for the N_1N_2 potential. Plotted as a function of stimulus frequency, those values of minimum sound level that give a neural response are the N_1N_2 audiogram for a particular animal. The audiogram thus measured may be slightly different from the psychoacoustic threshold of hearing.

Since the N_1N_2 potentials are the results of the excitation of receptors along the basilar membrane, and since the frequency of the stimulating sound determines which hair cells located at which specific points on the basilar membrane will respond, the integrity of the sensory epithelium at various points along the basilar membrane can be measured by seeing which responses are lacking. That is, if a range of stimulus frequencies is presented, the threshold of the N_1N_2 responses are not all normal and an elevated threshold shows us that the sensory epithelium is damaged. Information about where on the basilar membrane the damage is occurring can be obtained by observing the N_1N_2 threshold for different stimulus frequencies.

Examples of how the threshold N_1N_2 potential may be used to assess the effects of noise exposure on animals are shown in Fig. 3. Here, the threshold shift in rats that were exposed to octave bandpass-filtered noise is shown as a function of frequency for different noise levels and exposure times.

The experimental results shown in Fig. 3 were obtained in an effort to test the so-called "equal energy hypothesis," which states that the damage to the auditory

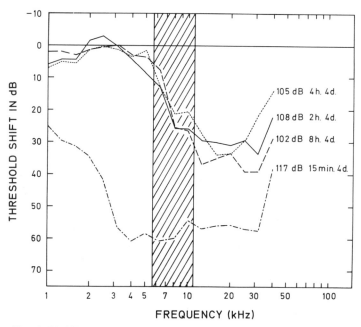

FIG. 3. Threshold shift for the compound action potentials recorded from the round windows of rats that were exposed to noises of different intensities. The duration of the exposure was so adjusted that the total noise energy was the same. The curves represent the mean value of the results obtained in 5 rats for each type of noise exposure. The test stimuli were bandpass-filtered clicks (⅓-octave bandpass filters were used) and the noise used to induce the hearing damage was bandpass-filtered white noise 1 octave wide, centered at 8 kHz (7).

system resulting from exposure to noise should be proportional to the level of noise times the length of exposure. As can be seen from the graph, the total energy (sound energy times exposure time) is the same for all five curves. For sound intensities between 105 and 111 dB sound pressure level (SPL), the degree of auditory damage was proportional to the sound energy level, but the highest sound intensity (117 dB SPL) produces a much larger degree of hearing loss than the lower intensities.

ASSESSING AUDITORY FUNCTION IN MAN

Neural potentials generated by the auditory nervous system are presently recorded to measure the threshold of hearing of patients who, for one reason or another, cannot participate in ordinary audiometric testing procedures. Such testing is done in two ways. One method consists of recording the compound action potentials from the auditory nerve in a fashion similar to that used in the animal experiments described above: an electrode is passed through the tympanic membrane and placed on the promontorium, and the cochlear potentials are then determined much as they are in animals (see, e.g., ref. 4). Since this method is invasive, and usually must be done under general anesthesia, its use has been limited.

Another method makes use of the farfield potentials from the ear and the auditory nervous system: the potentials that can be picked up by electrodes placed on the skin of the scalp (5). Such electrodes will record the potentials from different parts of the auditory nervous system. Since the transmission of activity along a nerve is relatively slow, and each synapse causes a discrete delay of about 0.7 msec, the potentials evoked by, for example, a click sound will consist of a series of peaks, each of which represents the activation of a different structure in the ascending auditory pathway (see, e.g., refs. 14 and 15). In clinical settings these potentials are usually recorded differentially from electrodes placed on the vertex or forehead and the ipsilateral mastoid, and are known as brainstem auditory evoked potentials (BSEP). Recorded in this way, the potentials are characterized by a series of five to seven vertex-positive peaks, each of which is labeled with a roman numeral to indicate where the potential was generated (5). Because of the long distance between the neural generators of the peaks and the points on the scalp from which these potentials are recorded, the potentials recorded are extremely small and the responses to a large number of stimuli must be averaged in order to be able to identify the different components of these potentials. When the hearing threshold is sought, the most convenient wave to observe is wave V, since this is the most robust of the waves and it decreases less in amplitude with decreasing stimulus intensity.

The BSEP are also studied as aids in diagnosing otoneurologic disorders. When used for this purpose all of the waves are important, and the most important parameter of the waves is their latencies, although it is now becoming apparent that their waveshapes and amplitudes are also significant factors. In all cases it is important to be able to identify the various waves with a high degree of certainty. For this purpose a recording as free of noise as possible is necessary. Because the amplitude of EEG activity is so high in comparison to that of BSEP, and because muscle activity also creates electrical interference, it is advantageous to use other methods of signal enhancement in addition to the averaging technique. When the ratio between the amplitude of the evoked potentials and the background noise is very small, signal averaging becomes a slow process for the purpose of signal enhancement. This is because the ratio between the potentials that bear a constant relationship to the stimulus (the evoked potential) and the activity that appears randomly only increases with the square root of the number of the responses that are averaged. Since the spectrum of the response usually does not coincide exactly with the spectrum of the unwanted background noise, spectral filtering becomes an attractive method for improving the signal-to-noise ratio.

The spectrum of the response is seldom separated totally from that of the noise, however, which makes the selection of filter setting a matter of compromising between attenuating as much as possible of the noise and as little as possible of the signal. If the filters attenuate energy within the frequency range in which the evoked potentials have significant energy, the result is distortion of the waveform of the signal. In addition, conventional electronic filtering not only distorts the waveform of the signal because of this, but it usually also causes a frequency-dependent phase shift that adds to the distortion, and, particularly, peaks of different width (thus different spectral content) may be shifted a different amount in time. Since it is the latencies of the peaks in the BSEP that are of the greatest diagnostic importance, such responses cannot be spectrally filtered to the extent that would optimally increase the signal-to-noise ratio.

So-called Bessel filters cause a linear phase shift that shifts all peaks an equal amount (2). When the degree of shifting is known, it is simple to compensate for the effect of these filters on the latencies. However, other aspects of the design of Bessel filters make them less attractive. Because digital filters can be designed to be more flexible than electronic filters, and because they can give a high degree of spectral suppression without causing variable degrees of time shift, digital filters are more suitable than electronic filters in filtering BSEP (3,10,16).

Digital filters perform mathematical operations on a digitized waveform, conveniently represented by the averaged response to many stimuli. The fact that digital filtering is performed after the responses are averaged is another advantage over electronic filters, because it makes it possible to subject one averaged recording to several different types of filtering. If filtering is done in the conventional way, using an electronic filter placed before the signal averager, only one type of filtering can be performed and a new recording must be made should another type of filtering be desired. This drawback is particularly serious when dealing with responses from patients in whom the signal-to-noise ratio may be poor and in whom it is inconvenient to prolong the recording to obtain a more satisfactory result.

We have used digital filters to interpret the results of clinical tests for about 5 years (10,16). Most of the patients tested have had otoneurological disorders. A signal is filtered digitally over time by convolving the averaged waveform with a weighting function. The actual mathematical operations are performed on a minicomputer. In Fig. 4 some examples of averaged BSEPs subjected to such filtering are shown. Figure 4A shows a "clean" BSEP recorded from a young person with no otoneurological abnormalities. Figure 5A shows typical BSEPs recorded from an elderly patient with a hearing loss. The advantage of filtering is obvious from this latter recording.

We use two different filters, one that reproduces all peaks and suppresses a moderate amount of noise (Figs. 4B and 5B) and one that only reproduces peaks I, III, and V of the BSEP but suppresses much more of the noise. As can be seen, the digital filter enhances the peaks for easier identification, and there is no shift of the peaks in time. A computer program identifies the peaks automatically and

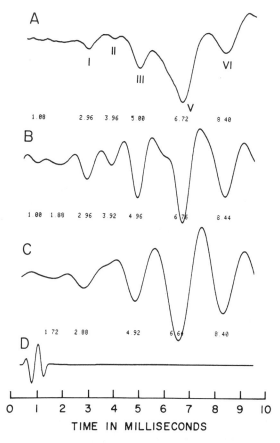

FIG. 4. Digital filtering of human BSEP. **A:** BSEP from a young, healthy subject without digital filtering (bandpass 11 to 3,400 Hz). **B:** Digital filtering that reproduces all peaks. **C:** After digital filtering that only shows peaks I, III, and V of the BSEP. **D:** The bottom curve shows the sound.

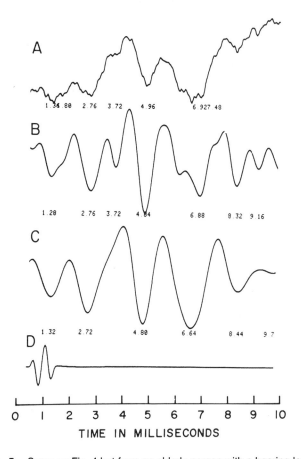

FIG. 5. Same as Fig. 4 but from an elderly person with a hearing loss.

prints out the exact values of their latencies. The weighting functions describing the digital filters illustrated in Figs. 4 and 5 are shown in Fig. 6. Digital filtering can also be performed in the frequency domain; in fact, the mathematical operations can often be done faster this way. However, we prefer to perform filtering in the time domain because there is almost no leakage of energy from sharp peaks when filtering is done in this way: filtering of 256 data points takes only 3 sec on a PDP 11/60 minicomputer.

The exact origins of the different peaks or waves of the BSEP have been studied in animal experiments (1), by observing the changes in the BSEP pattern that occur in patients with lesions at known locations along the ascending auditory nervous system, and, recently, by recording intracranially from different neural structures along the human ascending auditory pathway (11,12,14,15). We recorded from the auditory nerve, cochlear nucleus, vicinity of the superior olivary complex, and inferior colliculus during neurosurgical operations in the posterior cranial fossa.

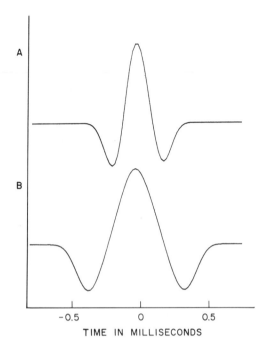

FIG. 6. A: Weighting functions of the digital filter used in Figs. 4A and 5B. **B:** Weighting function of the filter used in Fig. 4C and D.

TIME IN MILLISECONDS

The operations were performed to treat cranial nerve disorders, and the approach was through a retromastoid craniectomy. Recordings were made simultaneously from scalp electrodes placed in locations similar to those used to record BSEP in the clinical setting. An interpretation of BSEP based on results of intracranial recordings is shown in Fig. 7.

During the course of this work it became evident that recording the compound action potentials from the auditory nerve was useful in monitoring auditory function during neurosurgical operations, particularly during microvascular decompression operations for hemifacial spasm. These operations are associated with complications of hearing loss and we found that intracranial monitoring could substantially reduce this complication. By recording the compound action potentials directly from the auditory nerve instead of scalp BSEP during such operations, changes in the function of the auditory nerve can be detected instantaneously instead of waiting the relatively long time necessary to average enough responses from the scalp to be able to determine that a change has occurred. The instantaneous feedback to the operating surgeon provided by such intracranial monitoring allows him to change his approach early enough to avoid permanent injury to the acoustic nerve (13). We use a similar method to preserve hearing in patients undergoing surgery to remove small acoustic tumors (14).

Potentials that are directly recorded from the auditory nerve normally have a triphasic shape (Fig.8). The changes seen in these potentials as a result of insults to the nerve are usually an increase in latency and/or a decrease in amplitude of the negative phase (wave) of the potentials. When the insults to the nerve are

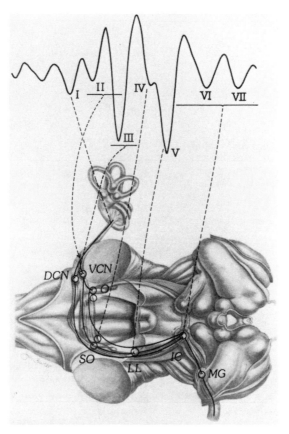

FIG. 7. Schematic outline of the neural generators of the BSEP in man (14). DCN, dorsal coch-lear nucleus; VCN, ventralcochlear nucleus; SO, superior olive; LL, lateral lemniscus; IC, inferior colliculus; MG, medial geniculate.

sufficiently severe, the only part of the potential that remains is the initial positive wave that appears as a broad positive wave. This indicates that the nerve no longer conducts neural activity and we feel that such a change in potentials calls for an immediate reversal of the procedure that caused the change (13). The most common cause of changes in auditory potentials is traction on the nerve from retraction of the cerebellum.

Figure 6 shows examples of recordings made during an operation for trigeminal neuralgia in which retraction of the cerebellum caused such a change in the compound action potential recorded from the auditory nerve, indicating blockage of conduction through the auditory nerve. From the sequence of recordings it is seen that the change occurred over a short period of time. The potentials recorded simultaneously from the scalp electrode (Fig. 9) showed changes that were not as easy to interpret as the potentials that were recorded directly. After about 2 min of averaging of the scalp BSEP there was a decrease in amplitude in the different peaks, which could no longer be identified. This was caused by alterations in the

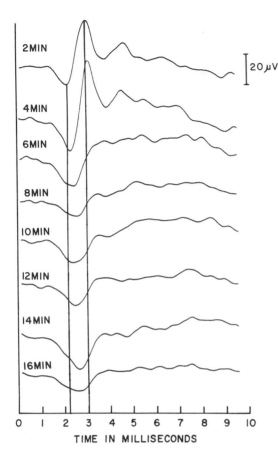

FIG. 8. Samples of recordings made intracranially from a distal location on the eighth nerve in a patient undergoing microvascular decompression surgery to relieve trigeminal neuralgia. The calibration applies to all curves, which show an average of 24 responses. The filter settings were 11 to 1,350 Hz. The stimuli were 2,000-Hz tonebursts of 1 msec duration delivered through an earphone inserted into the patient's ear and held in place with a standard earmold. The intensity of the sound was 100 dB SPL, corresponding to 90 dB peak equivalent hearing level. (The hearing level of the 1-msec tonebursts was 65 dB; ref. 13.)

latencies of the potentials resulting from the averaging process. Signal averaging of evoked potentials is an efficient method for enhancing evoked potentials that appear precisely at the same interval after the stimulus in a background of noise, but when the evoked potentials do not maintain a constant relationship over time with the stimulus (and maintain the same waveshape) the averaged response becomes meaningless. From the intracranial recordings shown in Fig. 8, it is evident that a change occurred in the potentials during the time when averaging was performed. This naturally also resulted in a change in the potentials that were recorded from the scalp, but this did not appear on the scalp-recorded BSEP until much later (Fig. 9). The potentials that were directly recorded stabilized after about 4 min but had a pathological waveshape. During the period when there was a stable but pathological auditory nerve potential the averaged potentials from the scalp electrodes rose in amplitude (because the potentials no longer changed, although they were still pathological). This increase in amplitude of the scalp-recorded potentials could have been interpreted as an improvement in auditory nerve function, which was obviously not the case as seen from the potentials that

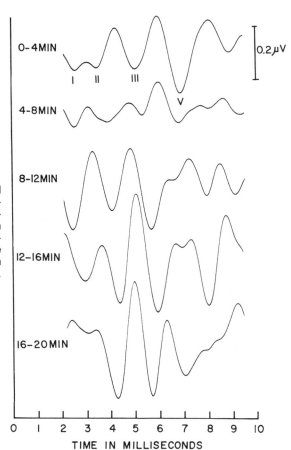

FIG. 9. Brainstem auditory evoked potentials (BSEP) obtained simultaneously with the recordings of responses from the eighth nerve seen in Fig. 8. Digital filtering was used to enhance the pattern of the BSEP. The calibration applies to all curves, which show an average of 2,048 responses.

were recorded directly. From this example it is evident not only that potentials recorded from the scalp are more difficult to interpret than are potentials that are directly recorded from the auditory nerve, but that potentials recorded directly give more accurate and more timely information about the status of the auditory nerve.

Another advantage of monitoring the potentials directly recorded from the auditory nerve is its value in teaching surgical procedures. The immediate feedback to the operating surgeon provided by this method clearly shows which step in the procedure has caused an insult to the auditory nerve. The value of monitoring the potentials recorded from scalp electrodes should not, however, be ignored: this is the only way of monitoring the function of the auditory system before the auditory nerve becomes directly accessible.

We use essentially the same stimuli to monitor auditory nerve function intraoperatively as we use to record BSEP clinically, namely, 2,000-Hz tonebursts of 1 msec duration at an intensity of about 95 dB SPL. This allows us to compare BSEP results obtained during the operation to those obtained clinically before the operation. We are aware that there may be more suitable stimuli with regard to providing a change in the response at the slightest change in neural function. However, the intraoperative monitoring technique we use has practically eliminated hearing loss as a complication in microvascular decompression operations for hemifacial spasm and vestibular disorders.

CONCLUSION

The techniques described in this chapter for studying and monitoring auditory nerve function electrophysiologically have provided us with much information about the functioning of the auditory nervous system. This information has been of benefit in increasing our general knowledge of this system, but perhaps more importantly, has also proven to be of immediate clinical value in decreasing the incidence of hearing loss associated with the treatment of lesions affecting the cranial nerves and auditory nervous system.

REFERENCES

1. Buchwald, J. S., and Huang, C. M. (1975): Far-field acoustic responses: Origins in the cat. *Science*, 189:382–384.
2. Doyle, D. J., and Hyde, M. L. (1981): Bessel filtering of brain stem auditory evoked potentials. *Electroencephalogr. Clin. Neurophysiol.*, 51:446–448.
3. Doyle, D. J., and Hyde, M. L. (1981): Analogue and digital filtering of auditory brainstem responses. *Scand. Audiol.*, 10:81–89.
4. Eggermont, J. J., Spoor, A., and Odenthal, D. W. (1976): Frequency specificity of tone-burst electrocochleography. In: *Electrocochleography*, edited by R. J. Ruben, C. Elberling, and G. Salomon, pp. 215–246. University Park Press, Baltimore.
5. Jewett, D. L., and Williston, J. S. (1971): Auditory-evoked far fields averaged from scalp of human. *Brain*, 94:681–696.
6. Møller, A. R. (1975): Latency of unit responses in the cochlear nucleus determined in two different ways. *J. Neurophysiol.*, 38:812–821.
7. Møller, A. R. (1982): Laboratory methods of assessing hearing loss. *Environ. Health Perspect.*, 44:87–92.
8. Møller, A. R. (1983): On the origin of the compound action potentials (N_1, N_2) of the cochlea of the rat. *Exp. Neurol.*, 80:633–644.
9. Møller, A. R. (1983): *Auditory Physiology*. Academic Press, New York.
10. Møller, A. R. (1983): Improving brain stem auditory evoked potential recordings by digital filtering. *Ear Hear.*, 4:108–113.
11. Møller, A. R., and Jannetta, P. J. (1981): Compound action potentials recorded intracranially from the auditory nerve in man. *J. Exp. Neurol.*, 74:862–874.
12. Møller, A. R., and Jannetta, P. J. (1982): Evoked potentials from the inferior colliculus in man. *Electroencephalogr. Clin. Neurophysiol.*, 53:612–620.
13. Møller, A. R., and Jannetta, P. J. (1983): Monitoring auditory functions during cranial nerve microvascular decompression operations by direct recording from the eighth nerve. *J. Neurosurg.*, 59:493–499.
14. Møller, A. R., and Jannetta, P. J. (1984): Neural generators of the brainstem auditory evoked potentials. In: *Evoked Potentials II: The Second International Evoked Potentials Symposium*, pp. 137–144, edited by R.H. Nodar and C. Barber. Butterworth Publishers, Inc., Woburn, MA.
15. Møller, A. R., Jannetta, P. J., and Møller, M. B. (1981): Neural generators of brainstem evoked

potentials. Results from human intracranial recordings. *Ann. Otol. Rhinol. Laryngol.*, 90:591–596.

16. Møller, A. R., Møller, M. B., and Millner, D. (1981): A computer system for auditory evoked responses. In: *Proceedings of the Fourteenth Hawaii International Conference on System Sciences* (Honolulu, Hawaii), edited by B. D. Shriver, T. H. Walker, R. R. Grams, and R. H. Sprague, *Vol. II*, pp. 430–438. Western Periodicals Company, North Hollywood, CA, 1981.

Toxicology of the Eye, Ear, and Other Special Senses, edited by A.W. Hayes. Raven Press, New York © 1985.

Psychophysical Methods for the Measurement of Somatosensory Dysfunction in Laboratory Animals

Patrick A. Cabe

Laboratory of Behavioral and Neurological Toxicology, National Institute of Environmental Health Sciences, Research Triangle Park, North Carolina 27709

As Arezzo (1) has noted, the great length of the peripheral nerve fibers makes them exquisitely sensitive to neurotoxicants. Motor function mediated by the long fibers innervating the hind limbs is frequently affected early in cases of neurotoxicosis (2).

The peripheral nerve trunks carry both motor and sensory impulses, and sensory dysfunctions also are widely reported neurotoxic signs. Maurissen (3) has tabulated the array of agents, both drugs and toxicants, known to yield somatosensory dysfunction. Decreased vibration sensitivity, altered temperature sense, impaired tactile ability, numbness, and a variety of subjective effects have been seen clinically.

Clinical effects are human health consequences of agent exposure, surely a crucial component of the total environmental health research effort. More important, however, must be the prediction of human health risks of agent exposure and the elucidation of mechanisms of injury (4). We want to know what effects may occur in exposed human subjects, and by what means such effects occur, without in fact exposing human subjects to potentially dangerous agents.

The general objective, then, is to demonstrate agent effects in nonhuman models in the laboratory under controlled conditions of maintenance and exposure. Because the somatosensory systems are affected early by a variety of agents, assessment of somatosensory function requires a high priority.

In this chapter I discuss aspects of the broad problem of testing nonhuman subjects for agent-induced somatosensory dysfunction, categories of somatosensory functioning, requirements for psychophysical assessment of sensory function, the logic of inferring agent effects on sensory functioning, and several general procedures for animal psychophysical testing.

CATEGORIES OF SOMATOSENSORY FUNCTION

Any major textbook or reference source can be consulted for an overview of somatosensory function (5–8). A convenient summary groups functions by anatomic locus (Table 1). Within each grouping, subgroupings of phenomenal or subjective experience can be identified. Thus, the cutaneous senses include touch-pressure, temperature, vibration, and superficial pain.

Cutaneous sensitivity has probably been most extensively studied, because the locus to be stimulated is easily accessible. What follows here is oriented toward the measurement of cutaneous sensitivity exclusive of pain. [The psychophysics of pain is discussed elsewhere by Weiss and Laties (9).]

Despite the ease of access to the body surface, tests of cutaneous sensitivity are complicated by a range of factors beyond the magnitudes of physical stimulation applied. A simple example is the variability in sensitivity to two-point stimulation as a function of locus of stimulation (8): the tongue, for instance, is very sensitive, the back and thigh much less so.

Other factors modulate the phenomenal experience of cutaneous stimulation. Spatial patterning is implied directly in the measurement of two-point thresholds: two points of contact are experienced as one if the two points are sufficiently close together. Simultaneous spatially distinct contacts may have inhibitory, summatory, or other effects (7).

Temporal interactions also occur. Adaptation to prior or cooccurring stimulation (for example, different temperatures) may alter the subjective magnitude of stimulation.

Temporal and spatial patterning may interact. A tactile phi phenomenon (7), in which cyclic stimulation of two spatially distinct loci yields the experience of a single contact moving between the two sites, is well known. Neurologists take advantage of spatial-temporal patterning in tests of recognition of letters drawn on the skin and of objects by touch (8).

Intermodal effects among the cutaneous senses yield higher-order experiences, as in "touch blends" (5). The experience of "oiliness," for instance, can be reduced to weak pressure plus warmth. The matching of objects examined tactually to samples presented visually is well known, even in nonhuman primates (10).

Kennedy (11), in a further interesting example of higher-order information available to skin senses, has reported that congenitally blind subjects are capable of identifying common objects depicted as raised ridges (the tactile equivalent of

TABLE 1. *Categories of somatosensory function*

Skin senses	Touch-pressure
	Temperature
	Vibration
	Superficial pain
Deep senses	Muscle, joint, tendon sensation
	Deep pressure
	Deep pain
Visceral senses	Organic sensation
	(hunger, thirst, nausea)
	Visceral pain

lines). Some blind subjects, asked to draw common objects, spontaneously invented line depiction conventions of interposition and linear perspective.

In summary, the experience of the environment available to the cutaneous receptors can occur on many levels, from those effects rather easily referred to the periphery to others that have complex cognitive components. Such effects pose challenging problems, and, in principle, any and all could be affected by exposure to toxic agents.

CHARACTERISTICS OF PSYCHOPHYSICAL ASSESSMENTS

In the examples cited above, the issues are psychophysical ones. The general psychophysical problem is to discover the relation between some varying character of physical stimulation and variations in the experience of such stimulation. Physical stimulation is often multivariate (e.g., vibration varies in frequency and amplitude), so psychophysical assessments often yield families of functions.

Every psychophysical experiment involves three components. First, the characteristics of the physical stimulation must be carefully controlled. Control of stimulation requires attention to details of stimulus generation, calibration of stimulus-generating devices, and, often, monitoring of stimulation parameters during presentation. Second, the locus of stimulation must be specified, both the specific body part and the extent and/or shape of the area stimulated. Locus is particularly important when repeated tests of function are intended, as across days, weeks, or months. Third, a means by which the subject can report his/her experience of the stimulation must be provided. Reports can range from very simple (a switch closure or a yes-no verbal report) to very complex (an introspective description).

Procedural details go beyond these three major components. The order of presentation of stimuli, their context (e.g., background or adaptation stimulation), and the kinds of comparisons to be reported all affect the design of particular investigations. Engen (12) provides a concise survey of these issues.

All three of the major components listed post difficulties for psychophysical assessments in animals. Perhaps the biggest hurdle is the requirement for a response mode that can vary with changes in stimulation. At best, one can get a crude categorical response (on the order of low-medium-high, or yes-no-not sure) from the animal, and most frequently investigators settle for some form of a yes-no response. Even so, guaranteeing that the response is being made appropriately, to the aspect of stimulation of interest and not to extraneous cues (e.g., apparatus noises), may require extensive preliminary training and/or a variety of control tests (13). The training investment, on the other hand, may purchase exquisite precision in the control of responding by the stimuli of interest.

Control of the locus of stimulation with human subjects is a relatively minor difficulty because we can enlist the subject's cooperation via verbal instructions. The animal subject either must be trained to maintain an orientation toward stimuli, be restrained in some manner, or both, in order that stimulation can be reliably applied to a specifiable body locus.

Always, precisely describable stimuli must be generated. The emergent problem here is that, in animal psychophysics, automation of the stimulus presentations, their order and variations, is desirable. The additional equipment required may increase the cost and complexity of animal psychophysical study.

ASSESSMENT OF AGENT EFFECTS ON SENSORY SYSTEMS

In general, a sensory dysfunction can be inferred from the observation that the psychophysical function for an agent-exposed subject is displaced relative to, or of a different shape than, the corresponding function in a nonexposed subject. Such evaluations are multivariate: while response change (or some derived measure, such as probability of response) is the single dependent variable, independent variables may include the parameters of the stimulus of interest (e.g., frequency and amplitude), yielding a family of curves, and must include a range of doses of the agent in question. Results reviewed by Stebbins and Moody (14) illustrate these points.

Since we infer altered sensory function from altered response, it is critical that nonsensory explanations for altered response be ruled out. Peripheral neuropathies, as a case in point, yield motor as well as sensory signs. Since some psychophysical procedures used with animals manipulate motivational levels (via food or water deprivation), and since ingestional changes often occur in toxicosis, motivational changes must be considered as a possible factor in response alterations.

Finally, modern psychophysical thinking invokes the concept of response bias, referred to an internal criterion for reporting detection of stimulation. Estimation of response bias is a central aim of signal detection theory (15). Signal detection methodology has been extended to the analysis of animal psychophysical studies in a number of cases. In principle, an effect of toxic agents may be to shift the subject's response criterion, an effect that would be reflected as a change in response bias, while detectability of the stimulus may or may not be affected.

OVERVIEW OF ANIMAL PSYCHOPHYSICAL TECHNIQUES

A variety of sources on animal psychophysical methods are available, with extensive bibliographies (13,16,17). My aim here is to critically review some of the available techniques for their usefulness in assessing agent-induced sensory dysfunction. The principal context is the evaluation of somatosensory function, but it must be stressed, on the other hand, that any of these methods could probably be applied to any sensory modality, given some ingenuity. Restrictions on applications are logistical and engineering problems rather than conceptual ones.

The overview presented here is summarized in Table 2, where candidate procedures are rated against major considerations in choosing a technique.

FACTORS IN EVALUATING ANIMAL PSYCHOPHYSICAL METHODS

Factors Related to the Psychophysical Function

There are three factors related to the psychophysical function: control of the parameters of the physical stimulation; control of the body locus, or sensory organ,

TABLE 2. *Comparison of animal psychophysical procedures*

	Method[a,b]						
Factors affecting choice	1	2	3	4	5	6	7
Control of stimulation parameters	0	+	0	−	+	+	+
Control of locus of stimulation	0	+	0	−	+	+	+
Precision of psychophysical function	−	+	0	−	+	+	+
Sensory-motor separation	−	0	+	−	+	0	0
Possibility of, need for response bias measurement	+	+	+	−	+	0	0
Motivational manipulation required	+	+	+	+	+	−	−
Amount of response training required	+	+	+	+	+	−	−
Amount of testing time required per function	−	+	−	−	+	0	−
Repeatability across time	+	+	+	+	+	+	+
Applicability to neonates	+	+	+	−	+	0	0
Labor intensiveness	−	0	0	0	0	+	+
Automatability	−	+	0	0	+	+	+
Equipment cost, complexity	+	0	0	+	−	−	−

[a]Methods are rated as follows: +, advantage; −, disadvantage; 0, no clear advantage or disadvantage.

[b]Methods are as follows: (1) reflex, orientation, or forced movement (kineses measures); (2) reflex modulation; (3) habituation/dishabituation; (4) preference, tropism measures; (5) classical conditioning; (6) operant conditioning; (7) conditioned suppression.

stimulated; and the precision of the psychophysical function(s) that can be obtained. The first two have already been discussed. The precision of the psychophysical function refers to the degree of variability resulting from any of a number of sources, perhaps the greatest of which is the "tightness" of the association between stimulus and response. Some methods are intrinsically more variable; others may provide for exquisite control of responding by stimulation.

Factors Related to Alternative Explanations for Altered Psychophysical Functions

Three factors (separation of sensory from motor components, response bias, and altered motivational milieu) have been discussed above. Psychophysical methods differ with respect to the degree that sensory and motor components of observed response change can be controlled or measured or come into play. Some methods, for instance, may utilize autonomic response, so that the motor component is negligible. In other cases, responses to varying stimuli may be evaluated as relative to one another; altered motor components, if they are homogeneous across the stimulus range being tested, may be taken out of consideration.

Response bias in some sense is an analytic entity. That is, under appropriate experimental designs it can be evaluated separately from detectability. Blough (18) provides an example of how such analyses can be performed. A range of designs lend themselves to response bias evaluation and the possibility of doing so is of some advantage.

Factors Related to Logistics and Design of Experiments

A prime motivation for listing this set of factors is that a large number of agents stand in need of some testing (19). Consequently, the time required to train and test subjects is an important consideration. Since dosing regimes that simulate environmental exposures are typically chronic and since the effects may be expected to be cumulative, methods that are repeatable across time (within-subjects designs) are most useful. Given the continuing strong interest in the evaluation of pre- and perinatal exposures, methods applicable (at least in principle) with very young organisms would be especially useful.

Economic Factors

No laboratory has infinite resources. Therefore, cost factors inherent in any method must be taken into account. The labor intensiveness and the level of such labor (e.g., kind and amount of training required) affect costs. Some methods may be automated, at some cost for development and for equipment, balanced off against labor costs saved, precision obtainable, and the possibility of testing more animals per unit of labor.

CANDIDATE PROCEDURES IN ANIMAL PSYCHOPHYSICS

Reflex, Orientation, and Forced Movement (Kineses) Measures

Reflexes are "prewired" motor or autonomic responses to stimuli, usually of a limited sort applied to a limited body region; the neurology literature provides numerous examples. Orientation measures refer to movements directed toward stimuli; these may be at a distance (sound, light, or chemical source) or on the body surface (a tactile stimulus applied to the skin). Kineses (20) refer to increases in activity as a function of imposed stimulation, e.g., increased movement at higher temperatures. Rough psychophysical functions can be derived by observing the variations in probability, amplitude, and/or latency of any such response as stimulus parameters are changed (19,21).

The major advantages of such methods are that, since the responses are built in, no training or motivational manipulations are necessary, and response bias is not a problem. Tests can be repeated in the same animals across time, so long as short-term effects (habituation) are allowed for. In principle, where appropriate reflexes can be identified, these methods should be applicable to neonatal animals. Equipment costs will probably be low.

The principal disadvantage is that, since reflexes are by definition sensory-motor arcs, sensory components may not be separated easily from motor effects. The functions obtained may be relatively imprecise, and the amount of hand labor required to derive functions may be quite large. These procedures are not readily automated.

Reflex Modulation

Hoffman and Ison (22) point out that the magnitude of a reflex (for instance, a startle response to a sharp noise) can be depressed by precedent or cooccurring stimuli, and that the reflex inhibition is related to the detectability of the precedent stimulus. This prepulse inhibition of reflexive response obviously can be incorporated into a psychophysical experiment. Russo (23) has reported the successful use of this technique to detect sensory dysfunction induced by environmental agents.

Reflex modulation holds great promise as a method for assessing agent-associated sensory dysfunction. Control of stimulation can be excellent, both in location and parametrically. The functions obtained (23) can be quite precise. Because the method is reflexive, response bias is not a problem and no motivational manipulation is required. Also, no special response training is necessary and the evaluation can be repeated across time. The method is useful with neonates (24) and can be automated, at least in some applications.

Habituation/Dishabituation

Presentation of a novel stimulus frequently can be seen to produce an orienting response, with both motor (startle) and autonomic (e.g., heart rate change) components (25). With repeated presentations, the orienting response wanes (habituation). Presentation of a second stimulus following habituation to the first may reinstate the orienting response (dishabituation). The habituation/dishabituation paradigm may be used as a psychophysical method.

An example of this approach is the work of Moffitt (26), who found that very young human infants could discriminate small speech sound differences. Infants showed habituation of a heart rate change to the syllable "ba" and dishabituation to a second syllable, "ga," which differed in one phoneme from the first.

Habituation/dishabituation has the potential advantage of separating sensory from motor effects of toxicants, in that autonomic measures can be used. This supports the method's use with neonates, too, where motor control may not be well developed. In fact, the method might be usable with some organisms prenatally. As with other reflex measures, response bias is not likely to compromise inferences of sensory dysfunction.

The major drawback is the amount of time likely to be required to derive a psychophysical function. Since the method employs (multiple) paired comparisons, testing may be quite time consuming.

Note that failure to observe dishabituation does not allow the inference of nondiscriminability of stimuli. Observation of dishabituation, however, is clear evidence for discriminability.

Preferences and Tropisms

Most organisms have multimodal preferences for a sensory context and, given the opportunity, will spend more of their time in the preferred context. For some organisms and some stimuli, the movement toward or away from the source of stimulation (e.g., heat, a chemical source) is highly reliable and predictable on the basis of knowledge about the gradient of stimulation present (20).

A typical preference experiment employs a choice box of some sort in which stimulus characteristics differ in two regions. By recording the relative proportion of time spent in the two areas, a rough psychophysical function can be generated.

In approximately the same fashion, tropisms may be tested: in this case, a gradient is constructed. For instance, a metal plate with one hot and one cold end specifies a temperature gradient. By noting the proportion of time spent in various zones of the gradient, again, a rough psychophysical function can be plotted.

These approaches have the advantage of relative simplicity. It is possible to automate them, for example, by using photocell arrays along a runway. Equipment cost and complexity generally will be low. Because the procedures depend on built-in preferences, no motivational manipulations are necessary and no special training is required. The method should be repeatable across time, too.

Control of the locus of stimulation will be difficult because the animal controls its own stimulation. The amount of time required to determine a psychophysical function may be protracted. The methods may be labor intensive, but the observations probably do not require a high degree of technical skill.

Since locomotor responses are typically employed, sensory and motor components will probably be confounded. Response bias (versus detectability) is not obviously measurable. As with habituation/dishabituation, absence of preference does not necessarily imply absence of discriminability.

Classical Conditioning

Classical conditioning can be used effectively in psychophysical experiments. The general procedure is to pair a signal, called the conditioned stimulus (CS), with an unconditioned stimulus (UCS), often mild electric shock. Usually the CS precedes or overlaps the UCS. The UCS elicits an unconditioned response or reflex (UCR), which may be overt, such as a limb flexion, or covert, such as a heart rate change. After some number of CS-UCS pairings, the CS alone comes to elicit a response like that elicited by the UCS. The response to the CS is called a conditioned response or reflex (CR). The ability of a stimulus to become a CS is *prima facie* evidence for its detectability.

Discriminative responses can also be established, in which case one stimulus is a CS +, paired with the UCS, and another is a CS −, paired with the absence of the UCS. By manipulating the difference between CS + and CS − pairs, their discriminability can be tested. Thus, measurement of thresholds for stimulus differences is possible.

Examples of classical conditioning in broadly psychophysical contexts are easily found in the psychology literature of the past century. Some recent applications that illustrate the potential of classical conditioning can be seen in the work of Kreithen and colleagues (27). The general problem Kreithen addresses is to discover the possible sensory bases for homing in pigeons.

His procedure is relatively straightforward. Stimuli of interest (the CS) are paired with mild subcutaneous electric shock (UCS) while heart rate is monitored. Heart rate acceleration (UCR) reliably follows shock. If the CS is detectable, it comes to elicit a heart rate acceleration. Conditioning is reported to occur after about 10 CS-UCS pairings; the remainder of a 50-trial session can then be devoted to varying stimulus parameters, during which a reliable psychophysical assessment can be made.

Using this procedure, Kreithen has studied sensitivity to magnetic fields, to barometric pressure changes, to the plane of polarized light, and to very low frequency sound (infrasound).

The only obvious disadvantage in this procedure is that equipment for recording and control of stimulus presentation may be relatively complex and expensive, but classical conditioning promises to be advantageous on most of the other factors listed.

Parenthetically, classical conditioning procedures are major components of Soviet behavioral toxicologic assessments (28), and are reported to be very effective in demonstrating neurobehavioral toxic effects.

Operant Conditioning

The methodology of operant conditioning in psychophysics is reviewed elsewhere (13,16,17,29). Operant procedures have been the most widely applied methods for the precise definition of animal psychophysical functions, for many reasons: The test apparatus can be tailored to the animal under test so that excellent control of stimulus parameters and locus of stimulus application are possible. The timing, location, type, frequency, and ultimate control of responding, coupled with the control of stimulation, can lead to extremely precise psychophysical functions. Functions have been shown to be highly repeatable across relatively extended periods of time. Operant methods have developed as highly automated technologies over the years; automation reduces labor costs but generally increases complexity of equipment and equipment costs.

Major disadvantages of operant procedures include the frequent requirement of motivational manipulation (e.g., food deprivation) and the fact that stable responding may only follow very extensive training.

Excellent examples of operant psychophysical methods in the somatosensory domain can be seen in the work of Maurissen (3), who is studying detectability of vibratory stimuli in monkeys, and in the approach reported by Burne and Tilson (30). The latter employ a relatively high probability response in restrained rats, a nose poke that is sensed by a photobeam interruption. Stepwise shock level changes are applied to the rat's tail, incrementing on a fixed-time schedule and decrementing contingent on the response. By monitoring the shock level increment-decrement reversals, the rat's threshold for reactivity to electric shock can be tracked.

The presentation of stimulation by itself can be a reinforcing event (31). In principle, this could be a foundation for psychophysical evaluation; it resembles the preference method mentioned earlier, with similar advantages and disadvantages.

For some purposes, the precision that can be obtained using operant methods may far outweigh the disadvantages. If, for example, correlations between histopathologic changes and functional disruption are the objective (14), the results achievable may justify the expense and time. At the other extreme, operant psychophysics may be prohibitively expensive for agent screening, at least as such methods are currently known. Given the flexibility that operant methods have demonstrated over the years, it may be that ingenious screening applications can be found in the operant psychophysical domain.

Conditioned Suppression

The operant and classical conditioning approaches have been combined in the conditioned suppression method. Animals trained under an operant schedule of reinforcement to emit a stable and moderately high rate of responding are exposed to a signal (CS) that precedes an unconditioned stimulus (UCS), often mild electric shock. Responding is interrupted (suppressed) by the UCS; then, suppression of response can be considered an unconditioned response. Over some number of CS-UCS pairings, the CS comes to suppress responding. Suppression of responding from a stable baseline in the presence of a CS, then, is evidence for detectability of the CS.

Typically, suppression is expressed as a ratio between pre-CS responses and CS responses, often calculated so that it can vary between 1.00 (complete suppression) and zero (no suppression). The suppression ratio increases toward 1.00 as conditioning progresses and varies directly with the detectability of stimuli. Applications of conditioned suppression to detectability problems have been reviewed by Smith (32) and have been used successfully in a variety of modalities, including cutaneous sensitivity.

Given that conditioned suppression is a hybrid operant-classical conditioning method, it tends to suffer from the disadvantages of both. Particularly, training and testing time, overall, may be excessive, and equipment may be relatively complex and expensive. The operant baseline will generally require motivational manipulation, though the suppression of responding itself will not.

Since the suppression ratio should be relatively insensitive to baseline shifts from session to session, the psychophysical functions derived should be relatively invariant, except for induced sensory changes.

SUMMARY AND CONCLUSIONS

The investigator interested in assessing agent-induced sensory function changes has a rather broad inventory of methods at his disposal. In general, selection of any psychophysical method entails tradeoffs, most frequently perhaps the precision-cost balance, where cost includes time, equipment, and labor expenditures. Simple, manual, quick procedures tend to yield imprecise psychophysical functions; more complex, automated, time-consuming techniques may lead to exquisitely precise functions.

A survey of animal psychophysical studies would demonstrate a preponderance of effort on the visual and auditory systems. Other modalities, from the familiar (taste, olfaction) to the exotic (barometric pressure, magnetic field sensitivity, sensitivity to electrical fields) have also been examined from time to time. It is easier to think in terms of the familiar modalities; those that are of less apparent immediacy to human life inspire less interest. However, where the interest exists, it seems that available psychophysical procedures (with some ingenuity) can be brought to bear.

The somatosensory domain is one of those in which animal psychophysical study has been relatively neglected. Maurissen's survey (3) of the overwhelming prevalence of agent effects on somatosensory function argues persuasively that the time is at hand to reverse this trend. For unknown agents, if they affect the nervous system at all, disruption of peripheral somatosensory function seems always to be a safe prediction.

Consequently, there is an urgent need for the application of existing animal psychophysical methods to the somatosensory area and for innovative new approaches, particularly where time and cost advantages can be found.

REFERENCES

1. Arezzo, J. C., Schaumberg, H. H., and Spencer, P. S. (1982): Structure and function of other somatosensory organs. *Eviron. Health Perspect.*, 44:23.
2. Cabe, P. A., and Tilson, H. A. (1978): The hind limb extensor response: A method for assessing motor dysfunction in rats. *Pharmacol. Biochem. Behav.* 9:133–136.
3. Maurissen, J. P. J. (1979): Effects of toxicants on the somatosensory system. *Neurobehav. Toxicol.*, 1 (Suppl. 1): 23–31.
4. Tilson, H. A., and Cabe, P. A. (1978): A strategy for the assessment of neurobehavioral consequences of environmental factors. *Environ. Health Perspect.*, 26:287–299.
5. Geldard, F. A. (1972): *The Human Senses*, 2nd ed. Wiley, New York.
6. Jenkens, W. L. (1951): Somesthesis. In: *Handbook of Experimental Psychology*, edited by S. S. Stevens, pp. 1172–1190. Wiley, New York.
7. Kenshalo, D. (1971): The cutaneous senses. In: *Woodworth & Schlosberg's Experimental Psychology*, 3rd edn, edited by J. W. Kling and L. A. Riggs, pp. 117–168. Holt, Rinehart and Winston, New York.
8. Ruch, T. C. (1965): Somatic sensation. In: *Physiology and Biophysics*, edited by T. C. Ruch and H. D. Patton, pp. 302–317. W. B. Saunders, Philadelphia.
9. Weiss, B., and Laties, V. G. (1970): The psychophysics of pain and analgesia in animals. In: *Animal Psychophysics*, edited by W. C. Stebbins, pp. 185–210. Appleton-Century-Crofts, New York.
10. Davenport, R. K., Rogers, C. M., and Russell, I. S. (1975): Cross-modal perception in apes: altered visual cues and delay. *Neuropsychologia*, 13:229–235.
11. Kennedy, J. M. (1980): Blind people recognizing and making haptic pictures. In: *The Perception of Pictures*, Vol. II, edited by M. A. Hagen, pp. 263–280. Academic Press, New York.
12. Engen, T. (1971): Psychophysics. I. Discrimination and detection. In: *Woodworth & Schlosberg's Experimental Psychology*, 3rd edn, edited by J. W. Kling and L. A. Riggs, pp. 11–46. Holt, Rinehart and Winston, New York.
13. Blough, D. S. (1966): The study of animal sensory processes by operant methods. In: *Operant Behavior: Areas of Research and Application*, edited by W. K. Honig, Prentice-Hall, Englewood Cliffs, NJ.
14. Stebbins, W. S., and Moody, D. B. (1979): Comparative behavioral toxicology. *Neurobehav. Toxicol.*, 1 (Suppl. 1): 33–44.
15. Green, D. M., and Swets, J. A. (1974): *Signal Detection Theory and Psychophysics*. Robert E. Krieger Publ. Co., Huntington, NY.

16. Blough, D. S., and Blough, P. M. (1977): Animal psychophysics. In: *Handbook of Operant Behavior*, edited by W. K. Honig and J. E. R. Staddon, pp. 514–539. Prentice-Hall, Englewood Cliffs, NJ.
17. Stebbins, W. E. (ed.) (1970): *Animal Psychophysics.* Appleton-Century-Crofts, New York.
18. Blough, D. S. (1967): Stimulus generalization as signal detection in pigeons. *Science*, 158:940–941.
19. Tilson, H. A., Mitchell, C. L., and Cabe, P. A. (1979): Screening for neurobehavioral toxicity: the need for and examples of validation of testing procedures. *Neurobehav. Toxicol.*, 1 (Suppl. 1): 137–148.
20. Fraenkel, G. S., and Gunn, D. L. (1961): *Orientation of Animals.* Dover, New York.
21. Marshall, J. R., and Teitelbaum, P. (1974): Further analysis of sensory inattention following lateral hypothalamic damage in rats. *J. Comp. Physiol. Psychol.*, 86: 375–395.
22. Hoffman, H. S., and Ison, J. R. (1980): Reflex modification in the domain of startle: I. Some empirical findings and their implications for how the nervous system processes sensory input. *Psychol. Rev.*, 87:175–189.
23. Russo, J. M. (1979): Sensation in the rat and mouse: evaluation by reflex modification. Unpublished Ph.D. dissertation, University of Rochester, Rochester, NY.
24. Kellogg, C., Tervo, D., Ison, J., and Parisi, T. (1980): Prenatal exposure to diazepam alters behavioral development in rats. *Science*, 207: 205–207.
25. Thompson, R. F., and Spencer, W. A. (1966): Habituation: a model phenomenon for the study of neuronal substrates of behavior. *Psychol. Rev.*, 173:16–43.
26. Moffitt, A. R. (1968): Speech perception by infants. Unpublished Ph.D. dissertation, University of Minnesota, Minneapolis, MN.
27. Kreithen, M. L. (1979): The sensory world of the homing pigeon. In: *Neural Mechanisms of Behavior in the Pigeon*, edited by A. M. Granada and J. H. Maxwell, pp. 21–33. Plenum Press, New York.
28. Ekel, G. J., and Teichner, W. H. (1976): An Analysis and Critique of Behavioral Toxicology in the USSR. Department of Health, Education and Welfare, National Institute of Occupational Safety and Health, Cincinnati, Ohio, Publication No. 77–160.
29. Blough, P. M., and Young, J. S. (1982): Psychophysical assessment of visual dysfunction. *Environ. Health Perspect.*, 44:47.
30. Burne, T. A., and Tilson, H. A. (1980): Titration procedure with rats using a nose poke response and tail shock. *Pharmacol. Biochem. Behav.*, 13:653–655.
31. Carlisle, H. J. (1970): Thermal reinforcement and temperature regulation. In: *Animal Psychophysics*, edited by W. C. Stebbins, pp. 211–230. Appleton-Century-Crofts, New York.
32. Smith, J. (1970): Conditioned suppression as an animal psychophysical technique. In: *Animal Psychophysics*, edited by W. C. Stebbins, pp. 125–159. Appleton-Century-Crofts, New York.

Toxicology of the Eye, Ear, and Other Special Senses, edited by A.W. Hayes. Raven Press, New York © 1985.

Environmental Factors Affecting Chemoreceptors: An Overview

Bruce P. Halpern

Department of Psychology and Division of Biological Sciences, Section of Neurobiology and Behavior, Cornell University, Ithaca, New York 14853

Vertebrate olfactory and gustatory receptors must be exposed to the fluids that are their relevant chemosensory environments. In terrestrial mammals, the sinuous and narrow nasal airways serve as protective accessory tissues for the olfactory receptors of the olfactory mucosa, which is hidden far inside the twisted passages. In contrast, taste receptors in all vertebrates, olfactory receptors in fish, and trigeminal chemosensory receptors (common chemical sense) in the epithelium of the nasal and oral cavities, and in the cornea, are directly exposed to the liquids and/or gases that bring chemosensory stimuli to them. The differentiated epithelial cells that form taste buds and the specialized neurons that are the vertebrate olfactory receptors are constantly replaced in normal adult animals, suggesting that chemosensory function per se is damaging to the receptors. Turnover of the sensory endings (but not the entire neurons) of the common chemical sense receptors is also likely, since trigeminal afferent terminals are in general quite dynamic.

Organic and sulfur-containing air pollutants may be among those which adversely affect olfactory receptors, but adequate data are not available. Certain metallurgical dusts and fumes are consistently associated with olfactory deficits, but the mechanism has not been elucidated. Studies of vertebrate respiratory system toxicology often do not examine the olfactory epithelium and rarely evaluate olfactory function.

Surfactants and metals can produce physiologic and/or morphologic damage in gustatory receptors. Some metals and other "antigeusic" substances are concentrated in saliva, a liquid which interacts closely with taste receptors. A general failure to evaluate potential chemosensory toxicants in relation to either human or nonhuman gustatory function accounts for the present inability to specify the incidence or severity of the problem.

The continued presence and operation of chemoreceptors indicate that mechanisms are available to cope with whatever morphologic and/or physiologic damage may be produced by common terrestrial and aquatic chemosensory environments. Additional environmental hazards derived from human culture (36,43,63,64,82,85) can, however, overwhelm the survival mechanisms of chemoreceptors (2,6). It is true that many of the pollutants that place chemosensory function at risk exist in nature. However, they usually occur at extremely low levels or in biologically inactive forms until industrial and/or urban activities concentrate, extract, and then liberate them.

OLFACTION

For terrestrial vertebrates, the environmental challenges to taste and olfactory receptors are rather different. Chemicals in solution or in suspension in air comprise the major chemosensory hazards for olfaction in terrestrial forms. Since solids and liquids need not arrive at the receptor sheet, olfactory receptors can be located so that "accessory tissues" of the nose permit access only to gases. In mammals, and in humans in particular, the sharp bends, narrow passages, and extensive ciliated mucosal surface of the turbinates and septum of the nasal airways cause almost all particles larger than 5 μm (82) to be deposited before they reach the olfactory receptor neurons of the olfactory mucosa (77), which are located on the most superior turbinate and associated septum (43).

During normal breathing, little of each inspiration flows above the middle turbinate, although a more even flow occurs during expiration. The large mucosal surface extending from the anterior nares absorbs over 90% of water-soluble vapors present in inspired air. Considerable adsorption of non-water-soluble gases also occurs. Thus the air flow pattern and mucosal sorption both tend to protect the olfactory receptors against exposures to high concentrations of chemicals (31,68,70,77). This mucosal sorption can be effective only when sufficiently low concentrations of the to-be-trapped particles, molecules, etc., are present in the mucus. To maintain these low concentrations, the cilia of the respiratory epithelium must move the mucus through the upper respiratory system and into the pharynx, where it is swallowed. This process is known as the mucociliary escalator (36). It results in replacement of the mucus about every 10 min (43). The mucociliary escalator is especially important for olfaction, since the mucus of the olfactory region *per se* is apparently not removed by direct ciliary action. Instead, the olfactory mucus is moved by adhesion to nonolfactory mucus.

Finally, the mucus-containing surface liquid and the rich blood supply of the nasal airways modulate the temperature and control the relative humidity of inspired air so that air temperature at the superior turbinate is within 5° of 37°C and the relative humidity is 100%, for a wide range of ambient temperatures (77). The resulting "constant temperature and humidity chamber" for the olfactory receptors, which is also well protected from the upper size-range of nonvapor input, might seem to be a benign environment (43).

If the olfactory receptors could interact with the chemosensory environment without incurring damage to themselves, we might expect these specialized neurons (40,75) to be relatively static structures. However, many studies have found that the olfactory receptor cells are constantly being replaced (39–43,69), and that the entire receptor neuron can regenerate from basal cells in adult vertebrates, including birds and mammals. The regeneration produces not only morphologic replacement but also functional recovery (58). These observations indicate that olfactory function is inherently damaging to the receptor. That is, the usual finding in healthy animals that have not been subjected to an intentionally polluted environment is constant replacement of the mucosal portion of the olfactory receptors. This receptor turn-over, which must have a considerable metabolic cost, can provide an adaptive advantage only if it is necessary for satisfactory olfactory function.

Olfactory damage caused by pollutants may result from an additional burden added to the challenge of normal olfaction. Structural and functional damage to the olfactory epithelium by ether or chloroform vapor was confirmed in the 1960s (2). Exposures to a sufficient concentration of either vapor for 6 to 10 min produced morphologic damage, but the same concentrations for less than 4 min resulted in only a brief depression of function. However, ether and chloroform are not common environmental pollutants (85). Therefore, they may be useful research tools and possible model agents rather than problem chemosensory toxicants.

Formaldehyde

Formaldehyde vapor (24,32,63) has become a common air pollutant. Olfactory deficits are reported to occur in humans exposed for some hours to formaldehyde vapor (3), but satisfactory psychophysical documentation is lacking. If formaldehyde vapor were an occupational hazard only for plastic, wood, and textile workers, as well as anatomists, formaldehyde olfactory toxicity would be a potential problem for only a small segment of the population (20,63). However, the development and commercial use of formalin-based synthetic polymers for phenolic and urea resins has brought the challenge of this possible chemosensory toxicant to the general population (20,63). These resins and related products are used in particle board and particle binders, plywood, and urea-formaldehyde foam insulation. Indoor air concentrations of formaldehyde can easily reach 1.2 mg/m^3 (1 ppm) in homes and offices when these formaldehyde-containing materials are used in construction (60). The major sources appear to be the urea-formaldehyde foam insulation (UFFI) and plywood. Thus homes without UFFI show a mean air concentration of formaldehyde of 0.04 mg/m^3, with an upper limit of 0.1 mg/m^3; homes with UFFI, a 0.14 mg/m^3 mean and a 4.1 mg/m^3 upper limit (60). It seems that the presence of UFFI raises the mean formaldehyde level by a factor of about 3 but may, in extreme cases, produce a 40-fold increase. Mobile homes can be a more severe situation. Here the mean concentration of formaldehyde in air is 0.41 mg/m^3, with an upper limit of 4.8 mg/m^3. Plywood, which has a very high daily emission rate, is thought to be a major source of the high formaldehyde levels in mobile homes. The problem may be more serious in urban settings, since formaldehyde occurs in gasoline and diesel engine exhaust and as a photodecomposition product in smog.

Irritant actions on the eyes and pulmonary airways in humans are observed at formaldehyde air concentrations of 2.4 to 6 mg/m^3 (2–5 ppm), a concentration no more than two or three times that needed to recognize by smell the presence of formaldehyde. The irritant concentration is very close to the 1976 National Institute for Occupational Safety and Health (NIOSH) recommendation of 1.2 mg/m^3 formaldehyde, is below the 1981 Federal Standard of 3.6 mg/m^3 (20), corresponds to the 1982 Code of Federal Regulations for 8-hr averages or ceiling concentrations (87), and is well below the Code of Federal Regulations "acceptable maximum peak" of 12 mg/m^3 (10 ppm) (87). These concentrations are only three to ten times the *mean* air concentrations of homes or offices with UFFI, or of mobile homes, and are below their observed upper limits. It should be noted that tissue damage from formaldehyde is known to occur at air concentrations of 30 mg/m^3 (25 ppm). It is recommended that if a formaldehyde odor is consistently recognized in one's environment, a problem is likely to exist (63). Of course, if formaldehyde damaged olfactory receptors, the recommended bioassay would be of limited value. Thus an adequate evaluation of the severity of the effects of formaldehyde on olfaction is needed, with reliable dose-response profiles.

Sulfur Compounds

Sulfur oxides and acids are major air pollutants (27,43,52,62,63,82). Irritant properties of sulfur dioxide are widely recognized (22,61). The upper respiratory system sorbs sulfur oxides very efficiently (52), although it is possible that the olfactory epithelium will be spared *(vide infra)*. Although the presence of such irritants does increase airway mucus secretion (72), sulfur dioxide concentrations of 2.61 mg/m^3 (1 ppm) or more impair nasal mucus flow (77).

For purposes of comparison, the United States Code of Federal Regulations maximum allowable 8-hr time-weighted average for an employee's exposure to sulfur dioxide is 13 mg/m^3 (5 ppm) (86). The United States Primary Air Quality Standard for sulfur dioxide is 80 μg/m^3 for annual arithmetic mean; 0.37 mg/m^3 (0.14 ppm) for maximum 24-hr average (87).

Surprisingly, continuous exposure to sulfuric acid aerosols with concentrations from 150 to 502 mg/m^3 for 7 days produced no nasal septum (or pulmonary) damage in rats or rhesus monkeys (79). Lesions were seen in guinea pigs, while in mice somewhat longer exposures resulted in ulceration in the larynx and upper trachea. Since the highest concentrations in this study were several times that found in industrial pollutant-induced smog, generalization of sulfur-induced nasal damage from rodents to primates may be equivocal. However, no evaluation of olfactory effects was made. It is also noteworthy that single 10-min exposures of humans to a 1-mg/m^3 H_2SO_4 mist, or 4-hr exposures of sheep or dogs to concentrations as much as 14 times higher, produced no immediate or delayed changes in lung function (52). Again, no olfactory evaluations were made. It may be that many of the consequences for humans of sulfur compounds dissolved or present as aerosols in inspired air involve sensory receptors. Both the olfactory system *per se* and intranasal termination of the trigeminal nerve, i.e., the common chemical sense (24,26), are likely to be affected.

Damage to the mouse trachea by inhaled sulfuric acid mist was confirmed by another study (57). In this instance, a 100-mg/m^3 mist, presented once for 3 hr, resulted in surface holes in tracheal epithelial cells, matted cilia, and very thick tracheal mucus coating when tissue samples were obtained 1 hr after the end of exposure. Unfortunately, the nasal cavity was not examined after this exposure.

The same study used a second sulfuric acid presentation technique: sorption onto carbon particles, which were then presented as an aerosol at 5 mg/m^3 (57). The acid-coated carbon particles had a mean diameter of 0.4 μm, which is within the size range of common fumes and/or mists produced by atmospheric dust, tobacco smoke, metallurgical dusts, and fumes, etc. (82). Concentrations of the sulfuric acid mist that was used to coat the particles were the same as that in the previously described mist-only techique (100 mg/m^3), as well as twice (200 mg/m^3) and one-half (50 mg/m^3) that concentration. Damage was seen in the nasal cavity after a single 3-hr exposure to the 100-mg/m^3 sulfuric acid mist-coated carbon particles. The external nares, anterior septum, and midseptum were all involved. Nonciliated cells showed holes, tears, and missing microvilli, while ciliated cells were tearing away at their cell edges. However, this damage did not extend to the posterior septum, where the olfactory mucosa is located. Only a mucus coating was observed in the latter area. Multiple (3–10) 3-hr exposures to the 100-mg/m^3-coated particles or to the 200-mg/m^3-coated particles led to heavier damage or to the appearance of macrophages in the anterior septum and midseptum, but did not produce significant involvement of the posterior turbinate. Twenty 3-hr presentations of particles coated with 50 mg/m^3 sulfuric acid mist yielded limited nasal damage, similar to that produced by a single exposure to the 100-mg/m^3-coated particles. No evaluation of olfactory function was made.

An absence of damage to the olfactory mucosa by sulfuric acid mists or coated particles is the general pattern (57,79), even when multiple presentations of concentrations almost 1,000 times the maximum 24-hr average permitted by U.S. Federal regulation (52) are used. However, this is not synonymous with an absence of damage to chemoreceptors. For the anterior septum and midseptum, damage is found with repeated exposures to 50-mg/m^3 (17.5 ppm)-coated particles, a concentration that can be approached in some large cities and in industrial settings (52). These turbinates have many trigeminal nerve endings, which provide nasal input for the common chemical sense (23). Consequently, damage to these turbinates, which do not carry olfactory mucosa, can produce a significant reduction in nasal chemosensory input (80). This loss could have important consequences for perceptions of nasal pungency and irritation (26) as well as for reflexes that are dependent upon normal nasal trigeminal function.

Cigarette Smoke

Cigarette smoke is a potentially damaging environmental factor that some humans voluntarily introduce into their respiratory system. Recent studies report that smokers have less nasal sensitivity than nonsmokers to a standard common chemical sense stimulus (23), CO_2 (26,33). Both the judged intensity of the CO_2 and a reflex apnea response to it were depressed in smokers. In contrast to these effects on response to the CO_2, responses to an olfactory stimulant, isoamyl butyrate, did not differ between smokers and nonsmokers. Since the filtering characteristics and fluid dynamics of the nasal airway would cause the olfactory epithelium to be less exposed to cigarette smoke than other regions of the upper respiratory system, "an explanation based on the mere location of the receptors in the nasal cavities" (26) is plausible.

Pathologic data relevant to a differential effect of cigarette smoke on olfactory epithelium versus other regions of the nasal cavity are provided by a study on hamsters (14). In this investigation golden hamsters *(Mesocricetus auratus)* were exposed to smoke from 8 cigarettes per day for 10 days. The exposure regimen was 10 puffs per cigarette, 1 puff every 58 sec, where each puff had a duration of 2 sec and was composed of 35 ml smoke diluted with 350 ml fresh air. The smoke-air mixture was present in the exposure chamber for 30 sec, and was then removed over the next 30 sec. The smoke-to-air ratio and puff volume were selected to resemble human smoking conditions.

This exposure to cigarette smoke in hamsters produced a large number of denuded ciliated cells in the epithelium of the anterior portion of the nasal cavity (nasoturbinate and maxilloturbinate bones), with broken and distorted cilia evident. Desquamating cells and focal hyperplasia of basal cells were also common in the smoke-exposed hamsters, but not in control groups. In contrast to these effects of cigarette smoke inhalation on the mucosa of the more anterior nasal cavity, "the olfactory epithelium appeared normal in all groups," except for hyperchromatic cell nuclei in 2 of the 20 hamsters exposed to smoke (14). Such differential damage to the anterior regions of the nasal cavity would produce selective effects on the common chemical sense. This would be the case because the sensory endings of trigeminal nerve origin, which provide nasal common chemical responsiveness, occur in the nonolfactory respiratory mucosa (23,43).

In contrast to the absence of damage to olfactory epithelium cells in golden hamsters, exposure to cigarette smoke in a carcinogenic agent-susceptible strain of mice (C57Bl/6J) produced damage to both receptor cells and supporting cells in the olfactory eithelium (65). The exposure regimen was 8 puffs per cigarette, 1 puff each minute, where each puff had a duration of 2 sec and was composed of 10% smoke. This is quite similar to the presentation sequence of the preceding study on hamsters (14). However, only 1 or 3 cigarettes were presented daily to the experimental-group mice, whereas 8 per day had been used with the hamsters. Both a dose-response relationship and a cumulative effect were observed in the C57Bl/6J mice. Only 17% showed olfactory epithelium damage after exposure to 1 cigarette per day for 6 days, while 78% had damage after a 9-day exposure. The daily dose effect was even more striking: All animals had olfactory epithelium damage after exposure to 6 cigarettes per day for 6 days. In general, changes in the olfactory receptor cells included diminished size and altered location of their "apical (distal) swellings (called olfactory vesicles), as well as a drastic reduction in the number of sensory cilia which normally protrude from each vesicle." For the supporting cells, alterations in mitochondria were noted, abnormal protrusions into the nasal cavity were seen, and few microvilli were present. None of these changes were found in SWR/J mice, which are resistant to tumor induction and skin pathology by carcinogens.

Metals

Toxic effects of excess or uncontrolled exposure to certain metals are often reported (36,83). Both heavy metals and others are involved. One source of such exposure is metallurgical dusts and fumes. The particle size of this source ranges from large particles, comparable in diameter to fine sand, to very small particles with a size similar to that of the smallest virus (82). This wide range can produce particle deposition throughout all parts of the nasal cavity, trachea, and lungs. Some toxic metal fumes, in particular lead fumes, are or have recenty been problems for the general population because of the use of tetraethyllead gasoline. However, most metallurgical fumes are encountered in particular industrial settings (22). Metals that tend to place chemosensory function at risk when inhaled include cadmium, manganese, mercury, nickel, and zinc (36,82,83). Specifically, human chemosensory deficits are directly associated with exposure to cadmium, mercury, and zinc; a "manganese pneumonia" has been seen in manganese workers, and inhalation of nickel dust or fumes has been shown to produce respiratory system damage in experimental animals (83).

Beating of respiratory cilia in hamsters is adversely affected subsequent to inhalation of an aerosol containing a cadmium or nickel salt (36). Sensitivity to cadmium is about 10 times that to nickel, but recovery may be faster with cadmium than after exposure to nickel. Manganese does not change ciliary activity under comparable conditions. As discussed earlier in the olfaction section of this chapter, any interference with ciliary action will depress the mucociliary escalator. This could change olfactory function because of alterations in the sorption on and in the mucus of respiratory mucosa, as well as because of changes in the patency of nasal passages that are triggered by irritation. Both the common chemical sense and olfaction, which involves the first cranial nerve, could be disrupted by these effects. In addition, to the extent that mucus movement at the olfactory mucosa is dependent on the mucociliary escalator of respiratory mucosa, an abnormal condition would develop at the olfactory mucosa. Finally, since the olfactory receptor cells have motile cilia, agents that are detrimental to ciliated cells may directly damage the olfactory neurons.

Cadmium

Cadmium is present as a vapor or powder during production of storage batteries, solders and other low-melting-point metals, and photoelectric cells and semiconductors, as well as during electroplating procedures and the processing of zinc ores (22,36,83). Complaints of olfactory deficits by workers in some of these industries had already appeared in reports published prior to 1950 (1,83). These complaints prompted several studies of olfactory competence. In one study (1), 106 workers in an alkaline battery factory were asked "What is your sense of smell like?", with the responses categorized as "good," "diminished," or "none." The same workers were tested for olfactory threshold to phenol dissolved in liquid petrolatum (mineral oil), with a concentration series intended to range from normal threshold to 200 times normal threshold. In addition, 85 of the workers received examinations of their nasal mucosa. An age-matched control group of 84 workers from a "neighbouring engineering factory in which there was no specific hazard" were both questioned concerning their sense of smell and tested for their phenol threshold. Examinations of the nasal mucosa of 75 of the control group were done.

Two metal-containing powders were in use in the alkaline battery factory. One contained 60 to 64% cadmium oxide; the other, 72% nickel hydroxide. Air samples analyzed for cadmium indicated 198 ± 186 $\mu g/m^3$ (mean $\pm$ SD), while samples analyzed for nickel showed 12 ± 19.9 $\mu g/m^3$. For purposes of comparison, the 1976 NIOSH limit was 40 $\mu g/m^3$ for cadmium; the threshold limit value (TLV) for nickel, 1 mg/m^3 (83). The 1982 U.S. Code of Federal Regulations specifies that cadmium dust shall not exceed an 8-hr time-weighted average of 200 $\mu g/m^3$; cadmium fumes, 100 $\mu g/m^3$ (88). However, "acceptable ceiling concentrations" are much higher, being 600 $\mu g/m^3$ for dust and 3 mg/m^3 for fumes (88).

Substantial differences in olfactory function existed between the cadmium-exposed and control groups (1). One-third of the cadmium group but only 8% of the control group had phenol thresholds 100 times normal threshold or higher; 27% of the cadmium group but only 5% of the control group were unable to smell the highest phenol concentration, which was designed to be 200 times normal threshold. None of the control workers, but 15% of the cadmium workers, reported that they had no sense of smell. Since age and cigarette smoking pattern might interact with these findings, the investigators compared subgroups of 51 control workers and 61 cadmium workers all of whom were cigarette smokers aged 35 and over. Phenol thresholds were significantly higher in the cadmium workers ($\chi^2 = 16.9, p < 0.001$).

For the examination of the nasal passages, the control and cadmium workers were presented randomly to an investigator who was not informed of the group status of each worker. Results of the examination were expressed as one of three categories: no indications of nasal irritation, mild irritation, or definite destructive changes. More than half the cadmium workers (52%), but only 37% of the control workers, were classed as showing mild nasal irritation. The majority (60%) of the control workers, but only 43% of the cadmium workers, had no irritation. Destructive changes were rare in both groups. In contrast to this pattern of mucosal changes, no statistically significant relationships were found between nasal examination status and either phenol threshold or report of olfactory ability. It should be noted that the olfactory mucosa *per se* is not mentioned and was not likely to have been visualized during a typical clinical examination.

Hazardous air concentrations of cadmium were not promptly eliminated when reports of problems appeared. For example, 25 years after the just-discussed study had been published, a 1976 NIOSH Health Hazard Evaluation (74) found that air concentrations of cadmium routinely exceeded 100 $\mu g/m^3$ in a plant producing nickel-cadmium batteries.

Metals and Aquatic Animals

Low concentrations of copper sulfate or mercuric chloride are chemosensory toxicants for olfaction in several fish genera (48). These salts, at concentrations below 1 μM, disrupt food-seeking behavior and/or migration. Histopathologic investigations indicate that the olfactory receptor cells of fish are selectively damaged by these metals. A 2-week exposure of rainbow trout *(Salmo gairdneri)* or lake whitefish *(Coregonus clupeaformis)* to 2.4 μM copper sulfate produced necrotic olfactory receptor neurons, while supporting cells were unaffected. An accumulation of metal in the olfactory mucosa occurs during such chronic exposure. At similar concentrations, mercuric chloride is slightly less damaging. Comparable effects have been observed in other genera. Since olfactory receptor cells do regenerate, recovery can occur if the fish are moved to clean water, but between 4 and 12 weeks are required.

Zinc and cadmium produce little histologically observable olfactory damage at micromolar concentrations. However, exposure to much higher concentrations of zinc sulfate, e.g., 200 μM, has produced olfactory neuron damage in a lamprey *(Entosphenus japonicus)*. Even higher concentrations of zinc, such as 10 mM or more, are usually required to yield histopathologic effects in fish.

Electrophysiologic measures from both the olfactory mucosa and the olfactory bulb confirm the behavioral and structural studies on toxic actions of copper and mercury. Threshold effects are seen at submicromolar concentrations, and a 50% reduction in neural responses to odorants is produced by a 30-min exposure to 2.2 μM copper sulfate. Silver and mercury salts are effective at similar concentrations. In contrast, the levels of cadmium, zinc, nickel, or lead required to produce olfactory deficits are above the lethal concentrations of these metals.

Olfactory Bulb

The central nervous system target of the olfactory receptor neuron axons, the olfactory bulb, apparently shows structural alterations in the rat as a function of the chemicals in inspired air (59). Initial reports suggested that bulb damage caused by overstimulation was being observed. However, replication of the changes using the original stimulus paradigm has been difficult. Some reports suggest that the anatomic changes are signs of normal function, with unchanged olfactory bulb regions reflecting a pathologic state caused by insufficient input from the olfactory receptors (43). Finally, some investigators, while finding transient behavioral changes, have observed no alterations in olfactory bulb morphology (28).

Summary: Olfaction

In general, olfactory systems of terrestrial animals respond to, and permit adaptive behavior in relation to, very low concentrations of a broad range of molecules in air (43,71). This high and differential sensitivity uses "accessory tissues," the nonolfactory portions of the nasal airways, to humidify, temperature control, and desaturate inspired air. The olfactory receptor neurons of the olfactory mucosa undergo constant turnover, and the entire neuron can develop in adult mammals from basal cells. These protective and replacement mechanisms may be insufficient to handle culturally produced air pollution. Chemosensory receptors of the trigeminal nerve-based common chemical sense are in more exposed locations. Formaldehyde vapor is potentially a serious olfactory receptor toxicant, but more data are needed. Sulfur oxides and acids are established problem sources, as are certain metals, such as cadmium. More broadly, any form of air pollution that adversely alters nasal mucosa, such as pH changes (85) or organic vapors (63), may also affect the nasal chemoreceptors.

The postsynaptic neurons of the olfactory bulb show histochemical changes following prolonged inspiration of air containing sufficient concentrations of a range of chemicals. Whether these changes, or their absence, are pathologic is not yet understood.

TASTE

Taste receptors of vertebrates occur in loci where contact with environmental chemicals in aqueous solution is a likely event (15). For fully aquatic forms, such as fish, these loci include, in addition to the mouth, the exterior surface of the body and sometimes appendages literally covered with taste buds (4,6,25). Other specialized "contact chemoreceptors," such as portions of the lateral line system and scattered chemoreceptors, are also found in fish and elasmobranchs. However, the receptor cells of these latter systems do not resemble those of taste buds, and the innervation may be either cranial or spinal nerves.

Since the fluid in which fish and other fully aquatic animals live is a liquid, olfaction and taste share the same stimulus solvent, and both can be affected by water pollution. For example, disruption of olfaction-dependent feeding and reproductive behavior in several invertebrate forms (48) and olfactory epithelium damage in fish (49), all caused by exposure to petroleum or petroleum extracts in water, have been reported.

Terrestrial vertebrates have taste receptors only within the mouth and pharynx. Adult humans and other mammals usually have taste buds on the tongue (generally on papillae located on the dorsal surface and sides of the tongue), the soft palate, and the epiglottis (15,46). Extensive protective and filtering accessory tissues comparable to the nasal airways are not found for vertebrate taste receptors. At best, a mucosal layer (5) covering external taste buds in aquatic forms (4,76) or a mixture of saliva and mucus (oral and pharyngeal taste buds) covers the receptor cell complex.

In humans and many other mammals, the tongue has a relatively thick and nonpermeable keratin layer (16). However, the keratin becomes very thin or disappears entirely in the vicinity of taste buds (46). An opening in the epithelium forms a pore (10,16,19,21) through which liquids, pastes, and particles less than 5 μm in diameter can approach the microvilli, which are the terminations of the receptor cells (37). These microvilli and the distal ends of the taste bud receptor cells from which they project are embedded in a matrix that may be a polysaccharide-protein mixture (5,21). The function of this pore chamber matrix is unknown, but it does not seem to present a substantial diffusion barrier (16,34). However, movement of chemicals from the pore chamber into either the taste bud cells or deeper into the taste buds does not readily occur (16), at least in living mammals (21). With prolonged contact, radiolabeled glycine, at least, can appear deep in the taste bud (45).

The relatively unprotected nature of taste receptors seems unavoidable if rapid but differential responses are to occur for a wide range of molecules and ions solvated in aqueous media. One would expect that such exposure, which also can involve a temperature range from 0 to almost 40°C (potential terrestrial environment ambient range for drinking water sources) and small particle abrasion, would quickly damage the receptors. This seems to be the case, since the taste bud receptor cells of vertebrates undergo constant replacement (16). These cells continuously develop from epithelial cells, enter the taste bud, follow a sequence of differentiation, and disappear. In poikilotherms the rate of cell turnover can be relatively slow (39) and is temperature-dependent. For mammals a typical taste bud receptor cell has a life span of 10 days (16).

Water Pollution

Water pollution is known to damage taste receptors in fish. Surface-active substances such as detergents appear to be one important factor (6,7); heavy metals, another (53,89). Mercurials reduce taste stimulus binding at relatively low concentrations, e.g., 100 μM $HgCl_2$. It may be that human taste receptors are also adversely affected by surfactants to which they are exposed. Situations such as detergents in water represent a pollution problem and are recognized as such. However, the surfactant sodium lauryl sulfate (dodecyl sodium sulfate), which is added to toothpaste (88), has been demonstrated to modify both human taste perception (30) and rat gustatory neural responses (84). Direct application of dentifrice to the tongue (51) has similar effects.

Saliva

Saliva is a major component of the environment of mammalian taste receptors (44). Sufficient variation in its composition or quantity alters taste function. Thus the ionic composition of saliva affects human taste judgments (9,10); a reduced supply modifies taste-dependent behavior (44), leads to altered neural responses, and is associated with structural changes in taste bud cells (37).

A number of metals and other elements are concentrated in saliva (17). This phenomenon includes the heavy metal mercury and perhaps lead, as well as copper and the halogen fluorine. It has given rise to the suggestion that saliva samples be used to monitor exposure to metal pollution in humans (17,18). Heavy metals have a variety of effects on living organisms (61). With reference to gustation, salivary metals may be significant because taste receptors are sensitive to topical application of metals (45). For example, 100 μM $CuCl_2$ depresses mammalian gustatory neural responses to sugars and amino acids. Since water supplies can be contaminated with heavy metals (35), human ingestion and subsequent salivary concentration are possible.

Taste Modifiers

Direct consumption of plants is practiced by many animals. In addition to the nutrients that are secured, this behavior brings a wide range of other organic molecules into the oral cavity. Some of these molecules are taste modifiers.

Taste modifiers have been defined as "natural substances of plant origin (which) modify the sense of taste by selectively changing the characteristics of gustatory receptors and/or primary neurons.... The action of gustatory modifiers (on taste receptors) can be (expressed as) primarily an alteration of classes or quality categories of responses or primarily a depression or enhancement of the intensity of otherwise unchanged quality categories. In either case, one, or more than one, quality category may be affected" (67).

Initial recognition of taste modifier action generally involves human taste judgments of foods after ingestion and/or mastication of plant components, such as leaves or fruits, which contain the active factor(s). This sequence, *per se*, could cause changes in behavioral gustatory responses because of habituation produced by central nervous system integration of successive taste inputs (47), or as a result of mixture interaction (8) between a residue in saliva of substances from the plant and the subsequently ingested food. Taste modification is distinguished from these phenomena because it will "continue beyond the time of compound/receptor interaction and (does not) involve central, rather than peripheral, nervous system processes" (54). Neurophysiologic measures of responses from primary gustatory neurons in invertebrates (54,56), anurans (45), and mammals (45,51), including humans (90), have provided the evidence for the assertion that taste modification occurs at the taste receptor.

A number of different types of molecules can produce taste modification (45). Some are saponins (29,55), while others are proteins (11,12,50). In addition, some of the catechins, flavanols, and flavins in tea (38,45,78) can produce taste modification (66,73), as can cynarin and chlorogenic acid, two compounds found in the artichoke (13). In all cases the effect is fully reversible, with a recovery time of minutes (81) to hours (11,66). It is likely that many other taste modifiers exist in the natural environment. In addition, there may be "artificial" taste modifiers in the array of chemicals that humans have created and now add to foods or other products. Sodium lauryl sulfate, which was discussed in the Water Pollution section, is one known example.

Summary: Taste

In general, the differentiated epithelial cells that make up vertebrate taste buds have little protection from the liquid-borne chemical and thermal events that are their stimuli. The constant and relatively rapid replacement of taste bud cells suggests a high likelihood of damage. Most gustatory stimuli probably do not penetrate further than the taste bud's pore chamber. Surfactants are known to affect and sometimes damage taste buds. They occur as pollutants in water supplies and are used as additives in oral hygiene products. Saliva has an important but not fully understood interaction with taste receptors. Since many heavy metals tend to concentrate in saliva, and taste responses can be altered or blocked by topical application of heavy metal solutions, exposure to heavy metal pollution may lead to gustatory damage.

OVERVIEW

Many potential environmental hazards exist for olfaction and taste. There has been a general failure to consider or evaluate chemosensory deficits as potential toxicologic problems. The importance of human chemosensory function and the many difficulties that result from chemosensory dysfunction have been recognized (86), but the incidence of chemosensory toxicants in the environment is largely unknown. Adequate testing of chemosensory function as part of industrial medical screening and as a component of more general examinations is needed. Our present ignorance may be obscuring a sizeable array of preventable or correctable chemosensory disorders. An active and aggressive program is needed to clarify the nature of environmental factors affecting chemoreceptors.

ACKNOWLEDGMENT

I thank W. S. Cain for discussions on the contents of this paper and P. C. Canney, P. A. Halpern, and S. T. Kelling for critical comments on the manuscript. Research support was from NSF grant BNS 8213476 and Army Research Office research contract DAAG29-82-K-0098 during preparation of this report.

REFERENCES

1. Adams, R. G., and Crabtree, N. (1961): Anosmia in alkaline battery workers. *Br. J. Ind. Med.*, 18:216–221.
2. Ai, N., and Takagi, S. K. (1963): The effect of ether and chloroform on the olfactory epithelium. *Jpn. J. Physiol.*, 13:454–465.
3. Andersen, I. (1979): Formaldehyde in the indoor environment—Health implications and the setting of standards. In: *Indoor Climate*, edited by P. O. Fanger and O. Valbjorn, pp. 65–88. Danish Building Research Institute, Copenhagen.
4. Atema, J. (1977): Functional separation of smell and taste in fish and crustacea. In: *Olfaction and Taste VI*, edited by J. LeMagnen and P. MacLeod, pp. 165–174. Information Retrieval, Inc., Washington, DC.
5. Bannister, L. H. (1974): Possible functions of mucus at gustatory and olfactory surfaces. In: *Transduction Mechanisms in Vertebrates*, edited by T. M. Poynder, pp. 39–48. Information Retrieval Ltd., London.
6. Bardach, J. E., and Atema, J. (1971): The sense of taste in fishes. In: *Handbook of Sensory Physiology, Vol. IV: Chemical Senses. Part 2: Taste*, edited by L. M. Beidler, pp. 293–336. Springer-Verlag, Berlin.
7. Bardach, J. E., Fujiya, M., and Holl, A. (1965): Detergents: Effects on the chemical senses of the fish *Ictalurus natalis* (le Sueur). *Science*, 148:1605–1607.

8. Bartoshuk, L. M. (1975): Taste mixtures: Is mixture suppression related to compression? *Physiol. Behav.*, 14:643–649.
9. Bartoshuk, L. M. (1977): Water taste in mammals. In: *Drinking Behavior: Oral Stimulation, Reinforcement, and Preference*, edited by J. A. W. M. Weijnen and J. Mendelson, pp. 317–339. Plenum Press, New York.
10. Bartoshuk, L. M. (1978): Gustatory system. In: *Handbook of Behavioral Neurobiology, Vol. 1: Sensory Integration*, edited by R. B. Masterton, pp. 503–557. Plenum Press, New York.
11. Bartoshuk, L. M., Dateo, G. P., Vandenbelt, D. J., Buttrick, R. L., and Long, L. (1969): Effects of *Gymnema sylvestre* and *Synsepalum dulcificum* on taste in man. In: *Olfaction and Taste III*, edited by C. Pfaffmann, pp. 436–444. Rockefeller University Press, New York.
12. Bartoshuk, L. M., Gentile, R. L., Moskowitz, H. R., and Meiselman, H. L. (1974): Sweet taste induced by miracle fruit *(Synsepalum dulcificum)*. *Physiol. Behav.*, 12:449–456.
13. Bartoshuk, L. M., Lee, C.-H., and Scarpellino, R. (1972): Sweet taste of water induced by artichoke *(Cynara scolymus)*. *Science*, 178:988–990.
14. Basrur, P. K., and Basrur, V. R. (1977): Surface alterations in the nasal mucosa of hamsters exposed to cigarette smoke. In: *Scanning Electron Microscopy/1977/II. Biological Applications of the SEM*, edited by O. Johari and R. P. Becker, pp. 507–512. IIT Research Institute, Chicago.
15. Beidler, L. M., editor (1971): *Handbook of Sensory Physiology, Vol. IV: Chemical Senses. Part 2: Taste*. Springer-Verlag, Berlin.
16. Beidler, L. M. (1978): Biophysics and chemistry of taste. In: *Handbook of Perception, Vol. VIA: Tasting and Smelling*, edited by E. C. Carterett and M. P. Friedman, pp. 21–49. Academic Press, New York.
17. Ben-Aryeh, H., and Gutman, D. (1979): Saliva for biological monitoring. In: *The Use of Biological Specimens for the Assessment of Human Exposure to Environmental Pollutants*, edited by A. Berlin, A. H. Wolff, and Y. Hagegawa, pp. 65–69. Martinus Nijhoff Publishers, The Hague.
18. Berlin, A., Wolff, A. H., and Hagegawa, Y., editors (1979): *The Use of Biological Specimens for the Assessment of Human Exposure to Environmental Pollutants*, p. 30. Martinus Nijhoff Publishers, The Hague.
19. Bernard, R. A., and Halpern, B. P. (1968): Taste changes in vitamin A deficiency. *J. Gen. Physiol.*, 52:444–464.
20. Brabec, M. J. (1981): Aldehydes and acetals. In: *Patty's Industrial Hygiene and Toxicology, Vol. 2: Toxicology. Part A*, 3rd edition, edited by G. D. Clayton and F. E. Clayton, pp. 2637–2646. Wiley-Interscience, New York.
21. Brouwer, J. N., and Wiersma, A. (1978): Location of taste buds in intact papillae by a selective staining method. *Histochemistry*, 58:145–151.
22. Burgess, W. A. (1981): *Recognition of Health Hazards in Industry: A Review of Materials and Processes*. John Wiley and Sons, New York.
23. Cain, W. S. (1981): Olfaction and the common chemical sense: Similarities, differences, and interaction. In: *Odor Quality and Chemical Structure. ACS Symposium Series, No. 148*, edited by H. R. Moskowitz and C. B. Warren, pp. 109–121. American Chemical Society, Washington, DC.
24. Cain, W. S., and Garcia-Medina, M. R. (1980): Possible adverse biological effects of odor pollution. Presented at the 73rd Annual Meeting of the Air Pollution Control Association, Montreal, Quebec, June 22–27.
25. Caprio, J. (1982): High sensitivity and specificity of olfactory and gustatory receptors of catfish to amino acids. In: *Chemoreception in Fishes*, edited by T. J. Hara, pp. 109–134. Elsevier Scientific Publishing Co., Amsterdam.
26. Cometto-Muniz, J. E., and Cain, W. S. (1982): Perception of nasal pungency in smokers and nonsmokers. *Physiol. Behav.*, 29:727–731.
27. Crocker, B. B., Novak, D. A., and Scholle, W. A. (1978): Air pollution control methods. In: *Kirk-Othmer Encyclopedia of Chemical Technology, Vol. 1*, 3rd edition, edited by H. F. Mark, D. F. Othmer, C. G. Overberger, and G. Seaborg, pp. 694–716. John Wiley and Sons, New York.
28. Cunzeman, P. J., and Slotnick, B. M. (1980): Olfaction after prolonged exposure to specific odors. Presented at 2nd Annual Meeting of the Association for Chemoreception Sciences, Sarasota, May 4–8.
29. Dateo, G. P., and Long, L., Jr. (1973): Gymnemic acid, the antisaccharin principle of *Gymnema sylvestre*. Studies on the heterogeneity of gymnemic acid. *J. Agr. Food Chem.*, 21:889–903.
30. DeSimone, J. A., Heck, G. L., and Bartoshuk, L. M. (1980): Surface active taste modifiers: A

comparison of the physical and psychophysical properties of gymnemic acid and lauryl sulfate. *Chem. Senses*, 5:317–330.

31. DeVries, H., and Stuiver, M. (1961): The absolute sensitivity of the sense of smell. In: *Sensory Communication*, edited by W. A. Rosenblith, pp. 159–167. John Wiley and Sons, New York.
32. Drago, N. P., Pruett, J. G., and Winslow, S. G. (1980): *Health Aspects of Urea-Formaldehyde Compounds. A Selected Bibliography with Abstracts. 1964–1980*. Federation of American Societies for Experimental Biology, Bethesda, MD.
33. Dunn, J. D., Cometto-Muniz, J. E., and Cain, W. S. (1982): Nasal reflexes: Reduced sensitivity to CO_2 irritation in cigarette smokers. *J. Appl. Toxicol.*, 2:176–178.
34. Faull, J. R., and Halpern, B. P. (1972): Taste stimuli: Time course of peripheral nerve response and theoretical models. *Science*, 178:73–75.
35. French, G. (1973): Water in relation to human disease. In: *Environmental Medicine*, edited by G. M. Howe and J. A. Loraine, pp. 40–71. William Heinemann Medical Books, London.
36. Gardner, D. E. (1982): Effects of gases and airborne particles on lung infections. In: *Air Pollution—Physiological Effects*, edited by J. J. McGrath and C. D. Barnes, pp. 47–79. Academic Press, New York.
37. Gomez-Ramos, P., and Rodriguez-Echandia, E. L. (1979): The fine structural effect of sialectomy on the taste bud cells in the rat. *Tissue Cell*, 11:19–29.
38. Graham, H. (1983): Tea. In: *Kirk-Othmer Encyclopedia of Chemical Technology, Vol. 22*, 3rd edition, edited by H. F. Mark, D. F. Othmer, C. G. Overberger, and G. Seaborg, pp. 628–644. John Wiley and Sons, New York.
39. Graziadei, P. C. C. (1974): The olfactory and taste organs of vertebrates: A dynamic approach to the study of their morphology. In: *Transduction Mechanisms in Chemoreception*, edited by T. M. Ponder, pp. 3–14. Information Retrieval Ltd., London.
40. Graziadei, P. C. C. (1977): Functional anatomy of the mammalian chemoreceptor system. In: *Chemical Signals in Vertebrates*, edited by D. Müller-Schwarze and M. M. Mozell, pp. 435–454. Plenum Press, New York.
41. Graziadei, P. P. C., and Monti Graziadei, G. A. (1979): Neurogenesis and neuron regeneration in the olfactory system of mammals. I. Morphological aspects of differentiation and structural organization of olfactory sensory neurons. *J. Neurocytol.*, 8:1–18.
42. Graziadei, P. P. C., and Monti Graziadei, A. G. (1983): Regeneration in the olfactory system of vertebrates. *Am. J. Otolaryngol.*, 4:228–233.
43. Grossblatt, N., editor (1979): *Odors from Stationary and Mobile Sources*. National Academy of Sciences, Washington, DC.
44. Halpern, B. P. (1967): Some relationships between electrophysiology and behavior in taste. In: *The Chemical Senses and Nutrition*, edited by M. R. Kare and O. Maller, pp. 213–241. The Johns Hopkins University Press, Baltimore.
45. Halpern, B. P. (1973): The use of vertebrate laboratory animals in research on taste. In: *Methods of Animal Experimentation, Vol. IV: Environment and Special Senses*, edited by W. I. Gay, pp. 225–384. Academic Press, New York.
46. Halpern, B. P. (1977): Functional anatomy of the tongue and mouth of mammals. In: *Drinking Behavior: Oral Stimulation, Reinforcement, and Preference*, edited by J. A. W. M. Weijnen and J. Mendelson, pp. 1–92. Plenum Press, New York.
47. Halpern, B. P. (1985): What to control in studies of taste. In: *Clinical Measurement of Taste and Smell*, edited by H. L. Meiselman and R. S. Rivlin. Macmillan, New York *(in press)*.
48. Hara, T. J., Brown, S. B., and Evans, R. E. (1983): Pollutants and chemoreception in aquatic organisms. In: *Aquatic Toxicology*, edited by J. O. Nriagu, pp. 247–306. John Wiley and Sons, New York.
49. Hawkes, J. W. (1980): The effect of xenobiotics on fish tissues: Morphological studies. *Fed. Proc.*, 39:3230–3236.
50. Hellekant, G. (1976): On the gustatory effects of gymnemic acid and miraculin in dog, pig, and rabbit. *Chem. Senses Flavor*, 2:85–95.
51. Hyde, R. J., Feller, R. P., and Sharon, I. M. (1981): Tongue brushing, dentifrice, and age effects on taste and smell. *J. Dent. Res.*, 60:1730–1734.
52. Jaeger, M. J. (1982): Toxic effects of SO_2 on the respiratory system. In: *Air Pollution—Physiological Effects*, edited by J. J. McGrath and C. D. Barnes, pp. 81–105. Academic Press, New York.

53. Jonsson, L. (1980): Chemical stimuli: Role in the behavior of fishes. In: *Environmental Physiology of Fishes*, edited by M. A. Ai, pp. 353–367. Plenum Press, New York.
54. Kennedy, L. M., and Halpern, B. P. (1980): Fly chemoreceptors: A model system for the taste modifier ziziphin. *Physiol. Behav.*, 24:135–143.
55. Kennedy, L. M., and Halpern, B. P. (1980): Extraction, purification and characterization of a sweetness-modifying component from *Ziziphus jujuba*. *Chem. Senses*, 5:123–147.
56. Kennedy, L. M., Sturchow, B., and Waller, F. J. (1975): Effect of gymnemic acid on single taste hairs in the housefly *Musca domestica*. *Physiol. Behav.*, 14:755–765.
57. Ketels, K. V., Bradof, J. N., Fenters, J. D., and Ehrlich, R. (1977): SEM studies of the respiratory tract of mice exposed to sulfuric acid mist-carbon particle mixtures. In: *Scanning Electron Microscopy/1977/II. Biological Applications of the SEM*, edited by O. Johari and R. P. Becker, pp. 519–526. IIT Research Institute, Chicago.
58. Kiyohara, S., and Tucker, D. (1978): Activity of new receptors after transection of the primary olfactory nerve in pigeon. *Physiol. Behav.*, 21:987–994.
59. Laing, D. G., and Panhuber, H. (1979): Application of anatomical and psychophysical methods to studies of odour interaction. In: *Progress in Flavour Research*, edited by D. G. Land and H. E. Nursten, pp. 27–46. Applied Science Publishers, Ltd., Barking, Essex, England.
60. Lebowitz, M. D. (1983): Health effects of indoor air pollutants. *Annu. Rev. Public Health*, 4:203–221.
61. Lee, S. D. (1977): *Biochemical Effects of Environmental Pollutants*. Ann Arbor Scientific Publishers, Ann Arbor, MI.
62. Lindvall, T. (1977): Perception of composite odorous air pollutants. In: *Olfaction and Taste VI*, edited by J. LeMagnen and P. MacLeod, pp. 449–458. IRL, London.
63. Loomis, T. A. (1979): Formaldehyde toxicity. *Arch. Pathol. Lab. Med.*, 103:321–324.
64. Martin, A. E. (1973): Air pollution in relation to human disease. In: *Environmental Medicine*, edited by G. M. Howe and J. A. Loraine, pp. 100–109. William Heinemann Medical Books, London.
65. Matulionis, D. H. (1974): Ultrastructure of olfactory epithelia in mice after smoke exposure. *Ann. Otol.*, 83:192–201.
66. Meiselman, H. L., and Halpern, B. P. (1970): Human judgments of *Gymnema sylvestre* and sucrose mixtures. *Physiol. Behav.*, 5:945–948.
67. Meiselman, H. L., Halpern, B. P., and Dateo, G. P. (1976): Reduction of sweetness judgments by extracts from the leaves of *Ziziphus jujuba*. *Physiol. Behav.*, 17:313–317.
68. Moulton, D. G. (1977): Minimum odorant concentrations detectable by the dog and their implications for olfactory sensitivity. In: *Chemical Signals in Vertebrates*, edited by D. Müller-Schwarze and M. M. Mozell, pp. 455–464. Plenum Press, New York.
69. Moulton, D. G., Celebi, G., and Fink, R. P. (1970): Olfaction in mammals—Two aspects: Proliferation of cells in the olfactory epithelium and sensitivity to odours. In: *Taste and Smell in Vertebrates*, edited by G. E. W. Wolstenholme and J. Knight, pp. 227–250. J. and A. Churchill, London.
70. Mozell, M. M. (1977): Processing of olfactory stimuli at peripheral levels. In: *Chemical Signals in Vertebrates*, edited by D. Müller-Schwarze and M. M. Mozell, pp. 465–482. Plenum Press, New York.
71. Müller-Schwarze, D., and Mozell, M. M., editors (1977): *Chemical Signals in Vertebrates*. Plenum Press, New York.
72. Nadel, J. A., Davis, B., and Phipps, R. J. (1979): Control of mucus secretion and ion transport in airways. *Annu. Rev. Physiol.*, 41:369–381.
73. Nakagawa, M., Anan, T., and Takayanagi, H. (1978): The relation of flavor depressor and chemical composition in summer green tea. *Chagyo Gijutsu Kenkyu*, 55:71–77.
74. NIOSH (1976): Health Hazard Determination Report No. 74-16-272, U.S. Department of Health, Education, and Welfare, Cincinnati, Ohio. Cited in reference 22, p. 168.
75. Pfaffmann, C., editor (1969): *Olfaction and Taste III*. Rockefeller University Press, New York.
76. Pfaffmann, C. (1978): The vertebrate phylogeny, neural code, and integrative processes of taste. In: *Handbook of Perception, Vol. VIA: Tasting and Smelling*, edited by E. C. Carterett and M. P. Friedman, pp. 51–123. Academic Press, New York.
77. Proctor, D. F. (1977): The upper airways. I. Nasal physiology and defense of the lungs. *Am. Rev. Resp. Dis.*, 115:97–129.
78. Sanderson, G. W. (1972): The chemistry of tea and tea manufacturing. In: *Recent Advances in*

Phytochemistry, Vol. 5: Structural and Functional Aspects of Phytochemistry, edited by V. C. Runeckles, pp. 247–316. Academic Press, New York.

79. Schwartz, L. W., Moore, P. F., Chang, D. P., Tarkington, B. K., Dunsworth, D. L., and Tyler, W. S. (1977): Short-term effects of sulfuric acid aerosols on the respiratory tract. A morphological study in guinea pigs, mice, rats, and monkeys. In: *Biochemical Effects of Environmental Pollutants*, edited by S. D. Lee, pp. 257–271. Ann Arbor Science Publishers, Ann Arbor, MI.
80. Silver, W. L., and Maruniak, J. A. (1981): Trigeminal chemoreception in the nasal and oral cavities. *Chem. Senses*, 6:295–305.
81. Smith, V. V., and Halpern, B. P. (1983): Selective suppression of judged sweetness by ziziphins. *Physiol. Behav.*, 30:867–874.
82. Sticksel, P. R., and Engdahl, R. B. (1978): Air pollution. In: *Kirk-Othmer Encyclopedia of Chemical Technology, Vol. 1*, 3rd edition, edited by H. F. Mark, D. F. Othmer, C. G. Overberger, and G. Seaborg, pp. 624–649. John Wiley and Sons, New York.
83. Stokinger, H. E. (1981): The metals. In: *Patty's Industrial Hygiene and Toxicology, Vol. 2: Toxicology. Part A*, edited by G. D. Clayton and F. E. Clayton, pp. 1493–2060. Wiley-Interscience, New York.
84. Sugihara, K., Yamamoto, T., and Kawamura, Y. (1977): Effect of detergents on taste nerve responses. *Jpn. J. Physiol.*, 19:463–468.
85. Tromp, S. W. (1973): The relationship of weather and climate to health and disease. In: *Environmental Medicine*, edited by G. M. Howe and J. A. Loraine, pp. 72–99. William Heinemann Medical Books, London.
86. Ward, P. H., chairman (1979): Report of the Panel on Communicative Disorders to the National Advisory Neurological and Communicative Disorders and Stroke Council. NIH Publication 79-1914, Bethesda, MD.
87. Whittemore, A. S. (1981): Air pollution and respiratory disease. *Annu. Rev. Public Health*, 2:397–429.
88. Windholz, M., editor (1983): *The Merck Index*, 10th ed. Merck and Company, Rahway, NJ.
89. Zelson, P. R., and Cagan, R. H. (1979): Biochemical studies of taste sensation. VIII. Partial characterization of alanine-binding taste receptor sites of catfish *Ictalurus punctatus* using mercurials, sulfhydryl reagents, trypsin and phospholipase C. *Comp. Biochem. Physiol.*, 64B:141–147.
90. Zotterman, Y. (1974): A taste modifier in primates and man. *Actual. Neurophysiol.*, 11:125–130.

Toxicology of the Eye, Ear, and Other Special Senses, edited by W. Hayes. Raven Press, New York © 1985.

Genetic Differences in Drug Metabolism Associated with Ocular Toxicity

*Hitoshi Shichi and **Daniel W. Nebert

*Institute of Biological Sciences, Oakland University, Rochester, Michigan 48063; and **Laboratory of Developmental Pharmacology, National Institute of Child Health and Human Development, National Institutes of Health, Bethesda, Maryland 20205

Other chapters in this book are concerned with drug toxicity and pathology related to tissues of the head and neck. This chapter deals more directly with the drug-metabolizing enzymes involved. These enzymes are responsible for toxification (i.e., potentiation of the toxic response by forming a reactive drug intermediate), as well as detoxication (metabolism leading to the excretion of innocuous products). This paper also emphasizes genetic differences in these enzymes, whereas genetics is not addressed in the other chapters. Although the genetic system described in detail here involves mice, there is ample evidence that the same system operates in man. It therefore should be obvious that, because of differences in genetic predisposition among individuals in the human population, a particular dose of an ophthalmic drug might be toxic to one person but not to another (and these two persons might even be siblings). Similar genetic differences in toxicity caused by drugs and other environmental pollutants are expected to be manifest among other tissues of the body, as well as in the eye.

We first describe the tissue localization and subcellular distribution of drug-metabolizing enzymes in the eye. Next, the genetic system called the *Ah* complex is introduced. Finally, genetic differences in acetaminophen- and naphthalene-induced cataract formation (lens opacification) and other ocular degeneration are shown to be related to the *Ah* locus.

CONCEPT OF EXTRAHEPATIC DRUG METABOLISM

Until the last two decades, it was generally accepted that the liver was the only important organ for drug metabolism. More recently, however, it has become clear that virtually every cell of every plant and animal (and certain bacteria) contains drug-metabolizing capability. At least part of this appreciation reflects the development of much more sensitive assays for drug-metabolizing enzymes. Toxification and detoxication of drugs and other environmental pollutants in extrahepatic tissues therefore can be very important (1).

The eye is no exception. For example, chloroquine retinopathy observed in malaria patients was attributed to an accumulation of unusually high levels of

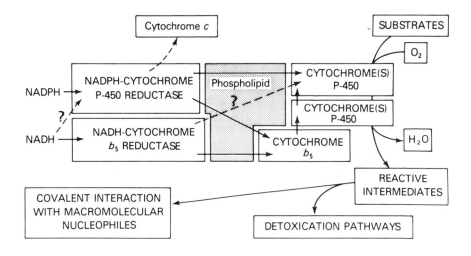

FIG. 1. Scheme for the membrane-bound multicomponent monooxygenase system(s) and the various possibly important pathways for hydrophobic substrates (8). For any given substrate, the relative balance between metabolic activation and detoxication likely would differ among different tissues, strains, and species. Age, genetic expression, nutrition, hormone concentration, diurnal rhythm, pH, saturating versus nonsaturating conditions of the substrate, K_m and V_{max} for each enzyme, subcellular compartmentalization of each enzyme, efficiency of DNA repair, and the immunologic competence of the animal may all be important factors affecting this balance.

chloroquine in the eye (2). Unless the eye possesses a mechanism for removing such drugs that enter ocular tissues via the circulating blood, therefore, accumulated chemicals of all types might exert adverse effects on photoreceptor cells, leading to visual impairment. Shortly after Bernstein's report on chloroquine toxicity (2), cytochrome P-450, a principal component of the drug-metabolizing enzyme system,[1] was detected spectrally in the pigmented epithelium of bovine retina (4). Although much progress has been made in studies on absorption, distribution, and clinical usefulness of ophthalmic drugs (5), information on ocular drug metabolism and toxicity remains quite scanty, in spite of obvious clinical importance.

Further, information about genetic differences in ocular drug toxicity is even more scarce. Steroid-induced glaucoma is a pharmacogenetic disorder, for example, although the etiology is unknown; about 5% of the United Sates population is homozygous for the recessive allele causing glaucoma induced by corticosteroid ophthalmic medications (6).

---

[1]In this chapter, cytochrome P-450 is defined as all forms of CO-binding hemoproteins associated with membrane-bound NADPH-dependent monooxygenase activities. We define cytochrome P_1-450 as all forms of CO-binding hemoprotein that increase in amount concomitantly with rises in induced aryl hydrocarbon hydroxylase activity following polycyclic aromatic inducer treatment. In view of the existence of more than one such form of P_1-450 (3), it is emphasized that this definition of P_1-450 is simplistic.

P-450-MEDIATED MONOOXYGENASE ACTIVITIES AND OTHER COORDINATED DRUG-METABOLIZING ENZYMES

Many environmental pollutants and other foreign compounds are chemicals that are so hydrophobic they would remain in the body indefinitely were it not for the metabolism resulting in more polar derivatives. These drug-metabolizing enzyme systems, which are localized principally in the liver, are usually divided into two groups: phase I and phase II. During phase I metabolism, one or more polar groups (such as hydroxyl) are introduced into the hydrophobic parent molecule, thus allowing a handle, or position, for the phase II conjugating enzymes (such as UDP-glucuronosyltransferase) to attack. The conjugated products are sufficiently polar that these detoxified chemicals can now be excreted from the body (7).

One of the most interesting of the phase I enzyme systems is a group of enzymes known collectively as the P-450-mediated monooxygenases (3,8). These membrane-bound enzyme systems metabolize polycyclic aromatic hydrocarbons such as benzo[a]pyrene (ubiquitous in city smog, cigarette smoke, and characoal-cooked foods) and biphenyl; halogenated hydrocarbons such as polychlorinated and poly-brominated biphenyls, insecticides, and ingredients in soaps and deodorants; strong mutagens such as N-methyl-N'-nitro-N-acetylarylamines and nitrofurans; numerous aromatic amines such as those found in hair dyes; nitro aromatics and heterocyclics; wood terpenes; epoxides; carbamates; alkyl halides; safrole derivatives; certain fungal toxins and antibiotics; many of the chemotherapeutic agents used to treat human cancer; most drugs; small chemicals such as benzene, thiocyanate, or ethanol; both endogenous and synthetic steroids; and other endogenous compounds such as biogenic amines, prostaglandins, indoles, thyroxine, and fatty acids.

Evidence is growing that metabolism to reactive intermediates by cytochrome P-450-mediated monooxygenase is a prerequisite for mutagenesis, carcinogenesis, and toxicity caused by numerous drugs, polycyclic hydrocarbons, and other envi-

TABLE 1. *Distribution of AHH, UDP-glucuronosyltransferase, and γ-glutamyltranspeptidase activities in various tissues of bovine eye*

Tissues	Enzyme activity, U/mg protein[a]		
	AHH	UDP-Glucuronosyltransferase	γ-Glutamyltranspeptidase
Retina	0.03	6	400
Lens	Not detectable	5	3
Cornea	0.02	8	320
Iris	0.15	23	640
Pigmented epithelium-choroid	0.31	84	430
Ciliary body	5.74	396	3,850

[a]Tissue homogenates were used for assay of enzymic activities. One unit of activity is the amount of enzyme protein that produces 1 pmol of product/min. Enzyme activities given here are specific activities, i.e., U/mg of tissue protein/min.

TABLE 2. *Subcellular activities of enzymes involved in mercapturate synthesis in the bovine eye[a]*

Subcellular fraction	Glutathione transferase[b]		γ-Glutamyltranspeptidase		Cystine aminopeptidase		N-Acetyltransferase	
	Ciliary body	Pigmented epithelium-choroid	Ciliary body	Pigmented epithelium-choroid	Ciliary body	Pigmented epithelium-choroid	Ciliary body	Pigmented epithelium-choroid
Tissue homogenate	5,210	480	3,850	430	100	8	13	2
Nuclei	780	230	270	67	1	Not detectable	7	1
Mitochondria	1,400	120	1,620	310	73	7	64	2
Microsomes	3,690	590	5,120	570	1,130	54	160	8
Supernatant	6,340	870	1,230	130	450	13	13	Not detectable

[a]Activities are expressed as U/mg protein. See Table 1 for definition of one unit of activity.
[b]With 1-chloro-2,4-dinitrobenzene as the substrate.

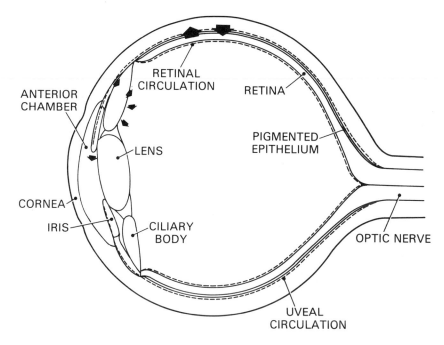

FIG. 2. Retinal and uveal blood circulation systems (shown as *dashed lines*). The retinal circulation provides nutrients for the retinal neurons, while the uveal circulation supplies nutrients for the pigmented epithelium (and visual cells), the ciliary body (and lens and cornea), and the iris. *Large arrows* denote entry of nutrients and exit of metabolic products between the uveal circulation (choroidal capillaries) and the pigmented epithelium. *Small arrows* indicate aqueous humor secretion by the ciliary body into the anterior chamber and aqueous humor.

ronmental pollutants. The steady-state levels of these reactive electrophilic intermediates, and consequently the rates at which they interact with the critical nucleophilic target, are dependent on a delicate *balance* between their generation and detoxication (Fig. 1). Changes in the balance between toxification and detoxication in any particular tissue of an individual may therefore affect his risk of tumorigenesis or toxicity.

SUBCELLULAR LOCALIZATION AND DISTRIBUTION OF DRUG-METABOLIZING ENZYMES IN THE EYE

The distribution (Table 1) and subcellular localization (Table 2) of several drug-metabolizing enzyme activities were studied in bovine eye. AHH activity[2] was chosen as an example of phase I metabolism (reflecting basal forms of P-450). UDP-glucuronosyltransferase, glutathione transferase, and *N*-acetyltransferase activities are typical phase II enzymes (9). γ-Glutamyltranspeptidase and cystine

---

[2]Abbreviations used include AHH, aryl hydrocarbon (benzo[a]pyrene) hydroxylase (EC 1.14.14.1); B6, the C57BL/6N inbred mouse strain; D2, the DBA/2N inbred mouse strain.

aminopeptidase are important in the pathway from glutathione conjugates of aromatic hydrocarbons to mercapturate formation (10). Most, if not all, of these six enzymes (Tables 1 and 2) are induced by various drugs or other environmental pollutants (3,9,10). Low levels of γ-glutamyltranspeptidase (11) and glutathione transferase (12) have been reported in the lens.

We conclude from Tables 1 and 2 that virtually all ocular tissues have detectable drug-metabolizing capability (13–16). The ciliary body and pigmented epithelium-choroid are by far the richest in these activities (see Fig. 2 for the location of these tissues in the eye). In fact, the specific activities of AHH and UDP-glucuronosyltransferase in the ciliary body are only about 10 to 20 times less than those in bovine liver. One of the glutathione transferases in the ciliary body was purified to homogeneity (Shichi and O'Meara, *unpublished*). The enzyme (molecular weight = 44,000) is an acidic protein (isoelectric point of about 5.7) with high affinity for chlorodinitrobenzene as substrate, and seems to be different from any of the glutathione transferase isozymes reported (17,18).

THE *Ah* LOCUS: GENETIC EXPRESSION OF INDUCED AHH ACTIVITY AND P_1-450 INDUCTION

The *Ah* locus is an experimental model system that has provided several good examples of a delicate balance between genetic and environmental factors in the etiology of cancer, drug toxicity, and birth defects (19). The *Ah* gene of the mouse regulates the induction (by polycyclic aromatic compounds such as 3-methylcholanthrene or benzo[a]pyrene) of numerous drug-metabolizing enzyme "activities" associated with several induced forms of cytochrome P_1-450.

At any given dose of inducer, the induction of AHH activity and at least two dozen other monooxygenase activities and associated forms of P_1-450 occurs in 3-methylcholanthrene-treated B6 and other genetically "responsive" inbred strains and is always much lower in 3-methylcholanthrene-treated D2 and other genetically "nonresponsive" strains. Besides the liver, this genetic expression is seen in such tissues as lung, kidney, intestine, lymph nodes, skin, bone marrow, pigmented epithelium of the retina (Table 3), brain, mammary gland, uterus, ovary, and testis.

TABLE 3. *Induction of ocular AHH activity in B6 and D2 mice by polycyclic aromatic compounds*

Intraperitoneal treatment	Specific AHH activity, U/mg protein[a]	
	B6	D2
Control	0.08	0.06
β-Naphthoflavone	0.36	0.07
3-Methylcholanthrene	0.39	0.08
2,3,7,8-Tetrachlorodibenzo-*p*-dioxin	0.47	0.10

[a]See Table 1. Tissue homogenates of the entire eye were prepared for the enzyme assay.

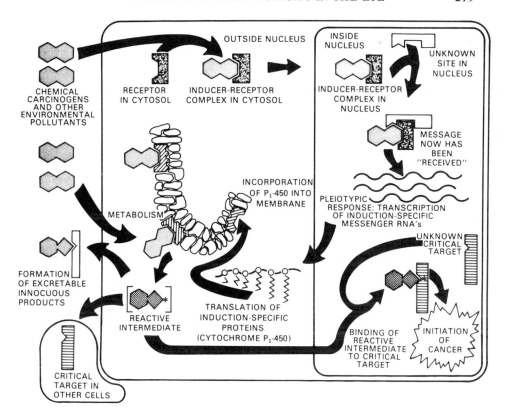

FIG. 3. Diagram of a cell and the hypothetical scheme by which a cytosolic receptor, product of the regulatory *Ah* gene, binds to inducer (20). Depending upon the half-life of the reactive intermediate, the rate of formation of the intermediate, and the rate of conjugation and other means to detoxify the intermediate, important covalent binding may occur in the same cell in which metabolism took place or in some distant cell. Although the "unknown critical target" is illustrated here in the nucleus, there is presently no experimental evidence demonstrating unequivocally the subcellular location of a "critical target(s)" required for the initiation of drug toxicity or cancer. (Courtesy of Dr. W. Junk.)

The genetic response is therefore called "systemic," or occurring throughout virtually all tissues of the animal. Responsiveness to aromatic hydrocarbons has been designated the *Ah* locus: *Ah*[b] is the dominant allele; *Ah*[d] is the recessive allele; the *Ah*[b]/*Ah*[d] heterozygote is phenotypically similar to the *Ah*[b]/*Ah*[b] mouse in terms of degree of responsiveness. The trait of *Ah*-responsiveness among crosses involving B6 and D2 mice is therefore autosomal dominant (19).

Several studies indicate that the fundamental genetic difference resides in the *Ah* regulatory gene (Fig. 3), which encodes the cytosolic receptor capable of binding to inducers such as 3-methylcholanthrene, benzo[a]pyrene, and 2,3,7,8-tetrachlorodibenzo-*p*-dioxin. To our knowledge, only certain foreign chemicals bind to this receptor with saturability and high affinity (apparent $K_D \cong$ nM). The B6 receptor appears to have at least 10 times better affinity toward inducers of P_1-450 than the

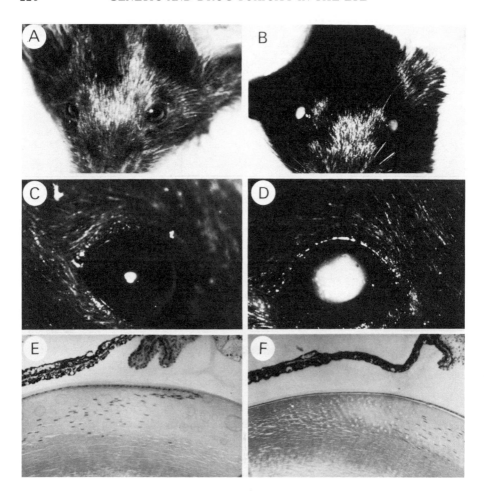

FIG. 4. (**A** and **C**) Genetically nonresponsive Ah^d/Ah^d homozygote, and (**B** and **D**) genetically responsive Ah^b/Ah^d heterozygous sibling from the B6D2F$_1$ × D2 backcross (26). These photographs were taken 5 hr after the mice had received acetaminophen and 53 hr after the mice had received 3-methylcholanthrene, an inducer of P$_1$-450. (**E** and **F**) Hematoxylin- and eosin-stained sections of ocular tissue from mice in (**A**) and (**B**), respectively (×325). The tissues from top to bottom are iris, cornea, and lens. Vacuoles seen in the subepithelial layer of the lens in (**F**) are the result of hydration of the lens cells and are always associated with cataract formation (27). Doses of more than 1,000 mg of acetaminophen/kg body weight were mostly fatal to Ah^b/Ah^d mice within the first 8 hr after acetaminophen administration, but in Ah^d/Ah^d mice these doses were not lethal, nor did they ever cause lens opacification. At lower doses of acetaminophen (400–800 mg/kg), the ocular opacity developed more slowly in Ah^b/Ah^d mice. If a cataract did not appear within 10 hr after acetaminophen administration, however, no cataract developed subsequently. The degree of opacification that had developed within these 10 hr was never reversible. (From ref. 26, with permission.)

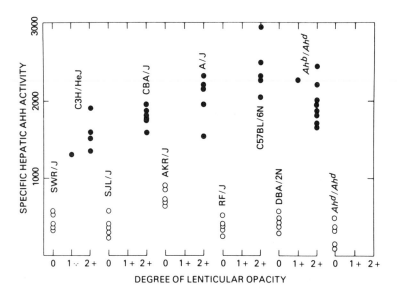

FIG. 5. Correlation between the hepatic AHH inducibility and cataractogenesis among five non-responsive inbred strains (○), four responsive inbred strains (●), and the responsive (Ah^b/Ah^d, ●) and nonresponsive (Ah^d/Ah^d, ○) progeny from the B6D2F₁ × D2 backcross (28). Each *symbol* represents an individual mouse. All mice had received 3-methylcholanthrene intraperitoneally 48 hr prior to intraperitoneal acetaminophen. The eyes were evaluated with an ophthalmic slit lamp 5 hr following acetaminophen treatment: 0 = No signs of opacification; 1 + = about 50% opacification; 2 + = complete opacification. The mice were then immediately killed, and the liver microsomal hydroxylase activity was determined. (From S. Karger, AG, with permission.)

Ah^d/Ah^d mouse (21). Translocation of the inducer-receptor complex into the nucleus has been demonstrated in the Ah-responsive heterozygote and homozygote (21) and requires a temperature-dependent step (22). Discrepancies between the dextran-charcoal adsorption assay and the sucrose density gradient assay have been recently understood via chromatographic studies of the Ah receptor (23).

What happens in the nucleus is not yet known (Fig. 3), but somehow the "information" (that these inducers of P_1-450 exist in the cell's microenvironment) is received; the response is transcription of specific mRNAs, translation of these mRNAs into specific enzymes such as P_1-450, and incorporation of P_1-450 into cellular membranes. These induced enzymes may aid in detoxication or they may generate increased amounts of reactive intermediates.

THE Ah LOCUS IN HUMAN POPULATIONS

In spite of shortcomings with the AHH assay in human cultured lymphoblasts (24), a growing list of clinical disorders appears to be associated with the human Ah gene. There clearly exists sufficient evidence that heritable variation of AHH inducibility occurs in man. Experimental difficulties, however, make it impossible at this time to be certain whether AHH induction is controlled by one or more genetic loci.

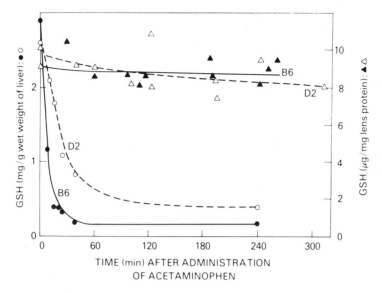

FIG. 6. Total glutathione (GSH) levels in the liver *(circles)* and lens *(triangles)* of 3-methylcholanthrene-treated B6 *(closed symbols)* and D2 *(open symbols)* mice following a large dose (1,000 mg/kg) of intraperitoneal acetaminophen (28). (From S. Karger, AG, with permission.)

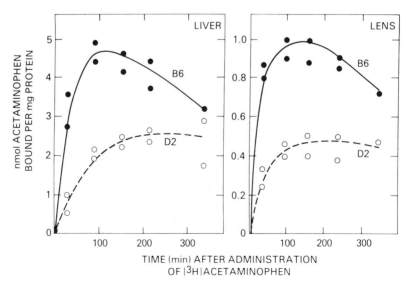

FIG. 7. Covalent binding of [³H]acetaminophen metabolite(s) to liver and lens proteins of 3-methylcholanthrene-treated B6 and D2 mice (28). (From S. Karger, AG, with permission.)

TABLE 4. Effect of oral acetaminophen or naphthalene on cataract formation in B6 and D2 mice

Inbred strain	Intraperitoneal P₁-450 inducer treatment[a]	Oral treatment[b]	Drug concentration, mg/ml[c]	Mean body weight[d]			Incidence cataracts, %	Comments
				Day 0	Day 21	Day 60		
B6	3-Methylcholanthrene	Acetaminophen	5	15.7 (15)	17.1 (13)	(0)	13.3	Two developed bilateral cataracts about day 10 and both died 1 to 2 weeks thereafter
D2	3-Methylcholanthrene	Acetaminophen	5	14.6 (15)	16.9 (15)	(0)	0	No cataracts at time of death
B6	3-Methylcholanthrene	Acetaminophen	10	16.2 (15)	17.6 (12)	(0)	13.3	Two developed bilateral cataracts about day 3 and both died within the next 2 weeks thereafter
D2	3-Methylcholanthrene	Acetaminophen	10	15.9 (15)	17.7 (15)	(0)	0	No cataracts at time of death
B6	β-Naphthoflavone	Acetaminophen	5	16.4 (15)	19.9 (15)	21.5 (15)	6.7	One developed a unilateral cataract about day 14; this was examined when mouse was killed 7 months later
D2	β-Naphthoflavone	Acetaminophen	5	15.4 (15)	20.5 (15)	22.8 (14)	0	No cataracts at time of death
B6	β-Naphthoflavone	Acetaminophen	10	15.9 (15)	20.8 (14)	22.3 (4)	13.3	One developed a unilateral cataract about day 11 and another developed bilateral cataracts about day 14; both died about day 36
D2	β-Naphthoflavone	Acetaminophen	10	16.9 (15)	21.6 (14)	23.9 (14)	0	No cataracts
B6	β-Naphthoflavone	Naphthalene	5	15.4 (15)	19.4 (14)	20.7 (13)	6.7	One developed bilateral cataracts about day 27; these were examined when mouse was killed 6 months later
D2	β-Naphthoflavone	Naphthalene	5	16.5 (15)	20.3 (15)	21.3 (15)	0	No cataracts
B6	β-Naphthoflavone	Naphthalene	10	15.4 (15)	17.2 (13)	18.8 (12)	6.7	One developed a unilateral cataract about day 8; this was examined when mouse was killed 7 months later
D2	β-Naphthoflavone	Naphthalene	10	16.5 (15)	16.7 (15)	19.4 (15)	0	No cataracts

[a] Injections twice weekly (28).
[b] The drug was dissolved in corn oil and the food was soaked in this solution of corn oil.
[c] Estimated drug concentration in corn oil in which the food was soaked.
[d] Mean body weights of group during feeding of the drug. The number of survivors is shown in parentheses.

CORRELATION BETWEEN THE Ah^b ALLELE AND LENS OPACIFICATION CAUSED BY INTRAPERITONEAL ACETAMINOPHEN

Acetaminophen, a widely used analgesic-antipyretic agent, is metabolized to a toxic intermediate largely by some form of polycyclic aromatic-induced P_1-450 (19). Therefore, we theorized that Ah-responsive mice—following treatment with polycyclic aromatic inducers to enhance P_1-450 levels—would display more acetaminophen toxicity than Ah-nonresponsive mice. This hypothesis turns out to be true not only in liver, where hepatic necrosis and covalent binding of acetaminophen metabolites occur (25), but also in the lens, where cataract formation was found (Fig. 4). An absolute correlation is found (Fig. 5) between lens opacification and the Ah^b allele among four Ah-responsive inbred mouse strains, five Ah-nonresponsive inbred strains, and among children of the $B6D2F_1 \times D2$ backcross.

Figure 6 illustrates the effects of acetaminophen on glutathione concentrations in the liver and lens of 3-methylcholanthrene-pretreated B6 and D2 mice. As expected, hepatic glutathione depletion is more pronounced in B6 than in D2 mice. Quite unexpectedly, however, lenticular glutathione levels are not depleted in either B6 or D2 mice following the large intraperitoneal dose of acetaminophen.

One possibility is that acetaminophen and its metabolites do not reach the lens and therefore glutathione is not depleted. This possibility was ruled out with the use of radiolabeled acetaminophen (Fig. 7). Similar kinetics of covalent binding occurs in both liver and lens protein, and in each case B6 tissues exhibit two to five times greater covalent binding than the corresponding D2 tissues.

How can covalent binding of acetaminophen metabolites occur in the apparent absence of any glutathione depletion? At least two possible answers come to mind. First, assuming glutathione depletion in the lens is necessary for cataract formation, one might envision some sort of compartmentalization of glutathione. In other words, although total lens glutathione concentrations are similar in B6 and D2 mice, a subcellular depletion of glutathione (directly in the anterior subcapsular region of the lens where the cataracts develop) might occur in B6 but not in D2. Such a localized depletion might be augmented by a sudden influx of reactive intermediates (generated by the liver, ciliary body, or whatever) so that local concentrations of the toxic agent far exceed local concentrations of glutathione in and near the anterior chamber. Alternatively, ocular toxicity may develop by a mechanism independent of glutathione levels. Electrophilic reactive intermediates

$\longrightarrow$

FIG. 8. Hematoxylin- and eosin-stained sections of ocular tissues from B6 mice that had received acetaminophen daily in the diet for more than 1 month (28).   **a:** Light micrograph showing ciliary body, iris, and trabecular meshwork. Note the presence of inflammatory cells in the angle *(arrowhead)* and the degenerative changes in the ciliary body. An atrophic iris and a certain amount of cellular infiltration of the episclera are observed. A peripheral anterior synechia is also seen. × 200.   **b:** Light micrograph showing the retina and choroid. Chronic degeneration of the choroid was frequently seen. The retina shows an almost normal appearance. × 200.   **c:** Light micrograph of the anterior cortical zone of the cataractous lens. Note the intermittent loss of epithelial cells from the epithelial cell layer *(arrowheads)*. × 184. (From S. Karger, AG, with permission.)

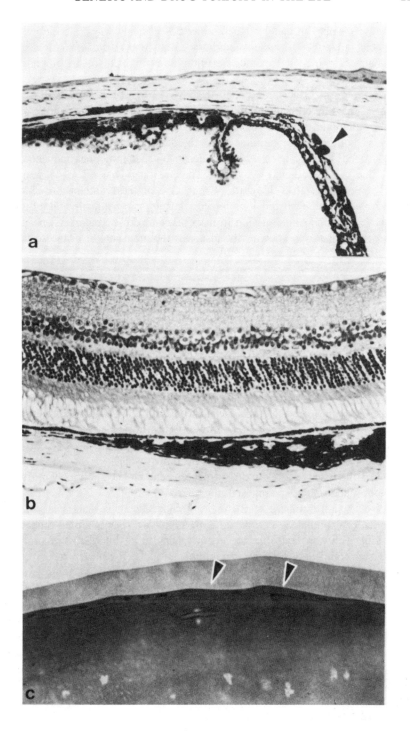

could cause changes in cellular macromolecules in many ways: alterations in oxidations and reductions of endogenous molecules, free radical formation, permeability changes in the lens membrane, alterations in metabolism of endogenous substrates, etc.

Very large doses of acetaminophen were used for the experiments illustrated in Figs. 4–7. The only clinical situation in which such large doses might be achieved would be attempted suicide. Relevant observations, however, have been recently reported. Upon hearing a seminar about the data in this report, Cohen and Burk (29) examined 10 patients showing evidence of acetaminophen-induced hepatotoxicity due to self-inflicted overdoses. The age range was 17 to 45 years, with only 2 women more than 23 years of age. One of these patients, a 45-year-old alcoholic about whom no previous medical history was available and who died 1 day later, was found on admission to have bilateral diffuse cataracts; no previous history of cataracts was known. She also was the only fatality in the series of 10 cases (29).

EFFECT OF DAILY ORAL ACETAMINOPHEN OR NAPHTHALENE ON CATARACT FORMATION

In additional experiments, we chose oral doses of acetaminophen, lower doses that are used clinically (Table 4). Oral naphthalene was also chosen for study because its monooxygenation is similarly catalyzed by some form of P_1-450 and associated with the Ah^b allele (19). Naphthalene-induced cataracts have been described (30) in workers from dye and chemical factories. The cataractogenic agent is claimed (31) not to be naphthalene itself but rather 1,2-naphthoquinone, which is formed from naphthalene-1,2-dihydrodiol. This diol of naphthalene reaches the eye via the bloodstream. Pathways of naphthalene metabolism have been extensively investigated both *in vivo* (32) and with liver microsomes *in vitro* (33–35). The phenol and the reactive arene oxide of naphthalene and acetaminophen are conjugated with glucuronide, sulfate, and glutathione.

Relatively small numbers of B6 mice develop detectable cataracts when acetaminophen or naphthalene is ingested daily (Table 4). Phenobarbital induces these conjugating pathways, and this fact may explain our finding (28) that oral phenobarbital can completely prevent acetaminophen-induced cataract formation. It is possible that the reactive intermediate of acetaminophen is an arene oxide or a quinone. No D2 mouse ever developed acetaminophen- or naphthalene-induced cataracts. All mice treated with 3-methylcholanthrene died within 6 weeks, apparently from the cytotoxicity of the chemical when injected twice weekly. On the other hand, β-naphthoflavone treatment was not very toxic; relatively few animals died during 60 days of daily oral acetaminophen or naphthalene combined with intraperitoneal β-naphthoflavone twice weekly. Of the 9 B6 mice that developed cataracts on these various oral regimens, 3 remained otherwise healthy for 6 or 7 months, at which time the animals were killed in order to examine histologically the lenticular opacities.

HISTOLOGY OF OCULAR TOXICITY INDUCED
BY ORAL ACETAMINOPHEN

Upon close microscopic examination, we found that tissue degeneration occurs not only in the anterior lens cortex but also in large areas of the uveal tract (Fig. 8a and c). The retina and pigmented epithelium are normal (Fig. 8b). The degeneration seen in the choroid, ciliary body, and iris appears to be of a chronic nature. Anterior synechiae and inflammatory cells at the angle are frequently observed. The number of epithelial cells is usually decreased in cataracts that were young (several hours or several days old). Intermittent loss of cells from the lens epithelial layer is seen in cataracts that had been present for at least 1 week (Fig. 8c). The gradual loss of the epithelial cells might result in metabolic derangements in the lens fibers, thereby leading to lens opacification. All lenses from D2 mice similarly treated do not show any evidence of ocular abnormalities.

POSSIBLE INTERRELATIONSHIP AMONG GENETIC DIFFERENCES
IN DRUG METABOLISM, DRUG-INDUCED CATARACTS, AND
SENILE CATARACTS IN THE HUMAN POPULATION

Cataracts induced by chemicals and drugs, especially naphthalene, have been extensively investigated because of their similarity to some forms of senile cataracts (31,36,37). It would be far more difficult to assess ocular toxicity in elderly patients receiving large daily doses of acetaminophen than to study patients attempting suicide with acetaminophen, because of the combination of genetic factors (i.e., the *Ah* locus in humans) and environmental factors (i.e., history of cigarette smoking, other drugs prescribed, dietary intake, etc.). Perhaps there exist other drugs in this same category, drugs that may cause ocular toxicity in a genetically determined small proportion of the total human population. We suggest that the ocular toxicity data shown in this report may be clinically important to certain patients receiving either a single large overdose of acetaminophen or high doses over an extended period of time.

REFERENCES

1. Gram, T., editor (1980): *Extrahepatic Metabolism of Drugs and Other Foreign Compounds.* SP Medical and Scientific Books, New York.
2. Bernstein, H. N. (1967): Chloroquine ocular toxicity. *Surv. Ophthalmol.*, 12:415–447.
3. Eisen, H. J., Hannah, R. R., Legraverend, C., Okey, A. B., and Nebert, D. W. (1983): The *Ah* receptor: Controlling factor in the induction of drug-metabolizing enzymes by certain chemical carcinogens and other environmental pollutants. In: *Biochemical Actions of Hormones, Vol. 10*, edited by G. Litwack, pp. 227–258. Academic Press, New York.
4. Shichi, H. (1969): Microsomal electron transfer system of bovine retinal pigment epithelium. *Exp. Eye Res.*, 8:60–68.
5. Zimmerman, T. J., Leader, B., and Kaufman, H. E. (1980): Advances in ocular pharmacology. *Annu. Rev. Pharmacol. Toxicol.*, 20:415–428.
6. Armaly, M. F. (1968): Genetic factors related to glaucoma. *Ann. N.Y. Acad. Sci.*, 151:861–875.
7. Williams, R. T., editor (1959): *Detoxification Mechanisms.* 2d ed. John Wiley and Sons, New York.
8. Nebert, D. W., and Negishi, M. (1982): Multiple forms of cytochrome P-450 and the importance of molecular biology and evolution. *Biochem. Pharmacol.*, 31:2311–2317.

9. Dutton, G. J. (1978): Developmental aspects of drug conjugation with special reference to glu-
   curonidation. *Annu. Rev. Pharmacol. Toxicol.*, 18:17–35.
10. Chasseaud, L. F. (1976): Conjugation with glutathione and mercapturic acid. In: *Glutathione:
    Metabolism and Function*, edited by I. M. Arias and W. B. Jakoby, pp. 77–144. Raven Press, New
    York.
11. Reddy, V. N., and Unakar, N. J. (1973): Localization of gamma-glutamyl transpeptidase in rabbit
    lens, ciliary process and cornea. *Exp. Eye Res.*, 17:405–408.
12. Awasthi, Y. C., Saneto, R. P., and Srivastava, S. K. (1980): Purification and properties of bovine
    lens glutathione-*S*-transferase. *Exp. Eye Res.*, 30:29–39.
13. Shichi, H., Tsunematsu, Y., and Nebert, D. W. (1976): Aryl hydrocarbon hydroxylase induction
    in retinal pigmented epithelium: Possible association of genetic differences in a drug-metabolizing
    enzyme system with retinal degeneration. *Exp. Eye Res.*, 23:165–167.
14. Shichi, H., and Nebert, D. W. (1980): Drug metabolism in ocular tissues. In: *Extrahepatic
    Metabolism of Drugs and Other Foreign Compounds*, edited by T. E. Gram, pp. 333–363. SP
    Medical and Scientific Books, New York.
15. Das, N. D., and Shichi, H. (1981): Enzymes of mercapturate synthesis and other drug-metabolizing
    reactions—Specific localization in the eye. *Exp. Eye Res.*, 33:525–533.
16. Saneto, R. P., Awasthi, Y. C., and Srivastava, S. K. (1982): Mercapturic acid pathway enzymes
    in bovine ocular lens, cornea, retina and pigmented epithelium. *Exp. Eye Res.*, 34:107–111.
17. Jakoby, W. B., and Habig, W. H. (1980): Glutathione transferases. In: *Enzymatic Basis of Detox-
    ification, Vol. 2*, edited by W. B. Jacoby, pp. 63–94. Academic Press, New York.
18. Reddy, C. C., Burgess, J. R., and Tu, C.-P. D. (1983): Isolation and characterization of an anionic
    glutathione *S*-transferase from rat liver cytosol. *Biochem. Biophys. Res. Commun.*, 111:840–846.
19. Nebert, D. W., and Jensen, N. M. (1979): The *Ah* locus: Genetic regulation of the metabolism of
    carcinogens, drugs, and other environmental chemicals by cytochrome P-450-mediated monooxy-
    genases. In: *CRC Critical Reviews in Biochemistry, Vol. 6*, edited by G. D. Fasman, pp. 401–
    437. CRC Press, Inc., Cleveland, OH.
20. Nebert, D. W. (1979): Multiple forms of inducible drug-metabolizing enzymes. A reasonable
    mechanism by which any organism can cope with adversity. *Mol. Cell. Biochem.*, 27:27–46.
21. Okey, A. B., Bondy, G. P., Mason, M. E., Kahl, G. F., Eisen, H. J., Guenthner, T. M., and Nebert,
    D. W. (1979): Regulatory gene product of the *Ah* locus. Characterization of the cytosolic inducer-
    receptor complex and evidence for its nuclear translocation. *J. Biol. Chem.*, 254:11636–11648.
22. Okey, A. B., Bondy, G. P., Mason, M. E., Nebert, D. W., Forster-Gibson, C., Muncan, J., and
    Dufresne, M. J. (1980): Temperature-dependent cytosol-to-nucleus translocation of the *Ah* receptor
    for 2,3,7,8-tetrachlorodibenzo-*p*-dioxin in continuous cell culture lines. *J. Biol. Chem.*, 255:11415–
    11422.
23. Hannah, R. R., Nebert, D. W., and Eisen, H. J. (1981): Regulatory gene product of the *Ah* complex.
    Comparison of 2,3,7,8-tetrachlorodibenzo-*p*-dioxin and 3-methylcholanthrene binding to several
    moieties in mouse liver cytosol. *J. Biol. Chem.*, 256:4584–4590.
24. Atlas, S. A., and Nebert, D. W. (1978): Pharmacogenetics: A possible pragmatic perspective in
    neoplasm predictability. *Sem. Oncol.*, 5:89–106.
25. Thorgeirsson, S. S., and Nebert, D. W. (1977): The *Ah* locus and the metabolism of chemical
    carcinogens and other foreign compounds. *Adv. Cancer Res.*, 25:149–193.
26. Shichi, H., Gaasterland, D. E., Jensen, N. M., and Nebert, D. W. (1978): *Ah* locus: Genetic
    differences in susceptibility to cataract induced by acetaminophen. *Science*, 200:539–541.
27. van Heyningen, R., editor (1975): *Cataract and Abnormalities of the Lens*. Grune and Stratton,
    New York.
28. Shichi, H., Tanaka, M., Jensen, N. M., and Nebert, D. W. (1980): Genetic differences in cataract
    and other ocular abnormalities induced by paracetamol and naphthalene. *Pharmacology*, 20:229–
    241.
29. Cohen, S. B., and Burk, R. F. (1978): Acetaminophen overdoses at a county hospital: A year's
    experience. *Southern Med. J.*, 71:1359–1364.
30. Hollwich, F., Boateng, A., and Kilck, B. (1975): Toxic cataract. In: *Cataract and Abnormalities
    of the Lens*, edited by J. G. Bellow, pp. 230–243. Grune and Stratton, New York.
31. van Heyningen, R. (1976): Experimental studies on cataract. *Invest. Ophthalmol.*, 15:685–697.
32. Boyland, E., Ramsay, G. S., and Sims, P. (1961): Metabolism of polycyclic compounds. 18. The
    secretion of metabolites of naphthalene, 1:2-dihydronaphthalene and 1:2-epoxy-1:2:3:4-tetrahy-
    dronaphthalene in rat bile. *Biochem. J.*, 78:376–384.

33. Jerina, D. M., Daly, J. W., Witkop, B., Zaltzman-Nirenberg, P., and Udenfriend, S. (1970): The role of the arene oxide oxepin system in the metabolism of aromatic substrates. *Biochemistry*, 9:147–156.

34. Oesch, F., and Daly, J. (1972): Conversion of naphthalene to *trans*-naphthalene dihydrodiol: Evidence for the presence of coupled aryl monooxygenase-epoxide hydrase system in hepatic microsomes. *Biochem. Biophys. Res. Commun.*, 46:1713–1720.

35. Bock, K. W., Van Ackeren, G., Lorch, F., and Birke, F. W. (1976): Metabolism of naphthalene to naphthalene dihydrodiol glucuronide in isolated hepatocytes and in liver microsomes. *Biochem. Pharmacol.*, 25:2351–2356.

36. Adams, D. R. (1930): The nature of the ocular lesions produced experimentally by naphthalene. *Br. J. Ophthalmol.*, 14:49–60.

37. Rees, J. R., and Pirie, A. (1967): Possible reactions of 1,2-naphthaquinone in the eye. *Biochem. J.*, 102:853–863.

Toxicology of the Eye, Ear, and Other Special Senses, edited by A. W. Hayes. Raven Press, New York © 1985.

A Review of Environmental Factors Affecting Hearing

John H. Mills

Department of Otolaryngology and Communicative Sciences, Medical University of South Carolina, Charleston, South Carolina 29425

This chapter reviews some of the environmental factors that are capable of producing an injury to the inner ear (cochlea) and auditory nerve. Hearing losses arising from a pathologic cochlea or auditory nerve are called sensorineural, as opposed to hearing losses arising from the middle or external ear, which are called conductive (34). The thrust of this paper is centered on the most common causes of sensorineural hearing losses, namely, noise exposure, aging, ototoxic drugs, and interactions between these agents.

EXPOSURE TO NOISE

Exposure to noise can injure the ear and produce a loss of hearing. The injury and hearing loss can be temporary or fully recoverable when the exposure or series of exposures is terminated. Temporary hearing losses can recover in a few minutes, a few hours, or as long as 2 weeks (33,73,92,93,138,139,141). Hearing losses that are measured 2 weeks or longer after the termination of an exposure are considered to be permanent because very little additional recovery occurs. The magnitude of a temporary or permanent hearing loss, or whether or not a temporary hearing loss becomes permanent, is determined by specific details of the noise exposures as well as the susceptibility of the individuals involved. An explanation of the details of noise-induced hearing loss is achieved most simply by considering three types of exposure: continuous exposures, intermittent exposures, and exposures to impulsive sounds.

Continuous Exposures to Steady-State Noise

Under the category of exposures to steady-state noise there are considerable data from both laboratory studies and field studies (73,74). In the former case, the experiments are concerned with temporary effects in humans (99,100,107,141) and both temporary and permanent effects in laboratory animals (41,53,93,94). Field studies are with humans and are mostly concerned with permanent threshold shifts produced in occupational settings (5,6,19,20,108). The laboratory studies, of course,

231

have the advantages of experimenter control of the noise exposure and repeated pre- and postexposure measurements of hearing. In occupational settings, the noise exposure is less well-defined, and the experimenter has less control over a large number of significant variables. In light of the uncertainty and the unavoidable lack of precision in field studies, there has been a considerable effort with laboratory investigations as well as an effort to relate laboratory results to the results of field studies.

Laboratory studies with human subjects, for obvious reasons, have studied temporary changes in hearing called temporary threshold shifts (TTSs). TTS experiments are straightforward. Audiograms (auditory thresholds for pure tones) are determined prior to one exposure or series of exposures. Then the subject is exposed for a minute or perhaps as long as a few days. In the case of lengthy exposures, quiet intervals of 5 to 10 min are interspersed within an otherwise continuous exposure and auditory thresholds are measured. The difference between one of these measurements and preexposure measures is called TTS.

The simplest way to describe the phenomenon of TTS may be in terms of the relation between TTS and characteristics of the exposure such as duration, frequency, and level. In regard to the duration of exposure, TTSs increase during the first 8 to 12 hr of an exposure and then reach an asymptote or plateau (7, 91,98,99,100,107). When the TTS at asymptote (ATS) is about 30 to 35 dB or less, the rate of growth is independent of the spectrum of the noise. That is, the relation between TTS and exposure duration is the same for low-frequency, high-frequency, and wide-band noise exposures (51,99,100). On the other hand, for exposures of a few minutes at high intensities, TTSs produced by high-frequency sounds ($\sim$1–4 kHz) increase more rapidly as a function of exposure duration than TTSs produced by low-frequency sounds ($<$1 kHz) (141). This frequency effect at high intensities may be explained by the effects of the acoustic reflex and by the fact that the acoustic reflex attenuates sounds below about 1 kHz more than sounds above about 1 kHz (138,139).

The relation between TTS and exposure intensity is complicated by the duration of exposure. For high-intensity sounds and short-duration exposures, small increases in level, e.g., 2.5 dB, produce substantial increases in TTS, e.g., 5 to 10 dB (33,37). In other instances, increases in exposure intensity produce decreases in TTS. For example, increases in level from 118 to 125 dB have resulted in decreases in TTS. These discontinuities in the relation between TTS and level have been attributed to a number of factors, including the acoustic reflex and changes in the vibratory mode of the ossicular chain (33,138). The relation between TTS and level is simplified greatly by defining or restricting the relation to ATSs or, in other words, to experiments in which the duration is greater than 8 to 12 hr. The relation between ATS and level is straightforward. ATS increases about 1.7 dB for every 1 dB increase in exposure level above a certain "critical level" (99). This so-called "critical level" is frequency-dependent, ranging from a low of 74 dB sound pressure level (SPL) for an octave-band noise centered at 4.0 kHz, to 78 dB at 2.0 kHz, and to 82 dB at 0.5 and 1.0 kHz. For a wide-band noise the level is 78 dBA

(99,100). Given these critical levels, one can estimate with accuracy the average ATS produced by a specific band of noise or a wide-band noise. For example, ATS at the test frequency of greatest effect will be 34 dB when the noise exposure is 8 hr or longer, the noise is centered near 2.0 kHz, and its level is 98 dB. Likewise, a wide-band noise of 100 dBA will produce an ATS of 37.4 [ATS = 1.7 (100 − 78)]. The frequency dependence of the critical levels, i.e., 74 dB SPL at 4.0 kHz decreasing to 82 dB at 0.5 kHz, indicates that high-frequency noises produce larger threshold shifts than low-frequency noises of the same SPL.

Laboratory investigations of ATS with chinchillas, gerbils, and monkeys (10, 12,21,41,53,93,94,96,101,102,105,132) show results that are qualitatively and quantitatively consistent with those observed in human subjects (3,91,98–100,107). That is, TTS grows to an asymptote as exposure duration is lengthened, and ATS increases about 1.7 dB for every 1 dB increase in noise level above a critical level. Critical levels are species-dependent with estimated values for monkeys very similar to those described above for humans (99). For gerbil and chinchilla, on the other hand, critical levels are 10 to 20 dB lower than those of humans and monkeys (99, and J. H. Mills, *unpublished data*). Thus noise exposures for different species can be equated in terms of ATS.

The major usefulness of measures of ATS may be in predicting the magnitude of permanent threshold shifts produced by repeated exposures to the same noise. It was hypothesized (98) that ATS produced by a given sound was an upper bound on any permanent threshold shift that can be produced by that sound regardless of the temporal characteristics of the exposure. This hypothesis is necessarily correct provided TTS grows to a true asymptote and not just a plateau, and provided hearing does not deteriorate further after the exposure is finally terminated. Research with animals shows that ATSs of about 50 dB are sustained (± 5 dB) for as long as 90 to 108 days (12,96,102) and perhaps even longer (J. H. Mills, *unpublished data*). Likewise, when these long exposures were terminated, hearing levels improved over a 2-week or longer period. Indeed, the only instances on record of hearing levels deteriorating further after cessation of a noise exposure involve impulsive sounds (52,79,80). In these cases the noise-induced hearing loss is an example of acoustic trauma, i.e., an acoustically-induced injury and hearing loss produced by one short-duration exposure. Thus a continuous or nearly continuous exposure to noise that produces an ATS of 5 dB or so will not produce a permanent threshold shift (PTS) in excess of 5 dB. Likewise, repeated exposures to noises at the "critical levels" described above will produce ATSs of 0 dB, and therefore PTSs of 0 dB. In other words, critical levels as defined here represent "acoustic injury thresholds" or "safe levels" of noise regardless of the temporal properties of the exposure. Critical levels have been measured for octave-bands of noise with center frequencies of 0.5, 1, 2, and 4 kHz; however, only estimates are available at frequencies below 0.5 kHz and there are no data available above 4.0 kHz.

Critical levels or acoustic injury thresholds are plotted on Fig. 1 along with audibility thresholds and discomfort thresholds (34). Three areas of interest become defined by these thresholds. The first area is bounded on the low side by the threshold of audibility and on the high side by critical levels or acoustic injury thresholds. This region thus describes sounds that are audible but present no risk of injury or hearing loss to humans regardless of the duration of the sounds or the number of times exposed. The uppermost region of Fig. 1 corresponds to the threshold of discomfort, which is estimated to be about 120 dB SPL. Nonimpulsive sounds in excess of discomfort thresholds present a high risk of acoustic injury and hearing loss regardless of duration or number of times exposed, particularly for sounds above 250 Hz. Sounds between the region of discomfort and critical levels are in the region of qualified risk. That is, the risk of acoustic injury and permanent hearing loss depends on the combined effects of level, duration, number of exposures, individual differences, and a virtually endless list of second-order variables

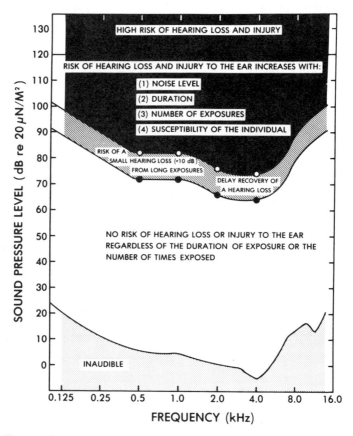

FIG. 1. The complete range of human audibility is categorized with respect to the likelihood of acoustic injury of the ear and noise-induced hearing loss (97).

(discussed later). An increase in any of the exposure characteristics increases the risk of injury and hearing loss, although the quantitative determination of the increase in risk is the subject of much debate. Figure 1 thus categorizes the range of human audibility into three regions, namely, no risk, qualified risk, and high risk.

Field studies of noise-induced hearing loss are mostly concerned with permanent threshold shifts caused by years of exposure to occupational noise. In these studies the criterion measure of permanent hearing loss is called noise-induced permanent threshold shift (NIPTS) and it includes a correction for hearing loss associated with aging. The accuracy of retrospective studies of NIPTS is not universally accepted. Debate usually is centered on the accuracy of the noise measurements and audiometric methods as well as the appropriateness of a control group that is used to correct for the effects of aging. While there may be many valid arguments about retrospective studies of NIPTS, there are, nevertheless, several field studies that are excellent in most aspects and have contributed significantly to the understanding of NIPTS (5,6,20,74,108,113,135). For exposures to nearly continuous noise for about 8 hr/day, these studies suggest that NIPTS begins at 4 kHz when the noise level exceeds 75 to 80 dBA. NIPTS at 4.0 kHz increases for about 10 years and then plateaus. NIPTS at 2.0 kHz increases for about 20 years while NIPTS at frequencies below 2.0 kHz starts after a "few" years and appears to continue throughout the working life of the individual. NIPTS increases as noise level increases above about 80 dBA for a test of 4.0 kHz, and about 85 dBA for other test frequencies. For test tones in the 4- to 6-kHz range, NIPTSs increase about 1.7 to 2 dB for each 1-dB increase in noise level. At levels in excess of about 95 dBA, the rate of change in NIPTS may increase abruptly. At levels in excess of 95 dBA, there is more uncertainty about the facts of NIPTS (19,46,100,135).

Of great interest is the relation, if any, between measures of TTS in the laboratory and measures of permanent threshold shifts (PTSs) in occupational settings. While there are a number of "coincidences" between TTS and PTS, there are also significant differences between TTS and NIPTS that are difficult to resolve. Rather than address all of these issues, here the effort shall be only to point out that the magnitude of TTS at 4 kHz after 8 hr of nearly continuous exposure to noise corresponds closely to that of NIPTS at 4.0 kHz produced by daily 8-hr exposures for 10 years to an occupational noise. This correspondence was first noted by Nixon and Glorig (108) and subsequently confirmed by others (20,74). This correspondence between NIPTS at 4.0 kHz and TTS after 8 hr of exposure also supports the concept of ATS and the hypothesis mentioned earlier, namely, that ATS is an upper bound on PTS. Thus, laboratory measures of ATS can indeed provide an accurate index of permanent effects that occur in the field.

Noncontinuous Exposures

Whereas the data base is massive for the effects of continuous exposure to steady-state noise of less than 95 dBA, the data base is less impressive for intermittent exposure to steady-state noise or exposure to noises with fluctuating levels (73,74). It is difficult to find occupational settings where the noise exposure can be clearly defined and measured accurately, and where there is a large number of employees who have worked for 20 to 40 years. Similarly, laboratory investigations must use humans (TTS) or animals, and the research is confronted with an almost endless list of variables. Moreover, because of regulatory efforts and the need for simplicity, there has been a fascination with the idea of a single-number correction factor. For example, one approach has been to equate noises with greatly varying temporal properties in terms of equal energy, equal pressure, or compromises on equal energy or equal pressure. Thus, a steady-state noise exposure for 8 hr with a sound pressure level of 90 dBA is assumed to be equal to an exposure of 4 hr at 96 dBA, 95 dBA, 94 dBA, or 93 dBA (135,139). In other words, there is great debate and confusion regarding the exchange of the intensity of the noise and the duration of the exposure. A compromise is the "5 dB rule" currently used by OSHA and the U.S. Department of Labor.

Our thesis is that a single-number correction factor that specifies a time-intensity trade-off in NIPTS or TTS is likely to be grossly incorrect at worst, or, at best, to have a very restricted range of application. This thesis is based on available literature and results in our laboratory. Our results (97, and J. H. Mills, *unpublished data*) indicate that a number to describe time-intensity trade ranges from 0 dB to as large as 8 dB. The situation is complicated in part because of the ability of the ear to use quiet periods to recover from the noisy periods. In other words, rest periods as short as a few seconds may be useful in protecting the ear, particularly in those conditions where the noise is present for only a few minutes. It is perhaps because of these quiet periods that rock musicians and others similarly exposed do not have large hearing losses (139).

At least two other approaches to the development of a single-number correction factor are currently under investigation. One of these involves predictions of NIPTS from TTS measures averaged across the periods of growth and recovery, and calculations of noise dose where noise dose is the time integral of the A-weighted sound pressure calculated over the exposure period. This method of predicting NIPTS at 4 kHz appears to be accurate (± 2 dB) in some instances and less accurate in others (± 10 dB). Another approach involves experimental animals in laboratory investigations in which the criterion measure of acoustic injury of the ear is the number of missing outer hair cells. Exposures can be controlled precisely and selected to test various schemes for predicting NIPTS. The validity of these animal experiments cannot be evaluated until more data are available (139).

Impulse Noise

The acoustic impulses produced by handguns and rifles are the cause of mild-to-severe sensorineural hearing losses (125,129). High-frequency hearing losses are typical of persons exposed to acoustic impulses with peak sound pressure levels in excess of about 145 to 155 dB SPL (55). Among hunters and military personnel,

PTS is usually largest in the left ear (129). The right ear (right-handed shooter) receives less acoustic energy than the left because of the head-shadow effect. The risk of NIPTS from acoustic impulses generally increases as the number of impulses increases, as the peak SPL of the impulses increases, and as the duration of each impulse increases (26,52,54–57,90,106,125,130). Also, specification of impulse duration is complicated, but apparently a critical factor (45,56,85). Detailed discussions of impulse noise and its effects on hearing are given elsewhere (46,52, 53,62,104,123–125,133,145).

It is worth noting that laboratory investigations of the effects of impulsive sounds with human subjects are very difficult to do without placing the subjects at risk. An impulse at a given level and repetition rate may produce very little in the way of measurable effects. However, a 10-dB increase in level may produce an unusually large shift in thresholds. In other words, the range of levels available to an experimenter is small, and individual differences are large. It is disconcerting to note many anecodotal and clinical reports that show severe hearing loss after exposure to one impulse (140) (acoustic trauma) or to a series of impulses (129). In fact, there are many reports documenting that acoustic impulses that had been innocuous on many previous occasions produce severe unilateral or bilateral PTS on a subsequent occasion.

The nature of the hearing loss produced by acoustic impulses is probably different from the nature of the hearing loss caused by continuous exposures to steady-state noise at moderate levels (10,52,79,121,126) (for example, 90 dBA). That is, the displacement of the basilar membrane by an intense acoustic impulse may be sufficient to produce "ripping and tearing" effects. Purely mechanical injuries may be produced by acoustic impulses (121,126), whereas injuries produced by lower-level acoustic signals may be caused by metabolic, biochemical, or vascular effects, including the depletion of energy stores, assembly of cell membranes, effects on proteins and lipids of the cochlea, mechanically induced changes in the shape of the tectorial membrane, vasoconstriction within the cochlea, and changes in the actin filament of the stereocilia of hair cells. Significant developments in the biochemical mechanisms of acoustic injury of the ear will probably be delayed pending significant developments in normal cochlear function, particularly the cochlear transducer mechanism and the identification of hair cell neurotransmitter.

INTERACTION AND MISCELLANEOUS EFFECTS

A significant result of the past few years or so has been identifying agents that interact with noise. An interaction or potentiation is said to occur when the injury or hearing loss produced by both agents is greater than that produced by either agent acting alone. Special cases of interaction are additivity and synergism. Additivity occurs when the total effect produced by both agents is equal to the sum of the effects of each agent. Synergism occurs when neither agent produces an injury by itself but injury occurs when the agents are combined.

A steady-state noise combined with an acoustic impulse can produce a significant synergism provided the two types of noise overlap in time and in spectral charac-teristics (9,46,49,110). Indeed, this dramatic example of a synergistic effect in noise-induced hearing loss was reported by Henderson and associates (53), who found that 157 dB (peak SPL) impulse by itself or a noise of 95 dB (by itself) produced no PTS or injury to the sensory cells, but the combined effect of the impulse and the noise was devastating to the cochlea. PTS ranged from 5 dB at 250 Hz, to 50 dB at 2.0 kHz, and to 35 dB at 8.0 kHz. Outer hair cells were totally destroyed over a 7-mm region of the basilar membrane. Injury to inner hair cells was nearly as severe. These results have been documented in a series of experiments with laboratory animals using other levels of impulses and continuous noise (53). There are other interactions between acoustic events that can either increase or decrease the risk of hearing loss. For example, noise combined with whole-body vibration (47,48,111,146) increases risk of hearing loss; however, a noise presented before an intense acoustic impulse can contract the stapedius muscle (acoustic reflex) and reduce the risk of hearing loss (44). The impulse is attenuated in the middle ear and the inner ear is thus protected. In the absence of the noise, the impulse travels through the middle ear before the reflex is activated (reflex latency, 10 msec) and injures the sensory cells of the inner ear.

Personal characteristics of individuals can affect noise-induced hearing loss. It appears that younger animals are more susceptible to acoustic injury than are older animals (8,25,29,32,42,58,75,114,147) and there is some evidence of a "critical period" at least in the mouse and the hamster (11,122). Melanization as evidenced by eye color (22–24) and race (119) has been thought to be a significant factor in noise-induced hearing loss (14,30); however, the evidence is equivocal at best (60,68,131). In large-scale studies of individual differences in noise-induced hearing loss (137), one factor has consistently been shown to be significant, namely, the preexposure hearing levels (audiograms) of the subject (15,61,94,109,138). Persons with poor hearing levels have less TTS or PTS from a given exposure than persons with excellent hearing levels. Also, males tend to show more effects from low-frequency (<1 kHz) noises than females, but the females have larger shifts from high-frequency noises (137). These results are explained by the acoustic properties of the middle ear, which are significantly different in males and females.

A large number of investigations have been directed at prophylactic or therapeutic treatment of noise-induced hearing loss (NIHL). The "treatments" from 1950 to about 1970 include vitamins A, B, and E, nicotinic acid, papaverium hydrochloride, nylidrin hydrochloride, thioctic acid, chlorpromazine, adenosine triphosphate, and ephedrine (138,139). None of these treatments were shown to be effective. More recent efforts have examined a large number of agents (25,39,40,83), including dextran 40 (65,69,70,86,87), a large number of vasodilators and vasoconstrictors (66,78,128), and a mixture of oxygen and carbon dioxide called carbogen (67,142). None of these treatments have been shown to be effective when rigorous control and evaluative methods are used. Initial results with carbogen, on the other hand, are not entirely negative, but more rigorous evaluations are required (142).

EXPOSURE TO NOISE AND AUDITORY PERCEPTUAL DEFICITS

Studies of auditory discrimination and reading skills of children living near freeways suggest deleterious environmental effects (28,95). In this study, where noise levels inside apartments ranged from 55 dBA to 75 dBA, the performance of second- to fifth-grade children on standardized speech discrimination and reading tests was correlated (0.48, 0.53) with noise levels for children who had resided in the apartment complex for at least 4 years. In other words, these data suggested that reading and listening skills were being affected negatively by freeway noise. Substantially more data are required to clarify all of the issues involved. Moreover, it remains unclear whether noise-related deficits in speech discrimination and reading are temporary and will be overcome by maturation and schooling, or are permanent. These data (28) may be the first to indicate that the development of important skills such as listening and reading is being affected by environmental noise.

AGING

Although it may not be legitimate to include aging as an environmental factor, the loss of hearing associated with aging is a major problem. It will become far more significant in the next decades; therefore, it is difficult to ignore in a discussion of causes of hearing loss.

The loss of hearing associated with aging is called presbyacusis. Presbyacusis has been subdivided into four categories: sensory, in which the major pathology is at the outer and inner hair cells; neural, where the major pathology is indicated by large losses of spiral ganglion cells (cell body of nerve VIII); metabolic, where major pathology is at the stria vascularis of the cochlea; and mechanical, where it is postulated that the elasticity or compliance of the basilar membrane and other structures is reduced. Of course, the central nervous system does not escape the effects of aging, nor does the sensitivity of other sensory systems, including gustatory, olfactory, and ocular (51,59).

Auditory sensitivity for pure tones (audiogram) and other auditory behaviors are affected in a manner that reflects to some extent the major pathology. For example, sensory and mechanical types of presbyacusis usually show moderate to severe losses in the high frequencies. In neural presbyacusis the audiogram may be normal or nearly so until greater than 50 to 80% of the spiral ganglion cells are missing. In cases of metabolic presbyacusis the hearing loss is moderate and affects all frequencies nearly equally.

While the quantitative facts of presbyacusis are important to clinical diagnosis and to patient management, they have significance as well to the problem of noise-induced hearing loss (82). That is, how much of a person's hearing loss is caused by noises of everyday living (sociocusis) and how much by previous infections, blows to the head, drugs, etc. (nosoacusis)? How do all of these causes of hearing loss interact and what is the nature of the interaction?

It is assumed that the effects of presbyacusis add linearly to the effects of occupational noise exposure. Moreover, presbyacusic control groups and occupational noise groups are assumed to have equal amounts of sociocusis and nosoacusis. Of course, these are extremely convenient assumptions, which are necessary to permit the calculation of NIPTS. For group averages, they may even have some accuracy. However, on an individual basis, gross errors probably occur. It is difficult, for example, to imagine that the additivity rules for neural presbyacusis are quantitatively identical to the additivity rules for mechanical presbyacusis.

The concept of presbyacusis has been altered by the results of studies completed in other cultures. Perhaps the most often quoted example is that of the Mabaan tribe of Africa (118). In this extremely quiet culture, the auditory thresholds of 80- to 90-year-old persons were approximately equal to 20-year-old persons in industrialized cities of North America and Europe. While some persons were quick to note the absence of noise, the authors pointed to the absence of cardiovascular disease, the absence of meat in the diet, the climate, the absence of stress, and the absence of peptic ulcers. It was concluded that hearing loss in old age is attributable not just to the effects of noise, drugs, and aging, but to the cumulative effects of these factors plus diet and stress–life-style factors. It is equally important to note that in Mabaans who had moved to Egypt, there was an unusually high incidence (for Mabaans) of hearing loss, cardiovascular disease, and peptic ulcers. In other words, auditory skills are affected directly by definitive agents such as noise and drugs, and by life-style as well.

OTOTOXIC DRUGS AND VIRAL INFECTIONS

Ototoxicity from aminoglycoside antibiotics is well known (2,50,51, 63,88,114,115,117,136). The aminoglycosides have a 2-decoxystreptamine as a central component. All are produced by the *Streptomyces* genus except the gentamycins, which are produced by a strain of *Micromonospora purpurea*. These antibiotics, which include kanamycin, gentamycin, neomycin, tobramycin, amikacin, sisomicin, netilmicin, and others, are bacteriocidal because they bind to proteins on the 30S segment of the ribosome (4).

Aminoglycoside antibiotics are indicated in the treatment of tuberculosis and serious gram negative infections with such bacteria as *Escherichia coli, Klebsiella, Proteus, Pseudomonas aeruginosa*, and *Serratia*, for example (4,43,50,63). Aminoglycoside antibiotics are used to treat at least one million people in the United States annually, and perhaps as many as four million (43).

Ototoxicity from aminoglycoside antibiotics may be cochleotoxic or vestibulotoxic. Tobramycin and amikacin are considered more cochleotoxic, whereas streptomycin and gentamycin are considered more vestibulotoxic. The incidence of ototoxicity varies from 2 to 25% and perhaps as high as 55% (18,43). In a prospective study of 38 courses of therapy in 113 patients (43), some significant associations with ototoxicity included high temperature, elevated hematocrit, high creatinine clearance, poor condition of the patient, and duration of therapy greater than 10 days. Serum levels, age, prior noise exposure, and use of other ototoxic drugs were not found to be significantly correlated with the incidence of aminoglycoside ototoxicity.

Cochlear toxicity from aminoglycoside antibiotics affects the inner row of outer hair cells first, followed by the outer rows of hair cells, then by the inner hair cells (43). The pathology has also been localized to the stria vascularis, spiral ligament, and spiral prominence. Several theories of the mechanism of damage have been proposed, including direct damage to the hair cells and disruption of the metabolism in the stria vascularis and spiral ligament, which leads to changes in cationic differences of the perilymph and endolymph (43). The mechanism of vestibular damage remains poorly defined.

Hearing loss produced by aminoglycoside antibiotics ranges from minimal to severe. It usually starts at high frequencies and progresses to low frequencies. Efforts at early detection of otoxicity are sometimes only marginally successful at restricting the magnitude of the hearing loss. By the time reliable changes in the audiogram are detected, the degenerative process is under way and may continue for weeks or months after termination of the antibiotic (7).

Of all the possible interactions, noise and drugs have received the most attention. Among all the drugs studied, one of the aminoglycosides, kanamycin (13, 16,17,36,37,84), has been studied extensively and shown to interact significantly with a variety of noises (120). The interaction is less than that predicted by an additive relationship. Moreover, noise exposure followed by the administration of kanamycin produces an interaction, whereas the reverse sequence does not (84,115,120). Additivity, by definition, is insensitive to order effects. Another aminoglycoside, neomycin, also interacts with noise (18). While aminoglycoside antibiotics interact with noise, the few data available on the loop diuretics ethacrynic acid (71) and furosemide do not show an interaction (134). Aspirin (sodium salicylate) interacts with noise (38,89) and appears to do so with sequential effects that are opposite to those observed with kanamycin (27). That is, the interaction is greatest when the drug is administered prior to the noise exposure. Effects of aspirin on hearing appear to be temporary rather than permanent (143,144).

A large number of viral infections have been associated with sensorineural hearing losses (76,77,81). Rubella and mumps are the classic examples. Hearing loss with mumps is usually unilateral, whereas the loss with rubella is bilateral. In both cases the temporal bone pathology includes extensive degeneration of sensory cells, stria vascularis, and tectorial membrane as well as the nerve supply (76,77). Recently, the cytomegalovirus (CMV), a member of the herpes group, has been isolated from the perilymph (35) and shown to cause congenital deafness (1,31, 35,103,127). Inclusion-bearing cells have been observed in the epithelium of the utricular and saccular macula, Reissner's membrane, and stria vascularis (103). It may possibly cause progressive hearing loss that starts at about 2 years of age (1,127). Severe middle ear infections are also associated with CMV (31).

Other viruses that have been implicated in both the gradual and sudden onset of sensorineural hearing loss include influenza, adenovirus, and herpes hominis (64).

Most viral infections of the inner ear are described as "endolymphatic labyrinthitis," with a pathology consisting of degeneration of the stria vascularis, organ of Corti, and tectorial membrane.

A large number of other factors are assumed to affect hearing (112). These include a long list of chemicals (116) and bacterial infections (112), as well as over 40 genetic and metabolic syndromes (72).

ACKNOWLEDGMENT

This manuscript was prepared under grant support from the National Institute of Environmental Health Services and under contract support (NO1-NS-1-2381) from National Institute of Neurological and Communicative Disorders and Stroke. Manuscripts in preparation by J. Saunders, R. A. Schmiedt, L. Humes, and W. Melnick on various aspects of noise-induced hearing loss were available and used to assist the author in the preparation of this manuscript. Nancy Topham and Janet Simmons aided in the preparation of the final document.

REFERENCES

1. Alford, C. A. (1974): Inapparent congenital cytomegalovirus infection with elevated cord IgM levels: Causal relationship with auditory and mental deficiency. *N. Engl. J. Med.*, 290:291–296.
2. Appel, G. B., and Neu, H. C. (1978): Gentamicin in 1978. *Ann. Int. Med.*, 89:528–538.
3. Barry, J. P. (1976): Asymptotic threshold shift. D.Sc. Thesis, University of Pittsburgh.
4. Barza, M., Lauerman, M. W., Tally, F. P., and Gorbach, S. L. (1980): Prospective, randomized trial of netilmicin and amikacin, with emphasis on eighth nerve toxicity. *Antimicrob. Agents Chemother.*, 17:707–714.
5. Baughn, W. L. (1973): Relation between daily noise exposure and hearing loss based on the evaluation of 6835 industrial noise exposure cases. EPA-USAF Aerospace Medical Res. Lab. AMRL-TR-73-53.
6. Berger, E., Royster, L. H., and Thomas, W. G. (1978): Presumed NIPTS resulting from exposure to an A-weighted Leq of 89 dB. *J. Acoust. Soc. Am.*, 64:192–197.
7. Bernard, P. A. (1981): Freedom from ototoxicity in aminoglycide tested neonates: A mistaken notion. *Laryngoscope*, 91:1985–1994.
8. Bess, F. H., Peek, B. F., and Chapman, J. J. (1979): Further observations on noise levels in infant incubators. *Pediatrics*, 63:100–106.
9. Blakeslee, E. A., Hynson, K., Hamernik, R. P., and Henderson, D. (1977): Interaction of spectrally-mismatched continuous and impulse-noise exposures in the chinchilla. *J. Acoust. Soc. Am.*, 61:S59.
10. Blakeslee, E. A., Hynson, K., Hamernik, R. P., and Henderson, D. (1978): Asymptotic threshold shift in chinchillas exposed to impulse noise. *J. Acoust. Soc. Am.*, 63:876–882.
11. Bock, G. R., and Seifter, E. J. (1978): Developmental changes of susceptibility to auditory fatigue in young hamsters. *Audiology*, 17:193–203.
12. Bohne, B. A., and Clark, W. W. (1982): Growth of hearing loss and cochlear lesion with increasing duration of noise exposure. In: *New Perspectives on Noise-Induced Hearing Loss*, edited by R. P. Hamernik, D. Henderson, and R. Salvi, pp. 283–302. Raven Press, New York.
13. Bone, R. C., and Ryan, A. F. (1978): Audiometric and histologic correlates of the interaction between kanamycin and subtraumatic levels of noise in the chinchilla. *Trans. Am. Acad. Ophthalmol. Otolaryngol.*, 86:400–404.
14. Bonnacorsi, P. (1965): Il colore dell'iride com "test" di valutazione quantiatativia, nell'uomo, della concentrazzione di melania nella stria vascolare. *Ann. Laryngol. Otol. Rhinol. Farengol.*, 64:725–738.
15. Botte, M. C., and Variot, M. H. (1979): Auditory fatigue in individuals having sustained an acoustic trauma. *Ann. Otolaryngol.*, 96:827–833.

16. Brown, J. J., Brummett, R. E., Fox, K. E., and Bendrick, T. W. (1980): Combined effects of noise and kanamycin. *Arch. Otolaryngol.*, 106:744–750.
17. Brown, J. J., Brummett, R. E., and Fox, K. E. (1980): Combined effects of noise and kanamycin. Cochlear pathology and pharmacology. *Arch. Otolaryngol.*, 106:744–750.
18. Brown, J. J., Brummett, R. E., and Meikle, M. B. (1978): Combined effects of noise and neomycin: Cochlear changes in the guinea pig. *Acta Otolaryngol.*, 86:394–400.
19. Burns, W., and Robinson, D. W. (1970): An investigation of the effects of occupational noise on hearing. In: *Sensorineural Hearing Loss*, edited by G. E. W. Wolstenholme and J. Knight. Williams and Wilkins, Baltimore.
20. Burns, W., and Robinson, D. W. (1970): *Hearing and Noise in Industry.* Her Majesty's Stationery Office, London.
21. Carder, H. M., and Miller, J. D. (1972): Temporary threshold shifts (TTS) produced by noise exposures of long durations. *J. Speech Hear. Res.*, 15:603–623.
22. Carlin, M. F., and McCroskey, R. L. (1980): Is eye color a predictor of noise-induced hearing loss? *Ear Hear.*, 1:191–196.
23. Carter, N. L. (1980): Eye colour and susceptibility to noise-induced permanent threshold shift. *Audiology*, 19:86–93.
24. Carter, N. L., Keen, K., Waugh, R. L., et al. (1981): The relations of eye colour and smoking to noise-induced permanent threshold shift. *Audiology*, 20:336–346.
25. Cazaubon, J., Padovani, P., and Vaillant, C. (1970): Clinical trial of EU 4200 in the treatment of acoustic trauma. *Med. Trop.*, 30:403–408.
26. CHABA (1968): Proposed damage-risk criterion for impulse noise (gunfire). Report of working group 57, NAS-NRC Committee on Hearing, Bioacoust. Biomech., Washington, DC.
27. Chen, C. S., and Aberdeen, C. C. (1980): Potentiation of noise-induced audiogenic seizure risk by salicylate in mice as a function of salicylate-noise exposure interval. *Acta Otolaryngol.*, 90:61–65.
28. Cohen, S., Glass, D. C., and Singer, J. E. (1973): Apartment noise, auditory discrimination, and reading ability in children. *J. Exp. Soc. Psychol.*, 9:407–422.
29. Coleman, J. W. (1976): Age dependent changes and acoustic trauma in the spiral organ of the guinea pig. *Scand. Audiol.*, 5:63–66.
30. Cunningham, D. R., and Norris, M. L. (1982): Eye color and noise-induced hearing loss: A population study. *Ear Hear.*, 3:211–214.
31. Dahle, A. J., McCollister, F. P., Stagno, S., Reynolds, D. W., and Hoffman, H. E. (1979): Progressive hearing impairment in children with congenital cytomegalovirus infection. *J. Speech Hear. Dis.*, 44:220–229.
32. Danto, J., and Caiazzo, A. J. (1977): Auditory effects of noise on infant and adult guinea pig. *J. Am. Audiol. Soc.*, 3:99–101.
33. Davis, H., Morgan, C. T., Hawkins, J., Galambos, R., and Smith, F. (1950): Temporary deafness following exposure to loud tones and noise. *Acta Otolaryngol. (Suppl.)*, 88:1–57.
34. Davis, H., and Silverman, S. R. (1975): *Hearing and Deafness*, 4th edition. Holt, Rhinehart and Winston, New York.
35. Davis, L. E., Fiber, F., James, C. G., and McLaren, L. C. (1979): Cytomegalovirus isolation from a human inner ear. *Ann. Otol.*, 88:424–426.
36. Dayal, V. S., and Barek, W. G. (1975): Cochlear changes from noise, kanamycin and aging: II. Potentiating effects of noise and kanamycin. *Laryngoscope*, 85 (Suppl.), 1:8–11.
37. Dayal, V. S., Kokshanian, A., and Mitchell, D. P. (1971): Combined effects of noise and kanamycin. *Ann. Otol. Rhinol. Laryngol.*, 80:897–902.
38. Eddy, L. B., Morgan, R. J., and Carney, H. C. (1976): Hearing loss due to combined effects of noise and sodium salicylate. *ISA Transactions*, 15:103–108.
39. Eibach, H., and Boerger, U. (1979): Acute acoustic trauma: The therapeutic effect of bencyclan in a controlled clinical trial. *HNO*, 27:170–175.
40. Eibach, H., and Boerger, U. (1980): Therapeutic results in acute acoustic trauma. *Otorhinolaryngology*, 226:177–186.
41. Eldredge, D. H., Mills, J. H., and Bohne, B. A. (1973): Anatomical, behavioral, and electrophysiological observations on chinchillas. *Adv. Otorhinolaryngol.*, 20:64–81.
42. Falk, S. A., Cook, R. O., Haseman, J. K., and Saunders, C. M. (1974): Noise-induced inner ear damage in newborn and adult guinea pigs. *Laryngoscope*, 84:444–453.
43. Fee, W. E. (1980): Aminoglycoside ototoxicity in the human. *Laryngoscope (Suppl.)*, Oct., 1–19.

44. Fletcher, J. (1976): The effect of the acoustic reflex on hearing. In: *Hearing and Davis*, edited by S. K. Hirsh, D. H. Eldredge, I. J. Hirsh, and S. R. Silverman, pp. 139–148. Washington University Press, St. Louis.

45. Hakanson, H., Erlandsson, B., Ivarsson, A., and Nilsson, P. (1980): Differences in noise doses achieved by simultaneous registrations from stationary and ear-borne microphones. *Scand. Audiol. (Suppl.)*, 12:47–53.

46. Hamernik, R. P., and Henderson, D. (1976): The potentiation of noise and other ototraumatic agents. In: *Effects of Noise on Hearing*, edited by D. Henderson, R. P. Hamernik, D. S. Dosanjh, and J. H. Mills, pp. 291–307. Raven Press, New York.

47. Hamernik, R. P., Henderson, D., and Coling, D. (1980): The interaction of whole body vibration and impulse noise. *J. Acoust. Soc. Am.*, 67:928–934.

48. Hamernik, R. P., Henderson, D., and Coling, D. (1981): Influences of vibration on asymptotic threshold shift produced by impulse noise. *Audiology*, 20:259–269.

49. Hamernik, R. P., Henderson, D., Crossley, J. J., et al. (1974): Interaction of continuous and impulse noise: Audiometric and histological effects. *J. Acoust. Soc. Am.*, 55:117–123.

50. Hawkins, J. E., Jr. (1959): The ototoxicity of kanamycin. *Ann. Otol.*, 68:698–715.

51. Hawkins, J. E., Jr. (1973): Comparative otopathology: Aging, noise and ototoxic drugs. *Adv. Otorhinolaryngol.*, 20:125–141.

52. Henderson, D., and Hamernik, R. P. (1978): Impulse noise-induced hearing loss: An overview. In: *Noise and Audiology*, edited by D. M. Lipscomb, pp. 143–166. University Park Press, Baltimore.

53. Henderson, D., and Hamernik, R. P. (1982): Asymptotic threshold shift from impulse noise. In: *New Perspectives on Noise-Induced Hearing Loss*, edited by R. P. Hamernik, D. Henderson, and R. J. Salvi, pp. 265–281. Raven Press, New York.

54. Henderson, D., Hamernik, R. P., and Hynson, K. (1979): Hearing loss from simulated work-week exposure to impulse noise. *J. Acoust. Soc. Am.*, 65:1231–1237.

55. Henderson, D., Hamernik, R. P., and Sitler, R. W. (1974): Audiometric and histologic correlates of exposure to 1-msec noise impulses in the chinchilla. *J. Acoust. Soc. Am.*, 56:1210–1221.

56. Henderson, D., Hynson, K., and Hamernik, R. P. (1977): Importance of the waveform of the impulse in formulating an impulse noise damage risk criteria. *J. Acoust. Soc. Am.*, 62:S34.

57. Henderson, D., Salvi, R. J., and Hamernik, R. P. (1982): Is the equal energy rule applicable to impact noise? *Scand. Audiol. (Suppl.)*, 16:71–82.

58. Henry, K. R. (1982): Age-related changes in sensitivity of the postpubertal ear to acoustic trauma. *Hear. Res.*, 8:285–294.

59. Hinojosa, R., and Naunton, R. F. (1980): Presbycusis. In: *Otolaryngology, Vol. II*, edited by M. Paparella and W. Shumrick, pp. 1777–1787. W. B. Saunders, Philadelphia.

60. Hood, J. D., Poole, J. P., and Freedman, L. (1976): The influence of eye colour upon temporary threshold shift. *Audiology*, 15:449–464.

61. Howell, R. W. (1978): A seven-year review of measured hearing levels in male manual steelworkers with high initial thresholds. *Br. J. Indust. Med.*, 35:27–31.

62. Hynson, K., Hamernik, R. P., and Henderson, D. (1976): B-duration impulse definition: Some interesting results. *J. Acoust. Soc. Am.*, 59:S30.

63. Jackson, G. G. (1977): Present status of aminoglycoside antibiotics and their safe, effective use. *Clin. Ther.*, 1:200–215.

64. Jaffe, B. F., and Maasab, H. F. (1967): Sudden deafness associated with adenovirus infection. *N. Engl. J. Med.*, 276:1406–1409.

65. Jakobs, P., and Martin, G. (1977): The treatment of blast trauma inner ear damage with Dextran 40. *HNO*, 25:349–352.

66. Jakobs, P., and Martin, G. (1978): The treatment of tinnitus resulting from blast injury. *HNO*, 26:104–106.

67. Jogelkar, S. S., Lipscomb, D. M., and Shambaugh, G. E. (1977): Effects of oxygen inhalation on noise-induced threshold shifts in humans and chinchillas. *Arch. Otolaryngol.*, 103:574–578.

68. Karlovich, R. S. (1975): Comments on the relations between auditory fatigue and iris pigmentation. *Audiology*, 14:238–243.

69. Kellerhals, B. (1977): Treatment of acute inner ear deafness (sudden deafness and acoustic trauma). *Laryngol. Rhinol. Otol. Grenzgeb.*, 56:357–363.

70. Kellerhals, B., Hippert, F., and Pfaltz, C. R. (1971): Treatment of acute acoustic trauma with low molecular weight Dextran. *Pract. Otorhinolaryngol.*, 33:260–264.

71. Kisiel, D. L., and Bobbin, R. P. (1982): Interaction of aminooxyacetic acid and ethacrynic acid with intense sound at the level of the cochlea. *Hear. Res.*, 6:129–140.

72. Konigsmark, B. W., and Gorlin, R. J. (1976): *Genetic and Metabolic Deafness.* W. B. Saunders, Philadelphia.

73. Kryter, K. D. (1970): *The Effects of Noise on Man.* Academic Press, New York.

74. Kryter, K. D., Ward, W. D., Miller, J. D., and Eldredge, D. H. (1966): Hazardous exposure to intermittent and steady-state noise. *J. Acoust. Soc. Am.*, 396:451–464.

75. Lenoir, M., and Pujol, R. (1980): Sensitive period to acoustic trauma in the rat pup cochlea: Histological findings. *Acta Otolaryngol.*, 89:317–322.

76. Lindsay, J. R. (1959): Sudden deafness due to virus infection. *Arch. Otolaryngol.*, 69:13–18.

77. Lindsay, J. R., and Hemenway, W. G. (1954): Inner ear pathology due to measles. *Ann. Otol. Rhinol. Laryngol.*, 63:711–754.

78. Lubomudrov, V. E., Dokukina, G. A., Kobets, G. P., Bondarenko, G. A., and Nikitina, C. A. (1973): Treatment of patients with acoustic trauma. *Voen. Med. Zh.*, 8:35–38.

79. Luz, G. A. (1970): Recovery from temporary threshold shift in monkeys exposed to impulse noise: Evidence for a diphasic recovery process. *J. Acoust. Soc. Am.*, 48:96(A).

80. Luz, G. A., and Hodge, D. C. (1971): The recovery from impulse noise-induced TTS in monkeys and man: Descriptive model. *J. Acoust. Soc. Am.*, 49:1770–1777.

81. Maasab, H. F. (1973): The role of viruses in sudden deafness. *Adv. Otol. Rhinol. Laryngol.*, 20:229–235.

82. Macrae, J. H. (1971): Noise induced hearing loss and presbycusis. *Audiology*, 10:323–333.

83. Maniero, G., and Molinari, G. A. (1975): Protective effects of brain cortex gangliosides from temporary hearing loss provoked by high intensity noise. *Riv. Med. Aernaut.*, 38:307–316.

84. Marques, D. M., Clark, C. S., and Hawkins, J. E. (1975): Potentiation of cochlear injury by noise and ototoxic antibiotics in guinea pigs. *J. Acoust. Soc. Am.*, 57:S1(A).

85. Martin, A. (1976): The equal energy concept applied to impulse noise. In: *The Effects of Noise on Hearing*, edited by D. Henderson, R. P. Hamernik, D. S. Dosanjh, and J. H. Mills, pp. 421–453. Raven Press, New York.

86. Martin, G., and Jakobs, P. (1977): Clinical comparison of dextran 40 and xantinol-nicotinate in the therapy of acoustic trauma. *Laryngol. Rhinol. Otol.*, 56:860–863.

87. Martin, G., and Jakobs, P. (1978): Blast trauma, a case of acute emergency treatment. *Therapiewoche*, 28:7758–7762.

88. McDowell, B. (1982): Patterns of cochlear degeneration following gentamicin administration in both old and young guinea pigs. *Br. J. Audiol.*, 16:123–129.

89. McFadden, D., and Plattsmier, H. S. (1983): Aspirin can potentiate the temporary hearing loss induced by intense sounds. *Hear. Res.*, 9:295–316.

90. McRobert, H., and Ward, W. D. (1973): Damage-risk criteria: The trading relation between intensity and the number of nonreverberant impulses. *J. Acoust. Soc. Am.*, 53:1297–1300.

91. Melnick, W. (1974): Human threshold shift from 16 hour noise exposures. *Arch. Otolaryngol.*, 100:180–189.

92. Miller, J. D., Watson, C. S., and Covell, W. (1963): Deafening effects of noise on the cat. *Acta Otolaryngol. (Suppl.)*, 176:1–99.

93. Mills, J. H. (1973): Temporary and permanent threshold shifts produced by nine-day exposures to noise. *J. Speech Hear. Res.*, 16:426–438.

94. Mills, J. H. (1973): Threshold shifts produced by exposure to noise in chinchillas with noise-induced hearing losses. *J. Speech Hear. Res.*, 16:700–708.

95. Mills, J. H. (1975): Noise and children: A review of literature. *J. Acoust. Soc. Am.*, 58:767–779.

96. Mills, J. H. (1976): Threshold shifts produced by a 90-day exposure to noise. In: *Effects of Noise on Hearing*, edited by D. Henderson, R. P. Hamernik, D. S. Dosanjh, and J. H. Mills, pp. 265–275. Raven Press, New York.

97. Mills, J. H. (1982): Effects of noise on sensitivity, tuning curves, and suppression. In: *New Perspectives in Noise-Induced Hearing Loss*, edited by R. P. Hamernik, D. Henderson, and R. Salvi. Raven Press, New York.

98. Mills, J. H., Gengel, R., Watson, C. S., and Miller, J. D. (1970): Temporary changes of the auditory system due to exposure to noise for one or two days. *J. Acoust. Soc. Am.*, 48:524–530.

99. Mills, J. H., Gilbert, R., and Adkins, W. Y. (1979): Temporary threshold shifts in humans exposed to octave-bands of noise for 16–24 hours. *J. Acoust. Soc. Am.*, 65:1238–1248.

100. Mills, J. H., Gilbert, R. M., and Adkins, W. Y. (1981): Temporary threshold shifts produced by wide-band noise. *J. Acoust. Soc. Am.*, 70:390–396.
101. Mills, J. H., and Talo, S. (1972): Temporary threshold shifts produced by exposure to high-frequency noise. *J. Speech Hear. Res.*, 15:624–630.
102. Moody, D. B., Stebbins, W. C., Johnson, L., and Hawkins, J. E., Jr. (1976): Noise-induced hearing loss in monkey. In: *Effects of Noise on Hearing*, edited by D. Henderson, R. P. Hamernik, D. S. Dosanjh, and J. H. Mills, pp. 309–325. Raven Press, New York.
103. Myers, E. N., and Stool, S. (1968): Cytomegalic inclusion disease of the inner ear. *Laryngoscope*, 78:1904–1914.
104. Nabelek, I. V. (1982): Advances in noise measurement schemes. In: *New Perspectives on Noise-Induced Hearing Loss*, edited by R. P. Hamernik, D. Henderson, and R. Salvi, pp. 491–509. Raven Press, New York.
105. Nielsen, D. W. (1982): Asymptotic threshold shift in the squirrel monkey. *New Perspectives on Noise-Induced Hearing Loss*, edited by R. P. Hamernik, D. Henderson, and R. Salvi, pp. 303–319. Raven Press, New York.
106. Nillson, P., Erlandsson, B., Hakanson, H., Ivarsson, A., and Wersall, J. (1980): Morphological damage in the guinea pig after impulse noise and pure tone exposures. *Scand. Audiol. (Suppl.)*, 12:155–162.
107. Nixon, C. W., Krantz, D. W., and Johnson, D. L. (1975): Human temporary threshold shift and recovery from 24-hour acoustic exposures. AMRL-TR-74. Aerospace Med. Res. Lab.
108. Nixon, J. C., and Glorig, A. (1961): Noise-induced permanent threshold shift at 2000 cps and 4000 cps. *J. Acoust. Soc. Am.*, 33:904–908.
109. Novotny, Z. (1975): Development of occupational deafness after entering into a noisy job at an advanced age. *Cesk. Otolaryngol.*, 24:151–154.
110. Okada, A., Fukuda, K., and Yamamura, K. (1972): Growth and recovery of temporary threshold shift at a 4 kHz due to a steady-state noise and impulse noises. *Int. Z. Angew. Physiol.*, 30:105–111.
111. Okada, A., Miyake, H., Yamamura, K., et al. (1972): Temporary hearing loss induced by noise and vibration. *J. Acoust. Soc. Am.*, 51:1240–1248.
112. Paparella, M. (1980): Sensorineural hearing loss in children—nongenetic. In: *Otolaryngology, Vol. II*, edited by M. Paparella and W. Shumrick, pp. 1707–1717. W. B. Saunders, Philadelphia.
113. Passchier-Vermeer, W. (1974): Hearing loss due to continuous exposure to steady-state broad-band noise. *J. Acoust. Soc. Am.*, 56:1585–1593.
114. Price, G. R. (1976): Age as a factor in susceptibility to hearing loss: Young versus adult ears. *J. Acoust. Soc. Am.*, 60:886–892.
115. Quante, M. (1973): Die Wirkung von Lärm und ototoxischen Substanzen auf vorgeschadigte Ohren. *Arch. Klin. Exp. Ohren. Naser Kehlkopfheilkd.*, 205:266–269.
116. Quick, C. A. (1980): Chemical and drug effects on the inner ear. In: *Otolaryngology, Vol. II*, edited by M. Paparella and W. Shumrick, pp. 1804–1827. W. B. Saunders, Philadelphia.
117. Reddy, J. B., and Igarashi, M. (1962): Changes produced by kanamycin. *Arch. Otolaryngol.*, 76:146–150.
118. Rosen, S., Bergman, M., Plester, D., El-Mofty, A., and Satti, M. H. (1962): Presbycusis study of a relatively noise-free population in the Sudan. *Ann. Otol.*, 71:727–729.
119. Royster, L. H., Thomas, W. G., Royster, J. D., et al. (1978): Potential hearing compensation cost by race and sex. *J. Occup. Med.*, 20:801–806.
120. Ryan, A., and Bone, R. C. (1978): Potentiation of kanamycin ototoxicity by a history of noise exposure. *Trans. Am. Acad. Ophthalmol. Otolaryngol.*, 86:125–128.
121. Salvi, R., Henderson, D., and Hamernik, R. P. (1979): Single auditory nerve fiber and action potential latencies in normal and noise-treated chinchillas. *Hear. Res.*, 1:237–251.
122. Saunders, J. C., and Bok, G. R. (1978): Influence of early auditory trauma on auditory development. In: *Prenatal and Neonatal Influences on Brain and Behavior*, edited by G. Gottlieb, pp. 249–288. Academic Press, New York.
123. Schmiedt, R. A. (1982): Differential effects of kanamycin and impulse noise exposure on responses of auditory nerve fibers. In: *New Perspectives on Noise-Induced Hearing Loss*, edited by R. P. Hamernik, D. Henderson, and R. Salvi, pp. 153–163. Raven Press, New York.
124. Schmiedt, R. A., Zwislocki, J. J., and Hamernik, R. P. (1980): Effects of hair cell lesions on responses of cochlear nerve fibers. I. Lesions, tuning curves, two-tone inhibition and responses to trapezoidal-wave patterns. *J. Neurophysiol.*, 43:1367–1389.

125. Smoorenburg, G. F. (1982): Damage risk criteria for impulse noise. In: *New Perspectives on Noise-Induced Hearing Loss*, edited by R. P. Hamernik, D. Henderson, and R. Salvi, pp. 471–490. Raven Press, New York.

126. Spoendlin, H. (1976): Anatomical changes following various noise exposures. In: *Effects of Noise on Hearing*, edited by D. Henderson, R. P. Hamernik, D. S. Dosanjh, and J. H. Mills, pp. 69–90. Raven Press, New York.

127. Stagno, S., Reynolds, D. W., Amos, C. S., Dahle, A. J., McCollister, F. P., Mohindra, I., Ermocrilla, R., and Alford, C. A. (1977): Auditory and visual defects resulting from symptomatic and sub-clinical congenital cytomegalovirus and toxoplasma infections. *Pediatrics*, 59:669–678.

128. Stipon, J. P., Guignard, J., Cudennec, R., and Soubeyrand, L. (1979): Utilization of nicergoline in the therapy of acoustic trauma. *Med. Armees*, 7,8:723–725.

129. Taylor, G. D., and Williams, E. (1966): Acoustic trauma in the sports hunter. *Laryngoscope*, 76:863–879.

130. Theopold, H. M. (1975): Degenerative alterations in the ventral cochlear nucleus of the guinea pig after impulse noise exposure. *Arch. Otorhinolaryngol.*, 209:247–262.

131. Tota, G., and Bocci, G. (1967): Importance of the color of the iris in the evaluation of resistance of hearing to fatigue. *Riv. Otoneurooftalmol.*, 43:183–192.

132. Trahiotis, C. (1976): Application of the animal data to the development of noise standards. In: *Effects of Noise on Hearing*, edited by D. Henderson, R. P. Hamernik, D. S. Dosanjh, and J. H. Mills, pp. 341–360. Raven Press, New York.

133. Tremolieres, C., and Hetu, R. (1980): A multi-parametric study of impact noise-induced TTS. *J. Acoust. Soc. Am.*, 68/8:1652–1659.

134. Vernon, J., Brummett, R., and Brown, R. (1977): Noise trauma induced in the presence of loop-inhibiting diuretics. *Trans. Acad. Ophthalmol. Otolaryngol.*, 84:407–413.

135. von Gierke, H. E., and Johnson, D. L. (1976): Summary of present damage-risk criteria. In: *Effects of Noise on Hearing*, edited by D. Henderson, R. P. Hamernik, D. S. Dosanjh, and J. H. Mills, pp. 547–560. Raven Press, New York.

136. Ward, P. H., and Fernandez, C. (1961): The ototoxicity of kanamycin in guinea pigs. *Ann. Otol. Rhinol. Laryngol.*, 70:132–142.

137. Ward, W. D. (1965): The concept of susceptibility to hearing loss. *J. Occup. Med.*, 7:595–607.

138. Ward, W. D. (1973): Adaptation and fatigue. In: *Modern Developments in Audiology*, 2nd edition, edited by J. Jerger. Academic Press, New York.

139. Ward, W. D. (1973): Noise-induced hearing damage. In: *Otolaryngology, Vol. II*, edited by M. M. Paparella and D. A. Shumrick, pp. 378–388. W. B. Saunders, Philadelphia.

140. Ward, W. D., and Glorig, A. (1961): A case of firecracker induced hearing loss. *Laryngoscope*, 71:1590–1596.

141. Ward, W. D., Glorig, A., and Sklar, D. (1959): Temporary threshold shift from octave-band noise: Application to damage-risk criteria. *J. Acoust. Soc. Am.*, 31:522–528.

142. Witter, H. L., Deka, R. C., Lipscomb, D. M., and Shambaugh, G. E. (1980): Effects of prestimulatory carbogen inhalation on noise-induced temporary shifts in humans and chinchillas. *Am. J. Otol.*, 1:227–232.

143. Woodford, C. M. (1974): Effects of noise and sodium salicylates on chinchilla evoked responses. Ph.D. Thesis, Syracuse University, Syracuse, New York.

144. Woodford, C. M., Henderson, D., and Hamernik, R. P. (1978): Effects of combinations of sodium salicylate and noise on the auditory threshold. *Ann. Otol. Rhinol. Laryngol.*, 87:117–127.

145. Yamamura, K., Aoshima, K., Hiramatsu, S., Hikichi, T., and Hiramatsu, S. (1980): An investigation of the effects of impulse noise exposure on man. (Impulse noise with a relatively low peak level.) *Eur. J. Applied Physiol.*, 43:135–142.

146. Yamamura, K., Takashima, H., Miyake, H., et al. (1974): Effect of combined impact and steady-state noise on temporary threshold shift. *Med. Lavoro.*, 65:215–223.

147. Yanz, J. L., and Abbas, P. J. (1982): Age effects in susceptibility to noise-induced hearing loss. *J. Acoust. Soc. Am.*, 72:1450–1455.

Subject Index

Cataract(s) *(contd.)*
  diabetic, 69
  drug-induced, 68
  formation, 11
    acetaminophen and, 223,226
    naphthalene and, 223,226
    galactose and, 10,69
    toxic, 11
    types of, 10
Catechins, 206
Cerebrospinal fluid, 17
Chemoreceptors, 195–211
Chloramphenicol
  optic neuropathy, 14
  ototoxicity, 156
Chlorogenic acid, 206
Chloroquine
  corneal toxicity, 5,66
  retinopathy, 7,70,71,76,213
Chlorpromazine
  corneal deposits, 5
  hearing loss and, 238
Choroid, 1,2
  drug metabolizing enzymes in, 215,216
  embryonic development, 57
Cigarette smoke, olfaction and, 199–201
Ciliary body, 1,2
  drug metabolizing enzymes in, 215,216
  embryonic development, 56
Clioquinol, 76
  axonopathy, 48
Clomiphene, 69
Clonidine, 64
Cocaine, 122,124
Cochlear function
  loss of
    aminoglycoside-induced, 240
    noise levels and, 147
Conjunctiva, assessing toxicity to, 112
Copper, 205
Cornea, 1,2,3–5
  acid injury to, 5
  adenosine triphosphatase in, 130–131
  alkali damage to, 5
  assessment of healing, 130
  curvature, 125
  damage to, assessing, 114,115
  drug metabolizing enzymes in, 215
  drug penetration into, 4,5
  edema, 125
  embryonic development, 57
  function, assessing, 125–130
  opacities, 66; *see also* Cataract

  permeability, 115–117
  structure, 3
  thickness, 125–128
    intraocular pressure and, 128
  toxicity to, 65–66
    determining, 112,114
  ulceration, 5
  vacuoles, 65
Coronary vasodilators, 71
Corticosteroids
  cataracts from, 11,77
  glaucoma from, 214
  intraocular pressure and, 10
  papilledema from, 13
Cutaneous sensitivity, 184
Cynarin, 206
Cystine aminopeptidase, 216
Cytochrome P-450, ocular
Cytomegalovirus, 241

D

Deafness, 76; *see also* Hearing loss
Descemet's membrane, 3,4
Desferrioxamine, 69
Diabetes mellitus, 10
Diazepam, 75
Digital filtering
  of brainstem auditory evoked potential, 175,176,180
  in otoneurological disorders, 174
Dimethyl sulfoxide, 68
Dinitrophenol, 11
Diquat, 69
Diuretics, 156
Doxorubicin, 44
Draize test, 104–112,138

E

Ear
  anatomy, 17–22
  embryonic development
    susceptibility to toxicity and, 145–153
  toxicity, *see also* Ototoxicity
    drug-induced, 82,84,156,240–241
    mechanism of, 22
Echothiophate iodide, 11
Edema, 65
  corneal, 125
  of eyelids, 64
  retinal, 73–74
Electrooculography, 7,135–136
Electroretinography, 7,72,134–135